About Children

Senior Editors

Arthur G. Cosby, PhD
Professor of Sociology,
Director,
Social Science Research Center
Mississippi State University

Robert E. Greenberg, MD
Chair, Board of Directors 1999-2003,
Center for Child Health Research
Professor of Pediatrics Emeritus,
University of New Mexico

Linda Hill Southward, PhD
Research Professor,
Coordinator,
Family and Children Research Unit,
Social Science Research Center,
Mississippi State University

Michael Weitzman, MD
Executive Director
Center for Child Health Research
Professor and Associate Chair of
   Pediatrics,
University of Rochester

Production Staff

Coordinating Editor
Holli C. Hitt

Design/Layout Editor
Jarryl B. Ritchie

Graphics/Data Coordinators
Jarryl B. Ritchie
Thomas Kersen, PhD

Contributing Editors
Heather Hanna
Pamela J. Cosby
Anne Buffington
Paige Tompkins, PhD

Layout Assistant
Dallas Breen

Reference Assistant
Destini D. Dunn

Internet Resources Coordinator
Megan Kavanaugh

AAP Publishing Staff

Director, Department of Marketing and Publications
Maureen DeRosa, MPA

Director, Division of Product Development
Mark Grimes

Manager, Product Development
Jeff Mahony

Director, Division of Publishing and Production Services
Sandi King

Manager, Editorial Services
Kate Larson

Manager, Print Production Services
Leesa Levin-Doroba

Director, Division of Marketing and Sales
Jill Ferguson

Manager, Consumer Product Marketing and Sales
Susan Thompson

Library of Congress Control Number: 2004102273

ISBN: 1-58110-142-2

MA0285

The views expressed herein are those of the authors, and no official endorsement by the American Academy of Pediatrics is intended or should be inferred. The recommendations in this publication do not indicate an exclusive course of treatment or serve as a standard of medical care. Variations, taking into account individual circumstances, may be appropriate.

The Social Science Research Center's Monitor Laboratory at Mississippi State University developed the maps and graphs found in this book. The maps were produced using ERSI's ArcGIS 8.3 and the graphs were created using Microsoft Excel. The majority of the data used in this book are publicly available via the Internet.

The Bower Foundation
and
The Phil Hardin Foundation

generously provided the support
that made this book possible.

Collaborating Centers for Child and Family Health Research

The Collaborating Centers for Child and Family Health Research is a joint venture of the Social Science Research Center of Mississippi State University and the Center for Child Health Research of the American Academy of Pediatrics. The researchers of the Collaborating Centers for Child and Family Health Research seek to create a comprehensive, multidisciplinary approach to child and family issues in all social and geographic components of our society. The collaboration is an intensive and responsible effort to define the primary research questions that lead to meaningful approaches to social and public policies regarding children, families, and communities. By combining the unique skills and attributes of each center, a fusion of complementary interests links child health professionals to the multiple disciplines and approaches that are essential for meeting the needs of children and families.

Editorial Board

Preface

What is the most critical information that parents, policymakers, advocates, teachers, child care providers, pediatricians, and scholars should know about children in the United States at the beginning of the new century and new millennium? How can this information be presented to reach the intended audience—namely, those who care *for* and those who care *about* children? Who can best provide this information? How will this information make a difference in the lives of children?

These questions were raised during a conversation between the leadership of the Center for Child Health Research of the American Academy of Pediatrics and the Social Science Research Center at Mississippi State University in the summer of 2000. This dialogue led to the establishment of the Collaborating Centers for Child and Family Health Research in March 2001. The rationale underlying the Collaborating Centers is the belief that the issues facing children are so profoundly complex that their exploration requires the collaboration of multiple professions, disciplines, and institutions. The Collaborating Centers provides a structure for these various entities to work together to further the understanding of the complexities of children's lives.

Soon after the establishment of the Collaborating Centers, *About Children* emerged as the signature project to address the fundamental issues by bringing together, in one volume, the voices of the country's foremost authorities on the most important topics facing children today. The goal is to present this information in a format and style accessible to a wide and diverse population. Inspired by the words of Joseph Pulitzer, creator of the Pulitzer Prize, *About Children* adheres to his guiding principle to "put it before them briefly so they will read it, clearly so they will appreciate it, picturesquely so they will remember it and, above all, accurately so they will be guided by its light."

About Children reflects the multifaceted dimensions of children's lives, and each of the following sections highlights one of five dimensions: their environments; their family life and well-being; their roles, hopes, and rights; their demographics and diversity; and their future. Within each of these sections, the authors provide the reader powerful, often poignant, and sometimes controversial portrayals of the various dimensions of children's lives in the hopes of stimulating discourse and encouraging discernment.

In describing *children's environments*, John de Graff cites symptoms of childhood "affluenza" as a "fever" for shopping and spending, swollen expectations about material needs, and a sense of self defined more by the labels on the inside of children's jackets rather than by an understanding of their inner selves. In contrast, Irwin Redlener informs the reader that families with children comprise 40% of the homeless population while Angie Vachio notes that women are the fastest-growing segment of all prison populations, and the majority of the women in prison are also mothers—often of very young children. Other equally intriguing and changing areas of children's environments include influences of media, advertising in schools, substance abuse, violence, urban housing, tobacco, and the post-9/11 world.

Nestled within children's environments are the important aspects of *their family life and well-being,* representing a kaleidoscope of care for children. The images are both striking and startling. The interplay between families' economic status and children's well-being is reinforced throughout this section. Helen Blank describes the ever-increasing need for and benefits of promoting quality child care throughout the country. Deborah Belle and Brenda Phillips reinforce the importance of appropriate care in children's after-school hours and the critical importance of these particular hours in a child's day. Donna Butts and Jaia Peterson weave statistics into their essay, emphasizing that 6 million children (1 out of every 12) live in households headed by a grandparent or other relative. Furthermore, 2 million children live in extended families without the presence of a parent.

Mary Edward Wertsch spotlights the lives of children who have a parent or both parents in the military. In doing so, she reflects upon her own experiences as a military child. Other very thoughtful analyses and stirring pieces include topics that affect children's lives such as turbulence, divorce, foster care, immigration, gender roles, and poverty. The final chapter in this section is written by Patrick Casey and presents an overview of food insecurity among children in the United States. The information in this essay becomes even more striking when contrasted with the essays in the next section about children's health—particularly the essay on the epidemic of overweight among children and adolescents.

Bernard Guyer and Alyssa Wigton begin the section on *children's health* and provide the reader with beacons of hope by spotlighting numerous accomplishments and improvements in child health over the last century and pointing the reader toward continuing and changing challenges of improving children's health today. Burton Edelstein's insightful analyses of how children experience tooth decay, framing the status of children's oral health as "the best of times and the worst of times," notes that tooth decay is the single most common chronic disease of childhood. This serves as a call to action as do other rampant child health concerns such as asthma, overweight, and attention deficit hyperactivity disorder. Bill Dietz stresses the importance of understanding overweight within the context of the child's family *and* their environment, given that the prevalence of overweight children has doubled and the prevalence of overweight adolescents has tripled in the past 20 years. Additional and equally important chapters examine the special health care needs, maltreatment, injuries, immunization, health insurance, and mental health of children. These chapters underscore the wide array of health concerns facing children and their families. While much has been done in many of these areas, the challenges to decreasing the incidence, severity, and prevalence of many child health issues are daunting. A common theme of this section deals with the critical role of primary and secondary prevention.

Despite these challenges, part of the answers to improving children's outcomes stem from increasing one's understanding and appreciation of *children's roles, hopes, and rights.* While not a panacea for reducing negative outcomes as many have hoped, John Bartkowski posits that religiosity of adolescents does serve as a protective factor in delaying the onset of many risk-taking behaviors. Paula Duncan and Emily Kallock's thoughtful essay encourages the reader to view adolescents from a strengths perspective as opposed to a deficit- and problem-based model. Shay Bilchik gives a succinct history of children's rights and guides the reader to consider the necessity of creating a system of justice based upon evidence-based practices for all children and youth.

The *demographics and diversity* of children and families are based on the latest available data with accompanying visualization of this data. Three of the country's leading demographers and social scientists, Daniel Litcher, Steve Murdock, and William O'Hare render compelling evidence of the changing demographic landscape of children and their families.

The final section, *looking toward their future,* describes promising practices for improving children's health and well-being by advancing technological and genetic understandings. It is particularly noteworthy that Judith Palfrey and Julius Richmond, whose combined careers have positively influenced and promoted the best of health care to countless children throughout the country, provide the reader with a rich perspective that spans more than 3 score years.

The authors are the country's foremost authorities on each of their respective topics. Their collective works include and highlight the need for important programs for children and youth; their research findings are cited in thousands of articles and hundreds of books and are often the basis of legislation and policies that have resulted in an improved quality of life for children and youth. Each author was asked to succinctly describe the most salient points about their topic that the public, parents, and policymakers need to know. *About Children* is the result of the authors' critical thinking to distill complex issues into an easily understood format. We are deeply indebted to the authors for their commitment to the process and their steadfast and timely work with our copyeditors.

About Children has become a reality because of the vision, support, enthusiasm, and encouragement of an array of individuals and entities. Because *About Children* is much more than an academic endeavor, we sought editorial board members whose individual contributions to the health and well-being of children are well-recognized and whose collective, interdisciplinary lens sharpens the vision of *About Children*. Our national search brought us the following stellar group of individuals: Arlene Bowers Andrews, Polly Arango, Rebeca Barrera, Shay Bilchik, Claude Earl Fox, Bernard Guyer, Robert Haggerty, Bill Isler, Kim Miller, and Paul Wise. We are indebted to each for the richness of their guidance, feedback, selection of chapter topics, and assistance in recruiting authors and editing the manuscripts.

Anne Buffington, Pam Cosby, and Heather Hanna were phenomenal in their roles as copyeditors, always demonstrating the epitome of professionalism. Destini Dunn provided valuable assistance in references. Our coordinating editor, Holli Hitt, held a pivotal role in keeping communication moving forward in all aspects of the project. The talents and expertise of Jay Ritchie and Tom Kersen to obtain and subsequently transform data into visual images are unmatched. Data were derived from a multitude of sources, with a particular focus on data that could be visualized as another mechanism to "tell the story" of various topics. In addition, these data were employed to heighten the awareness and understanding of regional and state differences across the country.

Megan Kavanaugh's annotated list of Internet sites greatly enhances and builds on the content of each chapter and section. The American Academy of Pediatrics Department of Marketing and Publications has been integral to the success of the project and making sure that deadlines for this volume were met.

The generous support of two Mississippi foundations, The Phil Hardin Foundation and The Bower Foundation, made *About Children* possible. The encouragement of Tom Wacaster (Phil Hardin Foundation) led to the initial grant and paved the way to the subsequent support of Anne Travis (Bower Foundation), which made this endeavor a reality. Truly, their belief and trust in the process and the product can never been overstated. The efforts of our coeditors, Robert E. (Bob) Greenberg and Michael Weitzman, have been superb. Bob Greenberg, in particular, has taken the adage of a "labor of love" to a new dimension.

About Children began as a conversation among the editors about the most important information our country needs to know about children. *About Children* provides a great deal of that information. Our hope is that the conversation that began among a few will turn into a national dialogue that raises additional questions and creates an awareness for individual or group calls to action, whether on a very personal level to increase one's understanding and share new insights with others or on a broader scale to provide succinct and timely information for policymakers, advocates, and all who care for and care about children.

Linda Hill Southward and Arthur G. Cosby

Web Site

About Children readers can now access an informative Web site offering a number of supplementary features. The Web site provides a PowerPoint presentation tailored to each chapter and ready for use, and each presentation incorporates the same high quality graphics and photos that appear in *About Children*. From multiple, hyperlinked Internet resources for each chapter topic to additional chapter tools, the companion Web site is a valuable asset for parents and professionals.

Visit today at: ***www.aap.org/AboutChildren***

Password: ***abochi3***

Contents

Part Four   **About Their Roles, Hopes, and Rights** **155**

Introduction

Purpose of This Book

Millions of children flourish in the United States, supported by stable, happy families. They grow to their potential, learn creatively, use diverse abilities, and come from all cultures and socioeconomic groups. Many neighborhoods support children and their families, create community, and build resources to support healthy child development. In these areas, schools enhance learning and facilitate children's mastery of both independence and social interactions. Local governments establish policies and programs that protect children and support their caregivers. Physical and mental health is optimized, with preventive services available to many.

Yet millions of other children flounder. Many face poverty, family chaos, deprivation, or violence in their homes and streets. Many fend for themselves, bewildered, hopeless, and depressed. Life challenges intrude on the private lives of families, threatening health, straining parents' abilities to cope, and making childrearing a struggle. Out-of-home supports, including early care and education and schools, often operate with woefully inadequate resources and may actually pose barriers to children who strive for success. The rocky roads impeding the lives of young children may become even more tortuous as the children enter adolescence. Learning may become irrelevant while behavior destructive to them and others may become the norm. A wasteland of unfulfilled potential exists in areas across the nation, marked by school dropouts, disrupted lives, and adults who fail to achieve competent responsibility. Inequalities in health status, opportunities, access to health care, and community resources as a function of income inequality, geography, and ethnicity have an immense negative impact on the lives of countless children and families. This tragic state reflects, in ways often unclear, the world we live in and the relationships between and among us.

Obviously, in the United States, we know how to promote healthy and happy child development. Yet, for many reasons, we often fail to ensure that every child benefits from our knowledge and resources. We often overlook the critical importance of the early years in a child's life and ignore children as societal priorities are debated and decided. We—our children and our families—are struggling to find direction, build our individual and collective futures, and feel the joy of reaching our potentials.

This book offers information to help citizens push harder for a unified vision of the good life for *all* children. The editors have gathered experts from around the country to state the facts, illustrate the trends, and offer opinions about the current quality of life for children in the United States.

Too often, we know what we do not want. We do not want all the negative conditions: poverty, preventable diseases, mental breakdowns, discrimination, violence, despair, ignorance, pollution, and exploitation. Rarely, we articulate what we do want. This introduction begins the book with a discussion of the good life for children. We offer a vision of the conditions of childhood that will promote healthy, happy lives for children and their families.

This book represents an attempt to display, in an easily understandable fashion, a wide array of factors that determine the health and well-being of children and their families. One goal is to help parents, teachers, child advocates, public officials, and professionals gain insight and information into the tapestry of factors that determine child well-being. We hope to help raise public consciousness about the lives of our children and enhance public demands for efforts to effectively respond to the needs of children and their families.

Our goal is that readers, excited to learn about factors that determine children's well-being, will seek more information and then take public action to solve the problems and create healthy alternatives. We trust that this book will enhance the readers' abilities and confidence as citizens who strive for the best possible life for both their own and all children.

Providing a Framework: *The Good Life for Children*

In attempting to understand and integrate those factors in our society that may enhance or compromise the lives of children, there is a clear need to frame what characteristics would, if present, make up the *Good Life for Children*. The sections below each provide an essential component of a happy and successful life for children and their families.

A Healthy Beginning

The National Academy of Sciences recently convened a network of early childhood development experts who reviewed current research-based knowledge and concluded, unequivocally, that all children are born wired for feelings and ready to learn; early environments matter and nurturing relationships are essential; and society is changing, and the needs of young children are not being met.[1] Recognizing that child well-being and health are determined by a vast array of factors—socioeconomic, psychological, environmental, genetic, cultural, and biologic—is not a new perspective. However, promoting comprehensive, systematic community and societal change to help families care for the full needs of their young, given the complex demands of our society, is new.

Human development is shaped by the mother and the infant's biology interacting dynamically with the broader physical and social environment. The well-being of an infant is determined, to a considerable degree, by events occurring during the gestational period. If the mother conceives while in good health, maintains a well-balanced and nutritional diet, exercises and rests appropriately, manages stress adaptively, and receives good health care, the infant's chances of starting life with vigor are enhanced considerably. Alternatively, exposure to tobacco, drugs (both recreational and therapeutic), or environmental toxins may all have negative effects on the developing fetus. Intrauterine growth retardation ("small-for-date babies") is seen under circumstances of maternal stress and poor maternal nutrition, as well as for reasons still to be defined. Being born prematurely may challenge the ability of the premature infant to successfully adapt to the extrauterine experience. A discrepancy in rates of intrauterine growth retardation between African American babies and those of other ethnic groups persists.

The outcome of pregnancy, in terms of the health and well-being of the baby, is enhanced through the provision of early and optimal prenatal care for the mother, even though the exact mechanisms whereby that beneficial effect occurs remain obscure. Maternal well-being is enhanced through the mother's practice of health behaviors, social support from people who care, material resources such as food and protection, and health care from skilled, accessible, culturally competent providers.

The Highest Attainable Standard of Health

Health has been defined by the World Health Organization as a "state of complete physical, mental, and social well-being, and not merely the absence of disease or infirmity."[2] his definition obviously creates an eternal and universal goal, one that has never been fully attained. Defining health in this manner indicates the breadth of the concept and the factors that determine it.

Access to comprehensive, preventive, compassionate, and continuous health care enhances children's health. However, being healthy is by no means determined by health care alone. Rather, the worlds in which children live—their families, their neighborhoods, their societies—have a much greater effect on their lives and their health. A child's nutrition, exercise, hygiene, rest, emotional expression, trust in caregivers, and self-perception are the foundations of health. They learn healthy ideas and practices from the adults around them. As they mature, their own behaviors affect their health. To achieve the highest attainable standard of health, we must raise every child to think of herself or himself as a health practitioner.

An Environment That Supports Rather Than Limits Health

The physical environment, including the mother's envirement during gestation, may dramatically affect the developing child. Clean air, light, space for motion, potable water, decent housing with utilities, and sanitary sewage and waste disposal are minimal requirements for healthy development. Exposure of the fetus or child to tobacco, drugs (recreational and therapeutic), bacteria from poorly preserved food or contaminated water, or environmental toxins imposes long-lived consequences. Lead-based paints, particulate content of urban air, uncontrolled use of pesticides, and food additives all may, under defined circumstances, lead to adverse consequences in both individuals and populations. When environments are not designed or controlled with children in mind, children run the risk of injuries from playgrounds, toys, access to weapons, traffic, or other hazards. Poverty is intimately related to the dangers in environmental exposures, since poverty-stricken communities are at much greater risk of environmental contaminations. Yet, aggressive social policies can and do lead to protection against environmental agents, and the struggle is ongoing to protect populations from environmental hazards and expose them to wholesome natural resources and built environments.

A Family Environment

The preamble to the United Nations *Convention on the Rights of the Child (CRC)* extols the significance of family for healthy child development. The *CRC* includes the following reasons:

> ...The family, as the fundamental group of society and the natural environment for the growth and well-being of all its members and particularly children, should be afforded the necessary protection and assistance so that it can fully assume its responsibilities within the community,
>
> The child, for the full and harmonious development of his or her personality, should grow up in a family environment, in an atmosphere of happiness, love and understanding....

Through the *CRC*, the United Nations has called upon all states to ensure that each child is raised in a family environment. Family environments may vary in terms of structure (i.e., number of people in the group, ages, gender, and other characteristics), processes (such as communication and time together), and resources (such as material goods and social networks). Some families share a single household; others are spread among more than one household, but have strong social interactions. Although families vary considerably, they all perform the core function that theorist Urie Bronfenbrenner[3,4] identified as essential to healthy development: Each person should be connected to at least one (preferably more) other person throughout life, starting at birth, and the connection should be characterized by irrational affection, reliability and stability over time, and positive interaction.

When children live with no consistent caregiver or unpredictable relations, they are at risk of developing attachment problems that can lead to serious emotional or behavioral conditions. With stable, caring families, children are more likely to thrive.

A Full and Decent Life if the Child Has a Disability

An evolving understanding of disabilities uses the following definitions: an *impairment* represents an alteration of body structure or function; a *disability* is the limitation that such an impairment exerts on the affected individual; a *handicap* refers to the limitations that society places on how individuals with disabilities can live their lives and flourish. Public policies and community resources that support comprehensive child development will focus on preventing any condition from becoming a significant handicap and limiting the extent to which an impairment disables a child. Achieving happier lives for affected individuals enriches everyone.

Freedom of Expression

The opportunity to tell others how and what one is feeling, thinking, understanding, or confused about is critical to the development of one's abilities, sense of self, and emotional self-regulation. Also, people must learn to respect the interests and needs of others, in childhood as well as adulthood. Learning to express emotions forms the foundation for developing friendships and interacting with the greater society. Thus, opportunities to express one's thoughts and feelings, as the capability to do so evolves during childhood, are critical developmental experiences.

For children to learn to express themselves, they must have adults and others who are willing to listen responsively. Through this interaction, children learn, in turn, to respectfully listen to others. The development of empathy and social responsibility are grounded in these processes.

Restorative Justice When Accused of Wrongdoing

Children experience the whole range of acts along the victimization and offending continuum. They make mistakes and hurt others, and they suffer the harm induced by others. When they do wrong, their caregivers and society have an opportunity to teach them to do right.

Unfortunately, children, particularly in the teen years, sometimes commit grievous wrongs, including murder and severe assaults. Many areas of the country have seen recent increases in arrest rates of youth. Most states have responded with retributive reactions that seem based on fear and revulsion. The age at which young people accused of violent crimes are adjudicated within the adult justice system is being progressively lowered. Sentences are long and harsh, and juvenile detention facilities are poorly staffed for rehabilitation. Some communities have developed preventive and restorative alternatives that address underlying causes and developmental needs, but in most areas, resources for such programs have been slow in developing. Justice for youth accused of wrongdoing becomes a clear marker of the quality of our civic life and the extent to which compassion and understanding control our legal responses.

Support for Recovery from Grief and Trauma

All children will experience losses, and some will face catastrophic trauma or harsh victimization. How a child copes with and recovers from these experiences depends considerably on the nature of support offered by others in the aftermath of the event or during the disclosure that loss or harm occurred. Many mental health problems have their origins in poorly resolved life events. Children need help making sense of negative life events, so their emotional energy can be channeled into typical developmental tasks, rather than drained into anxiety over lingering concerns and anticipation of potential threats. They need guidance about how to cope in adaptive, rather than maladaptive, ways.

Protection from Physical, Mental, and Sexual Violence and Exploitation

Perhaps no other obstacle to universally happy childhoods exceeds child maltreatment in its frequency or consequences. Too many children suffer maltreatment in all its forms: physical abuse, sexual abuse, psychological abuse, and neglect. In the United States, as in other countries, immense effort has been focused on detecting and responding to child maltreatment, preserving family structure and function, and preventing recurrence. Primary prevention of child maltreatment remains virtually an uncharted area, requiring careful, open, intensive studies of the epidemiology of various forms of child maltreatment so that preventive approaches can be effectively and rationally designed and implemented. Most instances of child maltreatment occur within family settings and require mobilization of community resources to assist in stabilizing the family while protecting the child from further abuse. Children must feel safe and be protected from injury in order to achieve healthy development.

Equal Opportunity for an Education That Optimizes Learning and Personal Growth

A person's educational level is a key predictor of life satisfaction. People of all ages who love learning and have mastered certain skills have advantages and freedoms that are unavailable to those with inadequate educational attainment. Education enhances personal growth and creates the substrate that leads to each person's ability to contribute to the larger community as a productive adult. If educational opportunities were uniform in all communities, inequities among people in differing life circumstances could be significantly reduced, and the fundamental goal of equality, inherent in any democratic society, could be approached. The struggle to achieve both quality and equity in public education continues, even while threatened by increasing flight to private and home schooling. Attempts to find answers to prevailing problems in public education abound, and new approaches are being taken in reducing class and school sizes, increasing involvement of all school personnel in classrooms, deriving learning motivation from the interests of students themselves, and finding new ways to increase the fiscal underpinnings of the educational system.

Protection from Economic Exploitation and from Discrimination Based on Race, Class, or Culture

Power always exists in any set of interactions between people. When used only for personal gain, such power unavoidably expresses itself in economic exploitation of those without power. When derived from the needs and interests of all people, power can be utilized for community gain and personal growth. Discrimination based on race, class, or culture, represents an agonizing legacy in the emergence and history of our country and still exerts its ugly consequences that limit the joy in the lives of children and compromises the opportunities of their parents. As the composition of our population evolves and changes over time, the nature of discriminatory practices also changes, yet persists. A major tenet of our political framework speaks to nondiscrimination and freedom for all. Achieving that goal represents perhaps the central task of our nation, and failure to improve our responses to each other represents a major obstacle to the lives of children.

A Standard of Living That Is Adequate for Physical, Mental, Spiritual, Moral, and Social Development

Childhood living conditions vary markedly between nations and, as is increasingly evident, within nations, including our own. The progression of income inequality in our own country matches most other countries in direction, but exceeds most in extent. Uncertainty regarding the precise relationship between living conditions and child development has raised concerns about the inadequacy of current definitions of the "federal poverty level." This has led to studies of what kinds of resources (i.e., living conditions) are necessary in order to enable children to grow in families where access to nutrition, housing, transportation, communication, and interaction with others is at a level that does not directly impede the growth and development of the child.[5] An immediate application of a concern for an adequate standard of living focuses on the lives of children themselves, in and of their own right, rather than viewing children only in the context of who and what they will become as adults and what role they may or may not play in the economic structure of the larger society. Children need to be viewed as human *beings* and not just as human *becomings*.[6] With that view, how the child's living conditions affect physical, mental, spiritual, moral, and social development can be more directly and effectively studied, and requisite changes can be implemented.

A Neighborhood That Supports Family Life

Humans are social creatures; we are meant to live in community with one another. As infants, we are born with the capacity to seek interaction with other humans. If we are nurtured, we develop the capacity to show care for others. Throughout life, people interact with family, friends, teachers, acquaintances, coworkers, neighbors, and fellow citizens. Our lives are influenced, directly and indirectly, by commerce and other economic forces, government, religious communities, nature, and the built environment. Humans develop from complete dependence on caregivers to relative autonomy and interdependence with other people. People give and they receive. Living in community is a natural part of being human.

Many of a child's contacts with community occur through their and their caregivers' interactions within their geographic neighborhoods. Neighborhoods can help or hinder children's access to the resources they need for survival, development, protection, and participation in society. In the best cases, neighborhoods offer safety, recreation, beauty, and help with the hectic pace of life. In the worst cases, they breed crime, addictions, exploitation, and despair. When families have problems, adequate neighborhoods help reduce stress and promote resilience. Various neighborhoods may optimize cooperative play or enhance the likelihood of accidents or injuries. Finding ways to give structure and strength to communities and neighborhood life represents an immense opportunity to enable all members of a neighborhood to support each other and to positively influence the development of each other's children. Enhancing neighborhood structure and function represents an exciting opportunity and responsibility.

Participation in Play and Recreational Activities, Cultural Life, and the Arts

It has been said that "understanding the atom is child's play next to understanding child's play." Play and recreation represent the primary way in which young children learn about the world, responsibilities towards others, and the role of cooperation as well as competition in their lives. Children have capacities for diverse expression through visual arts, body motion, drama, music, and the vast array of media through which they can share their imaginations. The opportunity to experience, as evolving skills allow, how the arts enhance personal excitement and joy and deepen respect for others makes access to the arts and culture an inviolate component of optimal child development.

The Good Life

The ideas in this introduction are adapted from the United Nations' *Convention on the Rights of the Child*.[7] The convention integrates civil, political, economic, social, and cultural rights. It has been proposed and generally accepted as providing a universally acceptable substrate for describing, assessing, and promoting early childhood, mid-childhood, and adolescent health and well-being. The intimate relationship between health and human rights has been both recognized and appreciated.[8]

The concept of the Good Life for children and the recognition that each child deserves to experience all of its components underpins the discussions that follow in this book. Each chapter is an attempt to examine the quality of life of children in the United States—the existing conditions that both support and impede access to the Good Life—in the hope that increased awareness will lead to both thought and action which, one day, will provide the Good Life for all children.

Arlene Bowers Andrews and Robert E. Greenberg

Part One: About Their Environments

With each passing year, we learn how complex and interactive the environments we live in have become. Our environments certainly encompass physical characteristics, such as air pollution or exposure to noxious chemicals. However, they also extend to our exposure to communication media, the nature of the neighborhoods in which we live, the type of housing we inhabit, or the substances that we allow to enter our bodies. We need to learn more about our environments in all of their complexity as a means of developing policies and practices that enhance the well-being of each of us—as individuals, as participants in a collaborative society, and as children or caregivers to children who live in an increasingly complex world.

Chapter 1

John de Graaf

Childhood
"Affluenza"

I can still remember the names and the games that rang out across the dusty playground "Red Rover, Red Rover, send Emerson Yazzie right over!" It was the fall of 1969, and I was teaching at a Navajo Indian boarding school in New Mexico. The 10-year-olds I taught grew up in one-room log dwellings scattered across the arid countryside. Their families earned less than a $1,000 a year. The children possessed scarcely more than the clothes they wore, and the school, nearly as poor, offered little to amuse them during recess periods.

Nonetheless, these lively boys and girls were always able to amuse themselves. More often than not, wide smiles illuminated their sunburned faces as they made up their own games and entertainment. Never did I hear them say they were bored.

At Christmastime that year, I returned to the suburban neighborhood where I'd grown up. My own 9-year-old brother and his friends were children of prosperity, with bedrooms resembling toy stores. Yet they continually complained to me that they had "nothing to do."

In the years since then—in a Guatemalan refugee camp in Mexico, or a landless peasants' settlement in Brazil, for example—I have seen poor children, cheerful and resourceful despite their lack of possessions. Meanwhile, their affluent American counterparts, awash in stuff, often feel deprived. They are the perpetually dissatisfied victims of an emerging, airwave-borne epidemic I now call "affluenza."

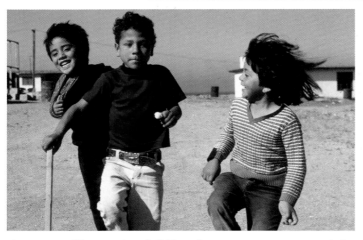

I have seen poor children, cheerful and resourceful despite their lack of possessions. Meanwhile, their affluent American counterparts, awash in stuff, often feel deprived.

Among affluenza's childhood symptoms one might include:

- a fever for shopping and spending,

- swollen expectations about material needs,

- decreasing immunity to the assaults of advertisers,

- self-concepts defined by brands of clothing, and

- a rash of debt by the time they leave college.

Polls consistently find that a wide majority of American parents today believe their children are "too materialistic." Psychologist Mary Pipher calls today's teenagers the "I want" generation. But that's no accident. Children have become the hottest targets of today's marketing dollars.

A generation ago, the Federal Trade Commission considered restricting advertising aimed at children, but, in 1980, Congress passed a law *preventing* such action. Since then, the amount of money spent by advertisers to reach children has increased by a factor of 20—from $100 million to $2 billion a year.

"Children are consumers in training, superstars in the consumer constellation," writes James U. McNeal, a leading expert on the youth market. Americans under the age of 12 now spend or influence the spending of an astonishing $565 billion a year. Alex Molnar, author of *Giving Kids the Business*, says many companies view children as "cash crops to be harvested." Those are harsh words, but even a quick visit to a marketing conference like Kid Power, held annually at Disney World, confirms Molnar's observation.

Speakers talk freely of "*owning*," "*branding*," and "*capturing*" children, seemingly without a second thought about what those words mean. "Connecting with kids in the face of moms is a constant challenge," says one Kid Power speaker. So marketers go behind Mom's back. They refer to parents as "*gatekeepers*" and offer tips to increase "*the nag factor*," so children will effectively pressure their folks to buy. They suggest rude and aggressive ads that make parents seem like fools. Paul Kurnit, founder of the KidShop marketing firm, teaches that "anti-social behavior in pursuit of a product is a good thing."

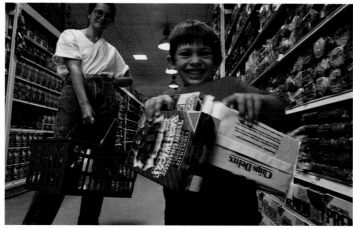

Ironically, the ad strategies come from highly paid psychologists who track children's spending behavior and responses to commercial messages through focus groups, questionnaires, and the Internet. This occurs despite the official commitment of the American Psychological Association to "improve the condition of both the individual and society" and to "help the public in developing informed judgments." "Psychology is a healing art. It's unethical to use it to trick or mislead children for commercial gain," says Gary Ruskin, director of Commercial Alert, an organization that monitors marketing to children.

Marketers continually seek ways to break through the "clutter" of other ads and make sure kids see theirs. In recent years, this has meant targeting relatively ad-free environments such as schools. A few years ago, I walked through the hallways of a high school in Colorado

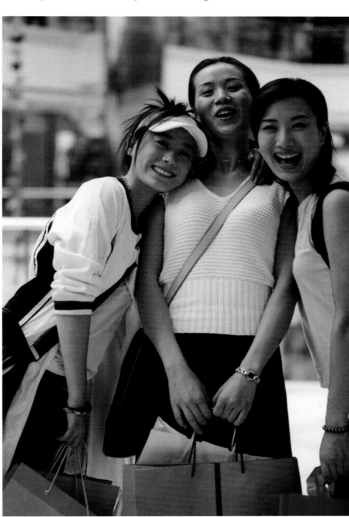

Springs, Colorado. From the walls, slick come-ons for junk foods competed for students' attention. "M & Ms are better than straight A's," read one ad. "Satisfy your hunger for higher education with Snickers," encouraged another. Most advertising in the schools is more carefully disguised as part of TV news programs or in math textbooks and other curricula.

From school, television, and numerous other sources, children see about 40,000 advertisements a year. Marketers say it is not a problem and claim they're only empowering children to be full participants in a material world. But child welfare experts suggest that training children to be caution-free consumers has serious consequences:

- It makes children feel like losers if they don't have the right brands. Seventy percent of American parents feel that advertising weakens their children's self-esteem. Again, that's no accident. Nancy Shalek, a kids' marketing guru, says that, *Advertising at its best* (italics added) is making people feel that without your product, they're a loser. Kids are very sensitive to that. If you tell them to buy something, they're resistant. But if you tell them they'll be a dork if they don't, you've got their attention. You open up emotional vulnerabilities, and it's very easy to do with kids because they're the most emotionally vulnerable."

- It encourages rude, aggressive, and sometimes even violent behavior, like the behavior displayed in the ads themselves. Video game ads often use violent imagery to sell, with headlines like "More Fun than Shooting Your Neighbor's Cat!"

- It encourages consumption of high-calorie, sugar-laden junk foods, exacerbating America's epidemic of childhood obesity.

- It leads to escalating debt problems among youth that carry over into adulthood. For the past 6 years, more Americans have declared personal bankruptcy than have graduated from college. College students often carry enormous credit card debt. One college president told me that credit card debt is now the number one cause of dropouts at his school and, probably, throughout the nation.

- It hasn't made our children happier. On the contrary, teenage suicides have tripled since the 1960s, and children's rates of depression have soared even more.

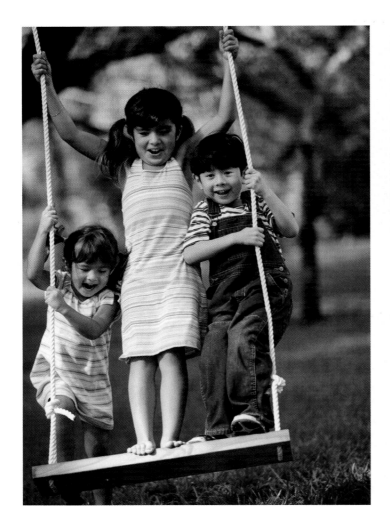

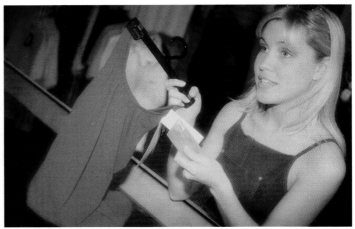

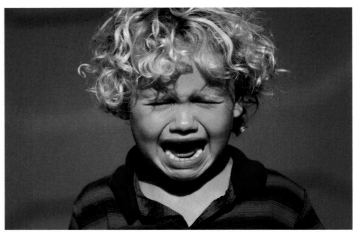

Since [1980], the amount of money spent by advertisers to reach children has increased by a factor of 20—from $100 million to $2 billion a year.

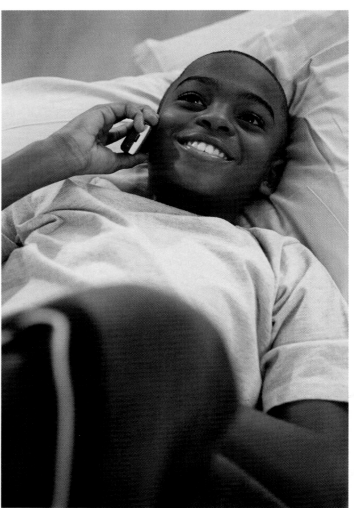

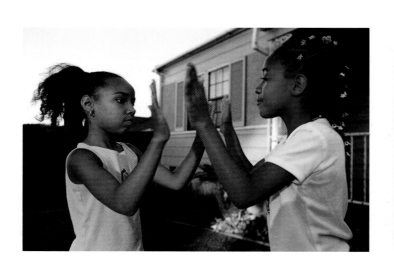

So what can we do to vaccinate our children against affluenza? Here are a few ideas:

- Turn off the TV, or sharply limit children's viewing. TV is a notorious "hot zone" for affluenza, with each ad a potential carrier of the virus. A recent study by Dr. Barbara Brock at Eastern Washington University found that 90% of kids who went without TV for 30 days reported that, while being subjected to far fewer marketing messages, they were happier, got more sleep, spent more time talking with their parents, and did better in school.

- Help keep advertising out of schools. A non-partisan coalition, including Ralph Nader on the Left and Phyllis Schlafly on the Right, is already working hard to achieve this. In Seattle, where I live, the school board recently agreed to begin phasing out commercial messages in city schools, including a news program, which includes 2 minutes of slick advertising in each day's 10-minute broadcast.

- Teach financial literacy and media literacy to children. In San Diego, Consumer Credit Counseling runs a program that begins in kindergarten, training kids to practice safe shopping and stay out of debt. It should be a model for other cities. Media literacy courses help kids see how TV ads manipulate them. Two Web sites that offer excellent financial and media literacy resources are *www.consumerjungle.org* and *www.pbskids.org/dontbuyit.*

- Consider legislation that restricts advertising that targets children. The province of Quebec and several European countries, recognizing that young children are often unable to separate facts from commercial appeals, prohibit television advertising to children under the age of 12. Sweden is seeking a European Union-wide ban on such advertising.

- Find time for meaningful one-on-one conversation with our children. Today, both parents and children are leading lives filled with overwork and over-scheduled activities. From 1979 to 2000, work time increased by 388 hours per year for dual-income households. Long work hours mean parents often don't have time for their kids, and what time they do have is frequently spent as a spectator or driver as children are shuffled from one activity to another. Child psychologists warn that children need more free time and unstructured play; their calendars are now commonly as filled up as those of their parents. A recent University of Michigan study found that the best predictor of students' success in college was having family meals together and real conversations with parents; yet, since 1970, the number of American families sharing dinners has dropped by a third. Parents often shower their children with things out of a feeling of guilt for not being able to give them enough time. It's wise for them to remember that "there's no present like the time."

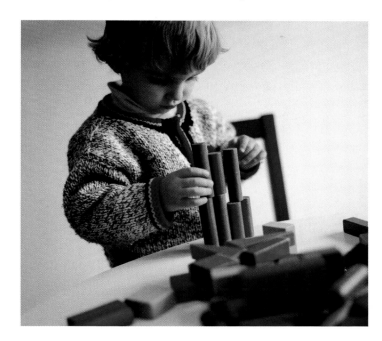

- Let children figure out for themselves what activities they can do to relieve boredom. "Boredom is the dream bird that hatches the golden egg of experience," wrote German social philosopher Walter Benjamin. Affluenza—the result of too frequently giving in to the nag factor—leaves children without the inner resources, and, often, the social supports and connections that are central to their becoming happy, well-adjusted adults.

The affluenza epidemic has struck deeply into American culture, infecting adults and children alike. But the disease can be cured if we recognize it and begin to vaccinate our children against it.

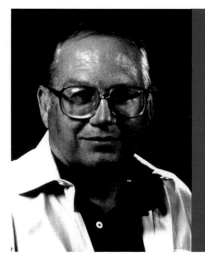

John de Graaf

John de Graaf is the coauthor of *Affluenza: The All-Consuming Epidemic* and co-producer of the popular *Affluenza* series on PBS. He has been producing television documentaries for 26 years. He is the national coordinator for Take Back Your Time Day (www.timeday.org) and the editor of *Take Back Your Time: Fighting Overwork and Time Poverty in America.* He is a member of the Simplicity Forum, the father of a 10-year-old son, and a resident of Seattle, Washington.

Chapter 2

Advertising in Schools

Alex Molnar

Schoolhouse commercialism takes many forms, from advertising on school property to the privatization of services such as lunch programs, school administration, and classroom teaching. Over the past three decades, advertising in schools has become increasingly pervasive and problematic.

Definitions of commercialism vary. The Oxford English Dictionary defines it as "the principles and practice of commerce; excessive adherence to financial return as a measure of worth."[1] In *Lead Us Into Temptation*, James Twitchell says commercialism consists of two processes: "*commodification*, or stripping an object of all other values except its value for sale to someone else, and *marketing*, the insertion of the object into a network of exchanges, only some of which involve money."[2]

Commercialism and childhood are a problematic combination. As marketing professor James McNeal notes, "Kids are the most unsophisticated of all consumers; they have the least and therefore want the most. Consequently, they are in a perfect position to be taken."[3] Marketing to children in schools is especially troublesome because students are a captive audience and are asked to believe that what they are taught in school is in their best interest.

Efforts by corporations to use schools to promote their points of view, address public relations or political problems, or sell products and services are not new. Over the last two decades, however, it appears that corporations have dramatically increased marketing activities directed at children in schools. Today, most large corporations and trade associations have some type of in-school marketing program. Marketing activities range from advertising on school buses, on scoreboards, and in lunchrooms to the creation of electronic and print "learning materials" for science, government, history, math, and current events classes.

Today, most large corporations and trade associations have some type of in-school marketing program.

The pervasiveness of schoolhouse commercialism raises serious issues about the impact on the lives and education of young people, including the potential for distorting and biasing children's lessons. Curriculum materials sponsored by corporate interests may offer self-serving information about controversial subjects. For example, a forest industry group, Pacific Logging Congress, distributes brochures and photos purporting to depict "environmentally responsible clear cuts." As one critic noted, "If you just start educating people at young ages around these facts, then they accept it as truth."[4]

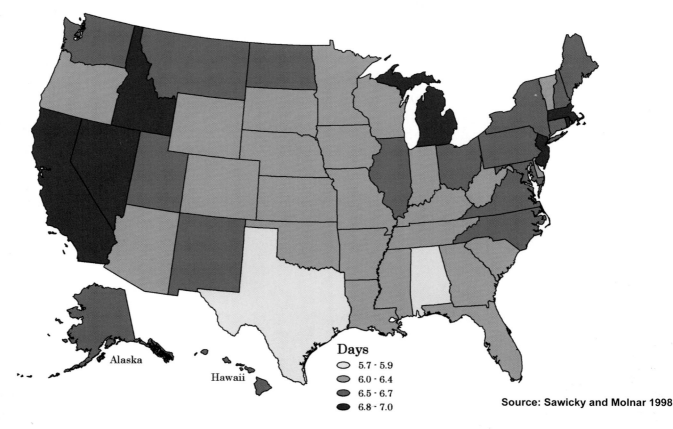

Days
- ◯ 5.7 - 5.9
- 6.0 - 6.4
- 6.5 - 6.7
- ⬤ 6.8 - 7.0

Source: Sawicky and Molnar 1998

Map 2.1: Estimated Number of Days of Instructional Time Annually Devoted to Channel One in a Subscribing School, 1998

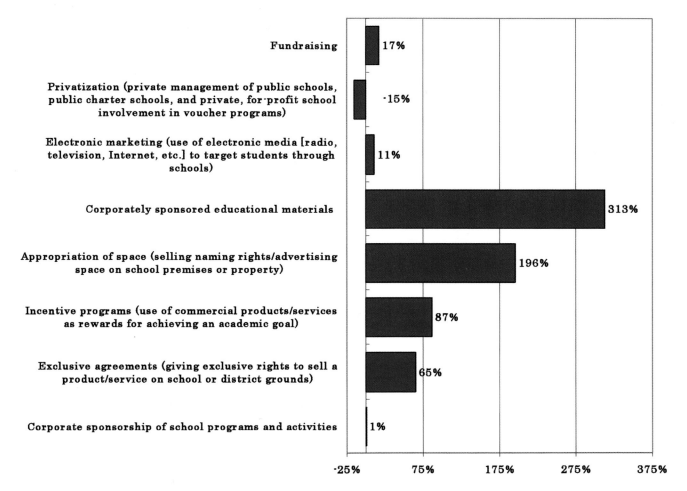

Fundraising — 17%

Privatization (private management of public schools, public charter schools, and private, for-profit school involvement in voucher programs) — -15%

Electronic marketing (use of electronic media [radio, television, Internet, etc.] to target students through schools) — 11%

Corporately sponsored educational materials — 313%

Appropriation of space (selling naming rights/advertising space on school premises or property) — 196%

Incentive programs (use of commercial products/services as rewards for achieving an academic goal) — 87%

Exclusive agreements (giving exclusive rights to sell a product/service on school or district grounds) — 65%

Corporate sponsorship of school programs and activities — 1%

-25%   75%   175%   275%   375%

Figure 2.1: Change in Commercial Activities in Schools, 2002-2003

Source: Molnar 2003

While no databases currently exist that allow the direct tracking of schoolhouse commercialism, the Commercialism in Education Research Unit at Arizona State University's Education Policy Studies Laboratory has devised a method of tracking schoolhouse commercialism indirectly through media references. Each year since 1998, the Commercialism in Education Research Unit has released a report on schoolhouse commercializing trends.[5-10] The 2003 report, *No Child Left Unsold*,[5] documents 5,264 media references to various school-based commercial activities between July 1, 2002, and June 30, 2003.

The rapid growth of commercially sponsored activities and materials promoting the consumption of foods of little or no nutritional value in public schools is attracting increasing attention. Schoolhouse marketing of such products raises fundamental issues of public policy. Schools are important venues for teaching students about health and nutrition. Exclusive marketing arrangements with soft drink and fast food companies; placement of vending machines offering candy and high-fat, salty snacks; "educational materials" sponsored by fast food outlets; incentive programs and contests that encourage the consumption of unhealthy foods; and direct advertising of junk food on Channel One (the ad-bearing TV channel shown in many schools) and other electronic marketing media constitute a pervasive, informal curriculum that sends children powerful and harmful health messages.

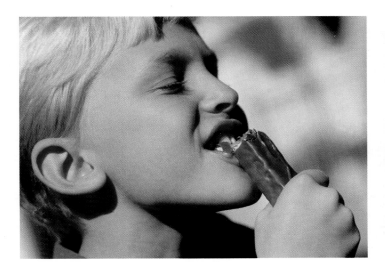

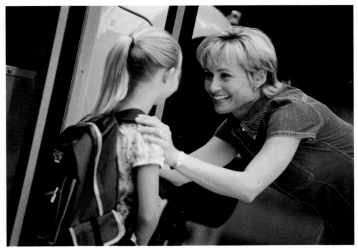

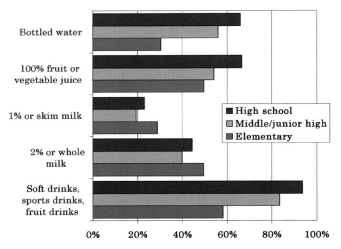

Figure 2.2: Percentage of Schools Selling Beverages by Type and School Level, 2000

Source: Centers for Disease Control and Prevention 2001

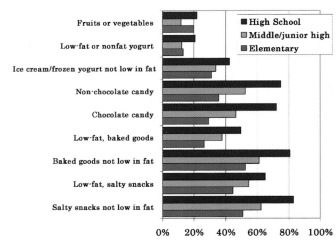

Figure 2.3: Percentage of Schools Selling Snacks by Type and School Level, 2000

Source: Centers for Disease Control and Prevention 2001

Accompanying the growth of such marketing practices has been a significant and alarming rise in obesity among young people. In October 2002, the U.S. Centers for Disease Control and Prevention (CDC) reported that rates of overweight in children have tripled in the last two decades. According to 1999 and 2000 data, 15% of children and teenagers (9 million) ages 6 to 19 were overweight with a body mass index at or about the 95th percentile.[11]

Soda consumption has increased dramatically. *The Washington Post* reports that, according to the Beverage Marketing Corporation, annual consumption per capita of soda increased from 22.4 gallons in 1970 to 56.1 gallons in 1998.[12] The Center for Science in the Public Interest found that a quarter of teenage boys who drank soda drank more than two 12-ounce cans per day, and 5% drank more than five cans per day.[13] Richard Troiano, a National Cancer Institute senior scientist, says the data on soda consumption suggest that there may be a link between childhood obesity and soda consumption.[12]

Soda consumption has additional health hazards, especially for girls. With soda displacing milk in their diets, an increasing number of girls may be candidates for osteoporosis. Harvard researchers found that physically active girls who drink soda are 3 times as likely to suffer bone fractures as girls who never drink soda. If the

soda of choice is cola, the risk increases 5 times.[14,15] With childhood obesity rates soaring, William Dietz, director of the Division of Nutrition at CDC, suggests that, "If the schools must have vending machines, they should concentrate on healthy choices like bottled water."[12]

School districts, teachers, parents, and policymakers have begun to look critically at corporate marketing and its impact on children's health. For example, PTA groups and citizens groups such as the Citizen's Campaign for Commercial-Free Schools (Seattle) and Parents Advocating School Accountability (San Francisco) have spoken out against school commercialism. Local school boards have also taken action. In Seattle, school-based advertising was severely restricted.[16] The Los Angeles school board has banned the sale of soft drinks beginning in 2004, citing an epidemic of adolescent obesity,[17] and has subsequently moved to ban junk food as well.[18] In Philadelphia, the schools' chief executive officer, Paul Vallas, sought a ban on soda in schools.[19] New York City schools banned soda, sweet snacks, and candy from vending machines.[20] The Texas Education Agency directed districts, as of the fall of 2002, to stop selling "foods of minimal nutritional value" in cafeterias, hallways, or common areas.[21] In January 2003, Aptos Middle School became the first school in San Francisco to implement the district's junk food ban.[22]

Professional organizations, including the National Education Association and the Society of Consumer Affairs Professionals in Business, have developed voluntary guidelines to help determine which, if any, corporate-sponsored materials have merit. Various organizations have adopted the Milwaukee Principles for Corporate Involvement in the Schools.[23] The National Association of State Boards of Education has developed sample policies to promote healthy eating.[24] The American Academy of Pediatrics has taken positions critical of advertising aimed at children in general and school-based advertising that promotes unhealthy lifestyle choices in particular.[25]

Legislators have begun to take note of school commercialism and its effects on children's health. In *Commercial Activities in Schools*, published in September 2000, the United States General Accounting Office reported that only seven states had laws or

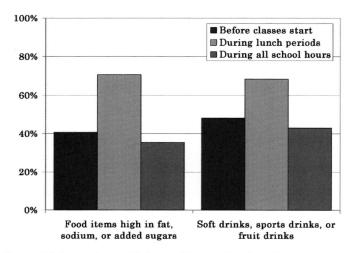

Figure 2.4: Percentage of Schools Allowing Food and Beverage Purchases by Time, 2000

Source: Centers for Disease Control and Prevention 2001

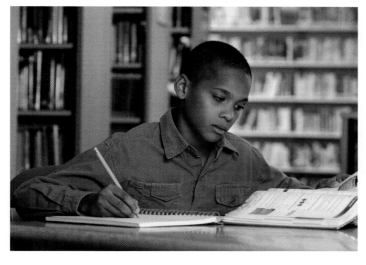

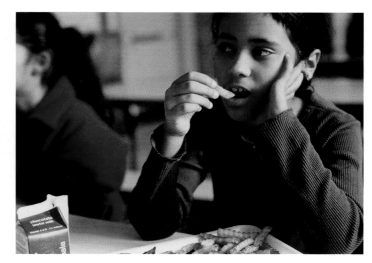

regulations that covered product sales, such as soft drink and snack food sales.[26] In October 2001, California Governor Gray Davis signed the Pupil Nutrition, Health, and Achievement Act establishing restrictions on the sale of soft drinks and candy in elementary and middle schools.[27] In September 2003, Davis signed the California Childhood Obesity Prevention Act that prohibits the sale of soft drinks during school hours to students in elementary schools beginning on September 1, 2005, and puts restrictions on the sale to middle and high school students beginning September 1, 2006.[27]

A review of 1999 to 2003 legislative activity by the Commercialism in Education Research Unit found 30 pieces of legislation and three resolutions that specifically addressed schoolhouse commercialism issues at the federal and state level. Three pieces of legislation actually enabled commercializing activities in the schools. Of the 30 pieces of legislation, 17 failed, 5 passed, and 8 were pending as of July 2003. Of the three resolutions introduced, two failed and one passed.[28]

Courts have become another avenue of opposition. In 2003, the Quality Beverage Association, joined by individual taxpayers and residents, filed a lawsuit in New York after the New York Education Commissioner authorized exclusive soft drink agreements. The

Curriculum materials sponsored by corporate interests may offer self-serving information about controversial subjects.

association claimed the commissioner violated state law concerning the after-hours use of school property, the state constitutional prohibition on using public property for the benefit of a private corporation, the state law governing competitive bidding of public contracts, and the regulation prohibiting commercialism on school property.[29] Also in 2003, an Oregon parent filed a suit against his child's school district for requiring his child to watch Channel One. The suit alleged that the district's contract with the broadcaster amounted to an unlawful delegation of powers to educate school-children reserved to the government under the Oregon Constitution.[30]

Despite increased opposition, commercialism in schools is so pervasive that it remains difficult for many people to see, blending seamlessly with the marketing maelstrom of American culture. Yet, the evidence suggests that parents and ordinary citizens are becoming much more concerned about the corporate exploitation of children in school.[5] Pedagogically marketing in schools undermines lessons such as those in nutrition. It allows curriculum content to devolve from material based on a serious professional assessment of what is best to teach, how best to teach it, and when best to teach it into a flea market in which anyone with enough money to buy a booth can present their story or pitch their product.

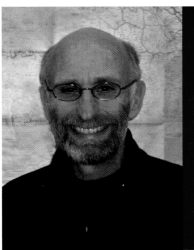

Alex Molnar

Alex Molnar is a professor of education policy and director of the Education Policy Studies Laboratory at Arizona State University. He has a BA in history, political science, and education; master's degrees in history and social welfare; a specialist's certificate in educational administration; and a PhD in urban education. Molnar's work has appeared in scholarly and professional journals as well as newspapers and magazines such as *The New York Times*, *The Wall Street Journal*, *USA Today*, *New Republic*, and *Education Week*. He has been a frequent guest on National Public Radio's *Market Place* and *The Nation*. He has appeared on television's *60 Minutes*, *The News Hour*, and *CNN Reports*, among others. Molnar is the editor or coauthor of several books, including *Changing Problem Behavior in Schools*, which is widely used by educators in the United States and has been translated into four languages; *Giving Kids the Business: The Commercialization of America's Schools*; *The Construction of Children's Character*; *Vouchers, Class Size Reduction, and Student Achievement: Considering the Evidence*; and *School Reform Proposals: The Research Evidence*.

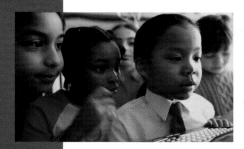

Chapter 3

Sandra L. Calvert

Interactive Media
and Well-being

In the information age, American children are growing up in a world of interactive computer media. These include personal computers, video games, and cell phones that link to the Internet. Access and usage patterns have expanded rapidly over the past two decades. While older youth have more options than younger ones, the use of computers begins for some infants in the first 2 years of life.

Although a mouse or a game controller requires hand-eye coordination for successful performance, a 2003 Kaiser survey documents that as many as 30% of 0- to 6-year-olds have played video games. Boys surpass girls in overall access to video game play as well as in daily use of video games. The Kaiser report also documents that as many as 11% of 0- to 2-year-

olds and 70% of 4- to 6-year-olds have used a computer at some point in their lives with 18% of 0- to 6-year-old children indicating they use a computer in a typical day. Parental attitudes about computer experiences are more favorable than their attitudes about video game play.[1]

Similarly, a survey of 8- to 12-year-olds (tweens) and 13- to 17-year-olds (teens) revealed that 88% of these children had access to a personal computer, and 76% had access to the Internet.[2] The researchers also found that video game equipment was accessible to 75% of this age group, and 50% had portable video games. Boys had more video game equipment than girls. Cell phones were available to 40% of teens, but to only 5% of tweens. Girls had more access to cell phones than boys.

For all American households, Nielsen reports that approximately 39 million homes (13%) have broadband access, allowing large amounts of information, including pictures, to be transmitted quickly from the Internet to the home, whereas approximately 70 million homes have narrowband access, providing much slower accessibility to online information.[3] In 2001, Jupiter Research documented that Asian American (63%) and Caucasian (62%)

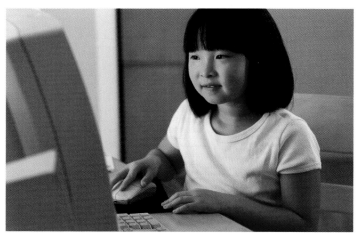

households were more likely to have Internet access than were African American (45%) and Latino (45%) households, and all groups' home access to the Internet was projected to expand rapidly.[4]

Uses and gratification theory examines the ways that children use different kinds of media and the kinds of needs those uses of media fulfill. While we have little data about why very young children use interactive computer

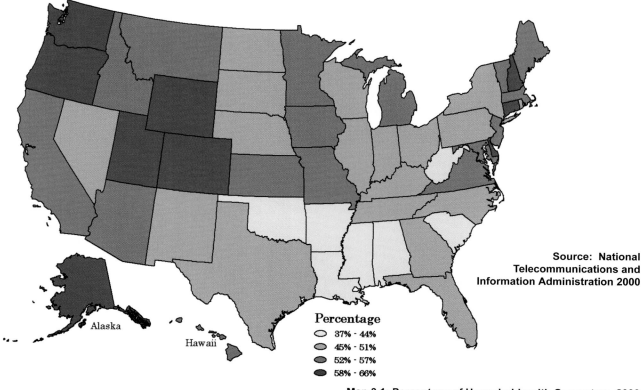

Source: National Telecommunications and Information Administration 2000

Alaska

Hawaii

Percentage
- ⬭ 37% - 44%
- ⬭ 45% - 51%
- ⬭ 52% - 57%
- ⬭ 58% - 66%

Map 3.1: Percentage of Households with Computers, 2000

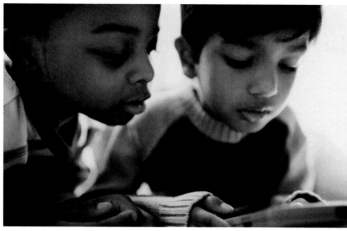

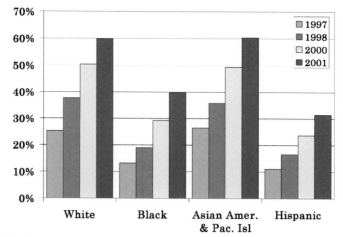

Figure 3.1: Overall Internet Use for Individuals Age 3 and Older by Race

Source: U.S. Department of Commerce 2002

technologies, tweens and teens say they use the Internet to master new skills, explore their identities, and make new friends.[2] Activities that make children feel proud about themselves include creating online journals, setting up and using cell phones, and playing games online. Children also report that creating personal Web pages, instant messaging, chatting online, sharing music, and making friends online allow them to explore and express who they are.

Cell phones are used primarily to meet communication needs, but they increasingly offer access to video game play and other online activities, making them a potential constant link to the Internet. When online, youth prefer instant messaging to e-mail for communications.[2]

> **Youth who explore their identities in multi-user domains sometimes work through issues that they face in real life.**

In the cognitive domain, there is a shift in children's thinking from iconic (visual) to symbolic (verbal) modes of thought that dovetails with the visual and verbal presentational forms of computers and video games.[5] Because of the increased use of pictorial displays, many computer technologies present content in forms that emphasize iconic modes of thought. Action, for instance, provides a visual way to think about and remember visually presented content that improves young children's memory of both visual and verbal material.[6] When examining the appeal of specific features, boys prefer action, whereas girls prefer musical rewards.[7] The data suggest that how a presentation is made affects children's memory of significant content.

Exposure to video games can also cultivate visuospatial skills. In a series of studies, Patricia Greenfield and her colleagues found that those who played video games well performed better on general tasks of spatial ability as well as divided attention tasks in which one has to perform more than one task at a time. While boys were generally better at video game play and spatial tasks than were girls, playing video games increased the spatial skills of those who were least proficient at these tasks (i.e., the girls).

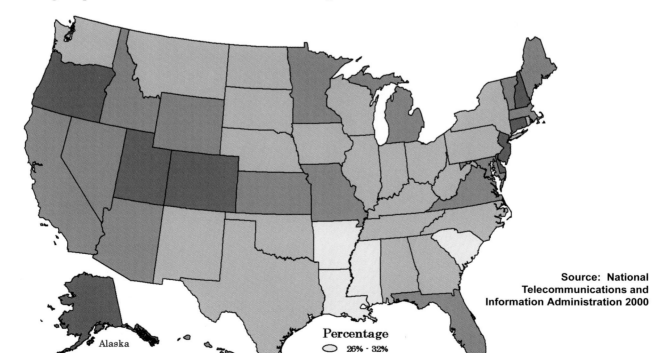

Source: National Telecommunications and Information Administration 2000

Percentage
- 26% - 32%
- 33% - 41%
- 42% - 47%
- 48% - 56%

Map 3.2: Percentage of Households with Internet Access, 2000

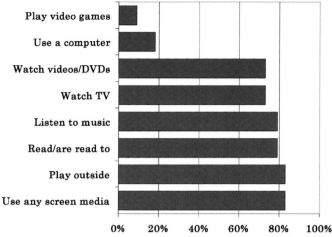

Figure 3.2: Typical Daily Activities for Chidren 0 to 6 Years Old, 2003
Source: Kaiser Family Foundation 2003

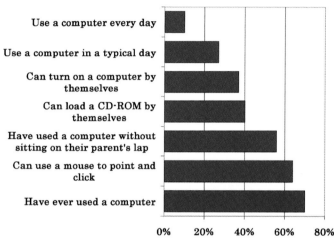

Figure 3.3: Computer Use and Skills of Children 4 to 6 Years Old, 2003
Source: Kaiser Family Foundation 2003

School systems often purchase and use software packages that facilitate children's learning. Computer-assisted instruction is generally effective in teaching educational content. These packages often take a step-by-step approach to teaching basic skills and reinforce successful performance each step of the way.

In the social domain, early fears that computer use would lead to social isolation are largely unfounded. Although one study found that adults initially gravitated to "weaker" online relationships rather than to "stronger" face-to-face interactions, follow-up studies revealed that, over time, adults returned to the stronger social interactions. Two

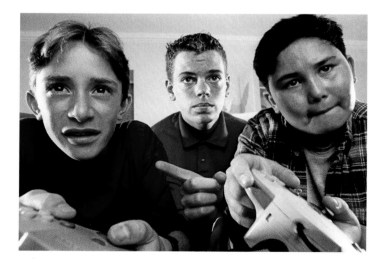

reasons may have accounted for this shift. One is that the novelty of the computer interactions has declined over time. The second is that online options have changed with the introduction of programs such as instant messaging. This allows users to interact with people that they know rather than with strangers who could possibly prey on them in some way.

Adolescents generally use instant messaging to stay in touch with friends and to be social.[8] One exception is youth with social adjustment problems who tend to interact with strangers.

Children and adolescents also experiment with their identity online, an activity that is a central developmental task for this age group. When youth are online, one advantage is that they can pretend to be anyone they desire. Multiuser domains, where fantasy worlds are constructed and explored; chat rooms; personal Web pages; and blogs, which are often diaries and running dialogues with others, are forums for such explorations. Avatars, which are animated or live depictions of a character, can be used to represent one's self.

Youth who explore their identities in multiuser domains sometimes work through identity issues that they face in real life.[9] When interacting with strangers, tweens tend to present themselves in ways that intertwine with their real-life identities. For instance, most children create avatars of their own biological gender. The online interaction style between two boys is more action-oriented and playful when compared to two girls, who tend to be more communicative as expressed via written exchanges. When boys and girls interact together in a pair, both sexes alter their communication styles with boys becoming less playful and more "talkative" and girls moving their avatars more and "talking" less.[10]

Cell phones allow youth to stay in touch with one another at all times via voice or text messages. In the future, cell phone communications will increasingly use the Internet as an interface.

The Internet allows advertisers to target youth through personal advertising strategies in which companies attempt to develop consumer brand loyalty through one-on-one interactions and the use of promotional materials that can be downloaded.[11] The Children's Online Privacy Protection

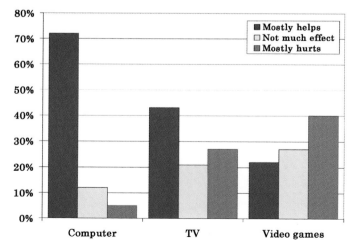

Figure 3.4: Video Game Activities for Chidren 4 to 6 Years Old by Gender, 2003
Source: Kaiser Family Foundation 2003

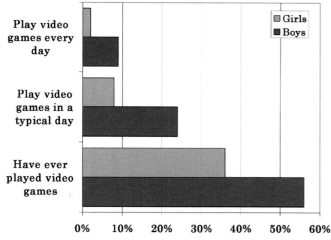

Figure 3.5: Parents' Views on Whether Media Helps or Hurts Children's Learning, 2003

Source: Kaiser Family Foundation 2003

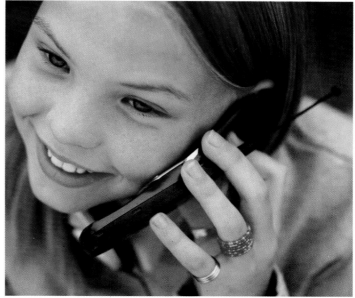

Act prevents some deceptive practices that are targeted at children who are under age 13.

Cell phones will increasingly become the avenue for interacting with children, and pop-up ads that suddenly appear in a small window of a computer or cell phone screen will become a new avenue for advertising to youth. The convenience of having a cell phone that can be used to purchase products will also track where the person is, providing companies with specific personal buying patterns that can be used to target individual consumers.

Interactive media use can benefit or harm children's health. Although negative effects of early exposure to media have not yet been documented, the American Academy of Pediatrics recommends no screen exposure until after age 2.

Video game play has been implicated in the development of aggressive behaviors. Playing aggressive video games can occur online and offline and can subsequently increase aggressive cognitions (e.g., thinking about words with aggressive meanings such as "kill" and "shoot") and aggressive behaviors (e.g., attacking or teasing others during play) as well as decrease constructive, prosocial behaviors (e.g., helping others).[12]

Repeated legislative efforts to restrict children's access to online sexually explicit content have generally failed

American children are growing up in a world of interactive computer media. These include personal computers, video games, and cell phones that link to the Internet.

because of the First Amendment rights of content providers. In a comprehensive report commissioned by the U.S. Congress, the National Academy of Sciences discussed a three-pronged approach to the online pornography issue: educational strategies, legislative strategies, and technological strategies such as filtering content. A related problem is the presence of online predators who target underage youth.

The Internet also provides a constructive forum for youth to explore their health-related questions. Adolescents use health-related sites to acquire information about their sexual health as well as to communicate with one another about illnesses.[13] In this way, the Internet provides a link to support groups that are not limited by spatial locations.

The past two decades demonstrated an explosion in children's access to, and use of, interactive computer technologies. In the future, two trends are notable. The first is the use of increasingly small mobile interactive wireless units that will be taken anywhere that children go. The second involves the phenomenon of convergence. Distinct media platforms of the future will merge, as seen already with cell phones becoming Internet links. Both trends will make interactive media an increasingly ubiquitous presence in children's daily lives.

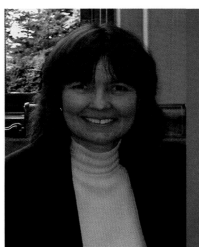

Sandra L. Calvert

Sandra L. Calvert, PhD, the director of the Children's Digital Media Center, is a professor of psychology at Georgetown University. She is author of *Children's Journeys Through the Information Age* (McGraw Hill, 1999), and coeditor of *Children in the Digital Age: Influences of Electronic Media on Development* (Praeger, 2002).

Dr. Calvert's research examines the role that interactivity and identity play in children's learning from entertainment media through studies conducted by the Children's Digital Media Center, which is funded by the National Science Foundation. She is also involved in media policy, recently completing research about children's learning from educational and informational television programs required by the Children's Television Act.

Professor Calvert is a fellow of the American Psychological Association. She has consulted for Nickelodeon Online, Sesame Workplace, *Blue's Clues*, and Sega of America to influence the development of children's television programs, Internet software, and video games.

Chapter 4

Thomas N. Robinson and James D. Sargent

Children and Media

Children spend a substantial share of their time watching various forms of popular media. In a 1998 nationwide survey,[1] parents reported that their 2- to 7-year-old children spent an average of about 2½ hours per day watching television, video game, computer, and movie screens. Eight- to 18-year-olds reported that they spent an average of about 4½ hours per day of "screen time." That translates into more than one-fourth of an average child's total awake life from age 2 to 18.[2] Clearly, any activities that account for such a large share of our children's lives should be of particular interest to child health and educational professionals.

Despite the rapid diffusion of new media technologies into family homes, the vast majority of media use continues to be television viewing. According to the 1998 survey, the television was on most of the time in 42% of homes, and it was on during meals in 58% of homes. Eighty-eight percent of children lived in homes with two or more televisions, and 32% of 2- to 7-year-olds and 65% of 8- to 18-year-olds had televisions in their bedrooms. Furthermore, African American and Hispanic children and children from families with lower socioeconomic status tended to watch even more television than other U.S. children. Adolescents also were reported to be avid readers of magazines, collectors of music CDs and MP3s, and users of the Internet an average of about a half hour per day.

Time spent with media may affect health through at least two mechanisms. From media, children and adolescents gain information about their world through the behaviors—which are often risky—of celebrities and other media figures. This information, when presented repeatedly, shapes children's attitudes toward these behaviors, softens resistance to engaging in risky activities, and enhances the perceived benefits of these behaviors, thereby contributing to the adoption and maintenance of the behaviors.[3] Risky behaviors thought to be affected by media include aggression, unhealthy eating patterns, physical inactivity, and substance use. In addition, media use is largely a passive activity. By substituting media use for play activities, children become more sedentary. Also, they decrease time spent actively socializing with others, potentially leading to poor social skills and a sense of isolation.

> **The most commonly cited adverse effect of media is the link between exposure to media violence and subsequent aggressive behavior. Violence is pervasive in television, movies, and video games.**

The most commonly cited adverse effect of media is the link between exposure to media violence and subsequent aggressive behavior. Violence is pervasive in television, movies, and video games. It has been estimated that by the age of 18 years, U.S. children witness more than 200,000 acts of violence on television alone.[4] The relationship between media violence and aggressive behavior has been the focus of more than 1,000 studies. Exposure to violent media seems to produce three effects: (a) direct effects, in which children become more aggressive and/or develop more favorable attitudes about using aggression to resolve conflicts, (b) desensitization to violence and the victimization of others, and (c) beliefs that the world around them is more dangerous than it truly is. Reviews of the research literature indicate a consensus that exposure to television violence increases children's aggressive attitudes and behaviors.[5] As a potential response, a recent controlled

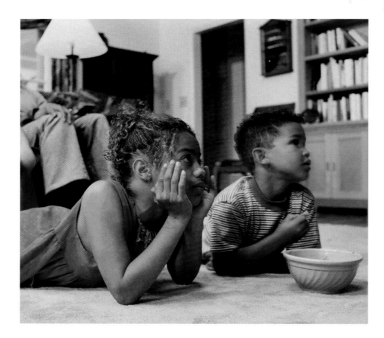

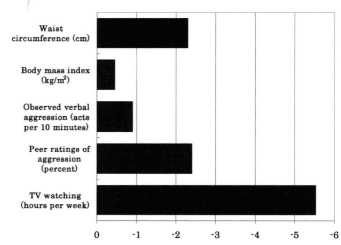

Figure 4.1: Effects of a Curriculum to Reduce 3rd- and 4th-Grade Television, Videotape, and Video Game Use Over 1 School Year, 1999
Source: Robinson, et al. 2001 and Robinson 1999

trial demonstrated that a curriculum designed to reduce 3rd- and 4th-grade children's television, videotape, and video game use decreased aggressive behavior, as rated by peers and directly observed on the playground.[6]

Another frequently cited adverse effect of media exposure is its impact on obesity.[2] Researchers hypothesize that media use contributes to obesity via one or more of three general mechanisms: increasing calorie consumption while watching or as a result of advertising, displacing physical activity, and/or reducing resting energy metabolism. Epidemiological studies from many different samples and settings have confirmed associations between television viewing and body fatness.[2] The results of several recent experimental studies have shown that reducing children's television viewing helps reduce the risk of obesity and helps promote weight loss in obese children.[2] One recent randomized, controlled trial demonstrated that a school curriculum designed solely to reduce 3rd- and 4th-grade children's television, videotape, and video game use produced a statistically significant and clinically significant reduction in weight gain.[7]

Research also suggests that media use increases the propensity to engage in other risk behaviors, such as alcohol consumption and tobacco use. Alcohol consumption is frequently portrayed in both entertainment programming and advertising, and alcohol is the most commonly shown beverage on television. Portrayals of alcohol use and alcohol ads are particularly common in prime time programming, music videos, and televised sports events. Content analyses indicate that alcohol use is usually portrayed favorably—often in association with sexually suggestive content, recreation, or motor vehicle use—and rarely in an unattractive manner or in association with negative consequences. A study that followed previously nondrinking, 14-year-old California 9th graders for 18 months indicated that watching more television and music videos substantially increased risks of subsequent initiation of drinking by the end of 10th grade.[8]

Media exposure has also been linked with smoking initiation. The typical movie contains five smoking depictions, and some contain a depiction every few minutes. A recent study examined adolescents' exposure to smoking in 601 popular contemporary movies. The average

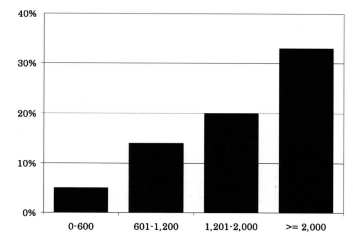

Figure 4.3: **Percentage of New England Adolescents (Ages 9-15) Who Tried Smoking by the Number of Smoking Scenes They Had Seen in Movies, 1999**

Source: Sargent, et al. 2001

adolescent had seen more than 1,000 smoking depictions in movies, and about 25% of the sample had seen more than 2,000.[9] It is not surprising that there was a strong relationship between higher exposure to movie smoking and adolescent smoking. Whereas only 5% of adolescents in a northern New England sample with low exposure to movie smoking had tried smoking, some 33% in a high-exposure group had.[10] After adjusting the analysis for more than 15 other variables, children in the highest category of exposure were almost 3 times more likely to have tried smoking. In addition, as might be expected, children who reported that their parents did not allow them to view R-rated movies had substantially lower rates of alcohol and tobacco use.[11] Based on this information, a professor of medicine at the University of California at San Francisco has developed a public health campaign with the aim of

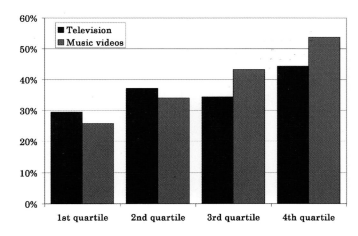

Figure 4.2: **Percentage of 9th Graders Starting to Drink Alcohol by End of 10th Grade by Exposure to Television and Music Videos from Lowest Exposure Quartile to Highest**

Source: Robinson, et al. 1998

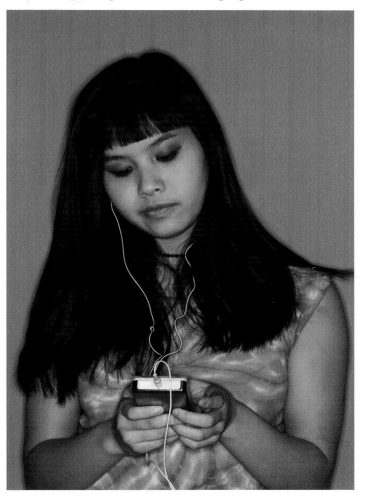

23

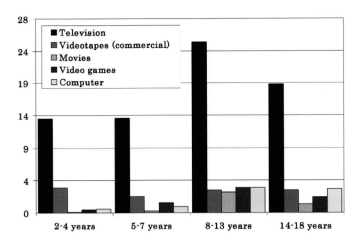

Figure 4.4: Hours of Media Exposure Per Week by Media Type and Age, 1999

Source: Kaiser Family Foundation 1999

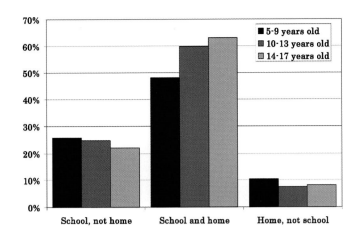

Figure 4.5: Percentage of Children Using Computers by Age and Location of Use, 2001

Source: U.S. Department of Commerce 2002

convincing the movie industry to give movies that show smoking an R rating.[12] The R rating and other policy solutions of the Smoke Free Movies campaign have been endorsed by the World Health Organization, the American Medical Association, and the American Academy of Pediatrics. From a public health perspective, rating smoking R could have a dramatic effect on children's exposure to smoking in movies by eliminating smoking from G, PG, and PG-13 movies.

Although there is a common perception that television and video games have an adverse effect on learning and school performance, research findings on the topic are not clear. Correlations between amount of television or video game use and academic achievement are generally small and become weaker when adjusted for socioeconomic status and IQ of the child. However, there is some evidence for a threshold effect, in which very heavy media users have substantially worse school performance.[13,14] Researchers hypothesize that television and video games either displace activities that would improve academic achievement, such as reading and homework, or that the formats of television shows and video games (e.g., rapid pace, scene changes, entertaining content) make children more easily distracted, making it harder for them to pay attention in school. On the other hand, just as media can "teach" undesirable behaviors, there is also evidence that properly designed educational media can improve reading, vocabulary, mathematics, problem solving, and creativity and even increase children's prosocial behaviors. This is an indication that it is the content, and not solely the media use, that makes the difference.

Many child health professionals and child advocates also are concerned about the large amount of advertising children see from a very young age. Some studies suggest that the average number of television commercials a child sees in a year has increased from about 20,000 to about 40,000 over the past three decades, now accounting for about one-sixth of children's television viewing time.[13,15] Additional viewing time is devoted to entertainment television programs and movies that are either based on specific products or promote an accompanying line of products. More recently, products are placed throughout entertainment programming as less conspicuous advertisements. Experimental studies demonstrate that advertising is successful at influencing children's

perceptions and choices, and meaningful regulatory attempts to limit advertising to children have repeatedly been resisted by the advertising and media industries.[16] Media literacy programs have been able to increase children's knowledge about advertising but have not resulted in skills that children use. The only method to show promise to date is to reduce children's total media exposure.[17]

With so much exposure, it is not surprising that media use has been tied to many different health, behavioral, and social effects in children and adolescents. Even small effects from brief exposures may be magnified substantially when multiplied over time and throughout such a large proportion of the population, potentially translating into very large effects among individuals,

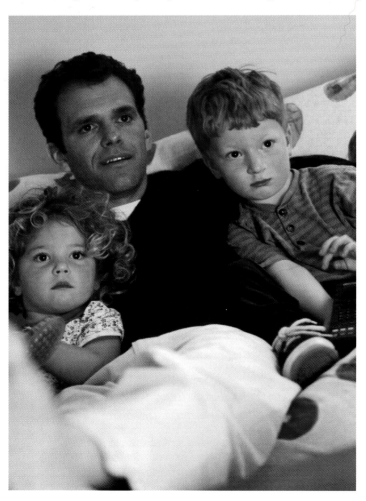

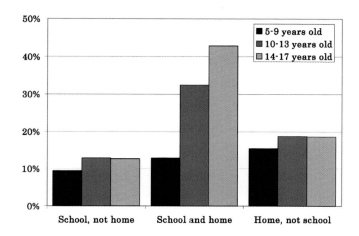

Figure 4.6: Percentage of Children Using the Internet by Age and Location of Use, 2001

Source: U.S. Department of Commerce 2002

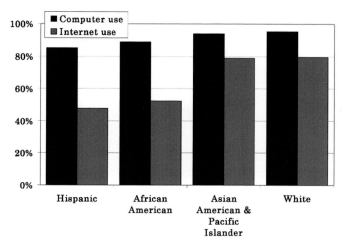

Figure 4.7: Percentage of Children Using Computers and the Internet by Race and Ethnicity, 2001

Source: U.S. Department of Commerce 2002

families, communities, and populations. There also are large variations in formats and content both within and between different media technologies. It should not be surprising, therefore, that both positive and negative effects may result from media exposure. As children's media environments continue to expand to include the Internet, electronic mail, instant messaging, digital recording devices, portable phones with cameras, etc., the impacts of media content on child health and behavior will grow.

To date, only reducing media exposure has been successful in mitigating the adverse effects of media content. Methods and technologies to reduce children's media use are becoming more available, but their diffusion has been slow. A number of educational and health organ-

> By substituting media use for play activities, children become more sedentary. Also, they decrease time spent actively socializing with others, potentially leading to poor social skills and a sense of isolation.

izations, including the American Academy of Pediatrics and the National Parent Teacher Association, recommend that parents limit their children's television and movie viewing and video and computer game playing to a maximum of 1 or 2 hours per day. Based on the evidence of media effects presented above, we recommend that child health, education, and welfare professionals (a) promote limits on children's media use (no more than 7 to 14 hours per week), (b) promote keeping television, video games, and the Internet out of children's bedrooms, and (c) advocate for tighter controls on media content and advertising directed at children, particularly content and advertising that contain substance use, including tobacco use.

Thomas N. Robinson and James D. Sargent

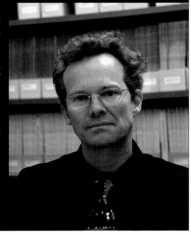

Thomas N. Robinson, MD, MPH, is an associate professor of pediatrics and medicine in the Division of General Pediatrics and the Stanford Prevention Research Center at Stanford University School of Medicine. His research focuses on the development and evaluation of health promotion and disease prevention interventions for children and adolescents, and he is principal investigator on numerous studies. Dr. Robinson also practices general pediatrics and directs the Pediatric Weight Control Program at Lucile Packard Children's Hospital. Dr. Robinson received his BS and MD from Stanford University and his MPH from the University of California, Berkeley. He completed his internship and residency in pediatrics at Children's Hospital in Boston and Harvard Medical School and returned to Stanford for postdoctoral training before joining the faculty in 1993.

James D. Sargent, MD, is a professor of pediatrics at Dartmouth Medical School. Dr. Sargent received his medical degree from the Tufts University School of Medicine. He completed his residency and a fellowship in pediatrics at Boston City Hospital before joining the Dartmouth Medical School faculty in 1989. He specializes in epidemiology and children's health. He is principal investigator of a study examining visual media influences on adolescent smoking behavior. In another study, he developed and implemented a tobacco use prevention intervention for rural schoolchildren in grades K through 12. In addition, he has conducted various studies in childhood lead poisoning, including an evaluation of calcium as a nutritional preventive agent, and several ecological studies identifying geographical predictors of lead poisoning.

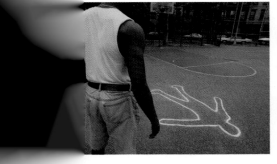

Chapter 5

Betsy McAlister Groves

Violence
in the Lives of Children

The book, *A Day in the Life of America*, chronicles a 24-hour period across the United States.[1] On May 2, 1986, two hundred of the world's leading photojournalists took pictures across the country from dawn through night. The book is a compilation of these photographs of family life and work and of people eating, socializing, and enjoying the outdoors.

However, this sanitized image of America is at odds with the current reality. In truth, there is no such thing as a day in the life of America's children without violence. If the photographers had been accurate, they would have included photographs of street fights, shootings, domestic assaults, and child abuse. For many children, violence and maltreatment create an America that is very different from the one depicted in the book.

Considering a range of indicators from homicides to gun ownership and violence in the media, the United States is more violent than most developed nations. Violence is a hallmark of U.S. culture and society. The United States has one of the highest homicide rates in the world. The homicide rate for young men is 73 times greater than the rate in similar industrialized nations. The proliferation of guns and other lethal weapons is directly linked to the increased homicide rates among children and to the numbers of violent incidents that children witness. Each day, 10 children in the United States are murdered by gunfire—approximately one every 2 1/2 hours. Homicide is the third leading cause of death among all children between the ages of 5 and 14 and the leading cause for Black youth.[2] This chapter will focus on violence in children's environments: violence in the media and real-life violence in the home or community.

Ninety-nine percent of American households have at least one television, making television the most ubiquitous source of exposure to violence for children.[3] The development and proliferation of television have revolutionized this society in a relatively short period of time. Fifty years ago, only a small percentage of households could afford a television. These televisions had small screens and produced black and white pictures. Networks were able to broadcast programs for only 2 or 3 hours in the evening. Now, the average preschooler watches 3 or 4 hours of television daily, viewing the programs on a large color screen using a remote control device to assist in choosing from dozens of channels. By the time preschoolers graduate from high school, they are likely to have seen more than 200,000 violent acts on television. In fact, children's commercial television programs contain more violent acts than programs for adults.[4] These statistics do not reflect children's increasing exposure to violent video games or movies accessed through VCRs or DVD players.

Television has profoundly changed the way young children receive messages about the outside world. Before the advent of television, parents could decide what to tell children about news from the outside world and when to tell them; they could monitor what was read to the child or what a child saw. However, television has greatly diminished parents' abilities to control these influences from the larger culture.[5] Some social scientists contend that television has destroyed the boundaries between adult knowledge and child knowledge.[6]

Hundreds of studies have made a compelling case for the extent to which media violence affects

> **Each day, 10 children in the United States are murdered by gunfire— approximately one every 2 1/2 hours.**

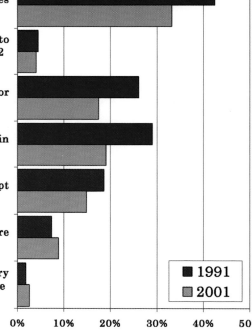

Were in a physical fight one or more times in last 12 months

Were injured in a physical fight and had to be treated by a doctor or nurse in last 12 months

Carried a weapon such as a gun, knife, or club in past 30 days

Seriously considered attempting suicide in last 12 months

Made a plan about how they would attempt suicide in last 12 months

Actually attempted suicide one or more times in last 12 months

Attempted suicide that resulted in an injury that had to be treated by a doctor or nurse in last 12 months

■ 1991
■ 2001

0%   10%   20%   30%   40%   50%

Figure 5.1: Percentage of 9th- through 12th-Grade Students Reporting They . . .

Source: Youth Risk Behavior Survey 1991 & 2001

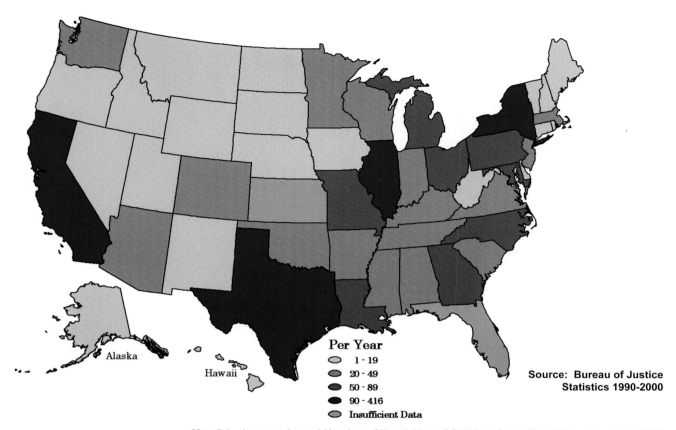

Per Year
- ⬭ 1 - 19
- ⬬ 20 - 49
- ⬭ 50 - 89
- ⬤ 90 - 416
- ⬬ Insufficient Data

Source: Bureau of Justice
Statistics 1990-2000

Map 5.1: Average Annual Number of Homicides of Children Ages 17 and Younger, 1990–2000

children.[7] Children imitate the violence they see on television. Exposure to television violence increases the viewer's apathy or desensitization to aggression.[8] Children who constantly observe violence in the media begin to see the world as a dangerous place. This worldview is a troubling message to give to young children and may discourage the kind of curiosity and exploration that leads to knowledge, self-confidence, and mastery. Finally, there is evidence that the effects of television violence on children persist into adulthood. A 15-year follow-up of children exposed to media violence shows that childhood exposure is predictive of aggressive behavior in young adult males and females.[9]

Real violence for children may include physical fighting, bullying, witnessing violence in the community, and witnessing violence in the home. Estimates show that nearly one-third of all high school students have reported being in a physical fight within the last year.[4]

Exposure to community violence includes crime, gang- or drug-related violence, school-related violence, and terrorist activities. While violent crime may be more prevalent in urban areas with a high concentration of poor families (one study in an urban health setting found that 10% of children had witnessed a knifing or shooting by the age of 6),[10] school violence and terrorist activities, such as the September 11 attacks, the Oklahoma City bombing, and the Columbine shootings, show no such class or geographic boundaries. School shootings have generally occurred in middle- or upper-class towns or suburbs, and virtually all children were affected by the September 11 attacks, regardless of where they lived. Recent studies of children's psychological symptoms after the September 11 terrorist attacks and the Oklahoma City bombings indicate many children in New York City and Oklahoma City had significant traumatic symptoms that were exacerbated by exposure to graphic television images.[11-13]

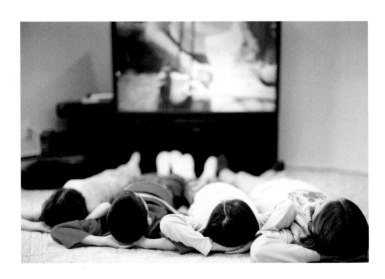

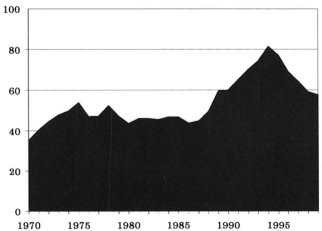

Figure 5.2: Rate of Violent Offense Arrest for Children Under Age 15 per 100,000

Source: Bureau of Justice Statistics 2004

27

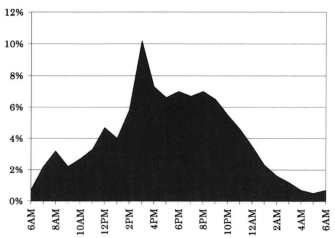

Figure 5.3: Percentage of Violent Victimization of Youth Under 18 by Time of Day
Source: Office of Juvenile Justice and Delinquency Prevention 1999

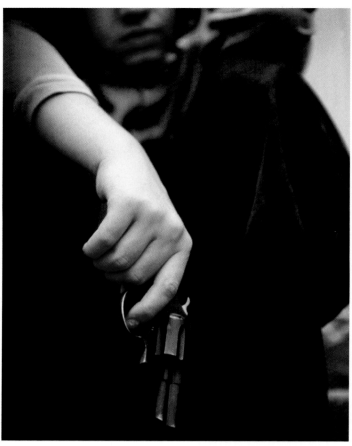

For this chapter, domestic violence is defined as abuse or threats of abuse between adult partners in the home. However, it could include child abuse, sibling abuse, and elder abuse—in other words, any violence or abuse among family members. Almost one-third of U.S. women are abused by a husband or a boyfriend.[14] Estimates of the numbers of children who witness domestic abuse vary from 3 million per year to 10 million.[15] The reason for the wide variation in estimates has to do with the differences in precise definitions of domestic violence, the sampling techniques used by the interviewers, and the ages of children included in the studies. Domestic violence occurs in rural and urban areas and among all classes and ethnicities. Evidence suggests that exposure to domestic violence may be profoundly damaging for children, especially young children.[16] Children depend on their parents for emotional safety and protection. When these parents are aggressive or victimized, they are less able to protect their children. In addition, children learn early and powerful lessons about the use of violence in intimate relationships, and because children imitate adults, they use this violence in their social relationships. Exposure to domestic violence has been associated with increased rates of juvenile delinquency, poor emotional health, and poor adult health outcomes.[17]

A child's age, gender, and ethnicity affects the type of violence a child is most likely to experience.[4] For young children, the most likely source of exposure to violence is

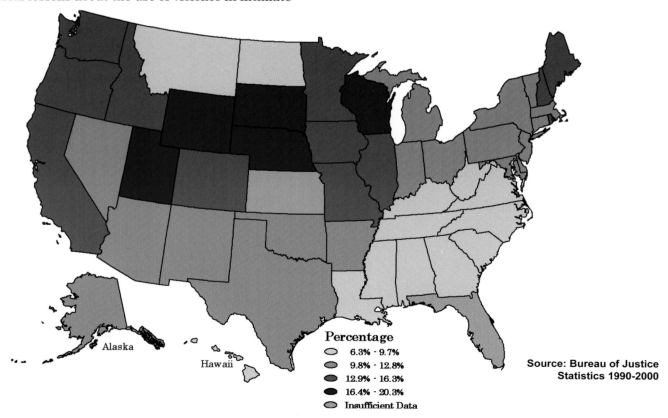

Percentage
- 6.3% - 9.7%
- 9.8% - 12.8%
- 12.9% - 16.3%
- 16.4% - 20.3%
- Insufficient Data

Source: Bureau of Justice Statistics 1990-2000

Map 5.2: Percentage of State's Homicide Victims That Were Children Ages 17 and Younger, 1990-2000

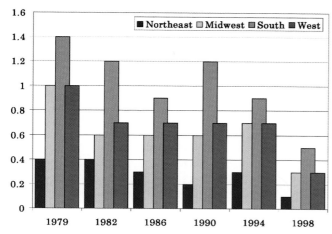

Figure 5.4: Rate of Death by Firearm for Youth Under Age 20 per 100,000 by Region

Source: Centers for Disease Control and Prevention 2003

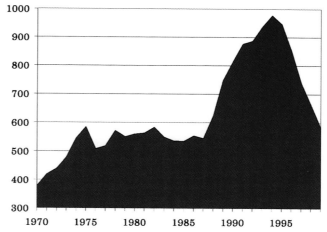

Figure 5.5: Rate of Violent Offense Arrest for Teens Ages 15 to 17 per 100,000

Source: Bureau of Justice Statistics 2004

the home, with parents or siblings being the perpetrators of that violence. As children grow up, they are more likely to encounter violence in schools or in the community. In addition, children ages 7 to 12 watch more television and, therefore, see more media violence. Homicide and suicide rates increase dramatically when children reach their teen years, as does dating violence. Females are more likely to be victims of sexual assault; males are more likely to be victims of homicide, aggravated assault, or robbery and more likely to carry a weapon.

The risk of violence varies by race and ethnicity. At all ages, Black children and youth are more likely to be victims of violence. The disparity by race is most dramatic for Black adolescents, who are 12.5 times more likely than their White counterparts to be victims of homicide. Hispanic adolescents are 6 times more likely to be homicide victims as White adolescents.[4] These disparities reflect several contributing factors, particularly poverty. When people at the same income level are compared, there are few differences among races. This finding suggests that violence is a function of poverty, not race.[18]

While the type of violence a child may be exposed to varies by age, ethnicity, and gender, the effects of this violence

By the time preschoolers graduate from high school, they are likely to have seen more than 200,000 violent acts on television. In fact, children's commercial television programs contain more violent acts than programs for adults.

are more uniform. There is no age at which a child is immune to the effects of exposure to violence, especially real-life violence. Recent studies show that infants and toddlers are acutely aware of trauma in their environments and show symptoms of stress that are quite similar to symptoms seen in older children and adults.[19,20]

For older children, exposure to violence may result in chronic anxiety, fear, increased aggression, and preoccupation with the violence. These symptoms, in turn, affect a child's school performance, social relationships, and basic ability to trust adults. In short, exposure to violence changes the landscape of childhood, sometimes permanently.

In summary, we see that children's exposure to violence is not solely an urban problem. Violence touches the lives of families and children across the country: in rural areas, in middle-class or affluent suburbs, and in inner cities. As politicians, policymakers, and leaders become more aware of the impact of violence on children, there is increasing urgency to begin the process of restoring safety and security in communities and homes. While the specific steps for restoring this safety may be the subject of political discussion, the moral urgency to act is beyond debate.

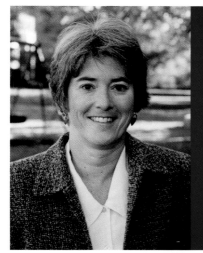

Betsy McAlister Groves

Betsy McAlister Groves, MSW, LICSW, is the founding director of the Child Witness to Violence Project at Boston Medical Center and assistant professor of pediatrics at Boston University School of Medicine. She is the past recipient of a fellowship from the Open Society Institute and has been a fellow at the Malcolm Weiner Center of Social Policy at Harvard University. Her publications include a book, *Children Who See Too Much: Lessons from the Child Witness to Violence Project*, published in 2002, and articles in the *Journal of the American Medical Association, Pediatrics, Harvard Mental Health Letter*, and *Topics in Early Childhood Special Education*. She has served on the Massachusetts Governor's Commission on Domestic Violence and the Massachusetts Juvenile Justice Advisory Committee. In addition, she has served as a consultant to Family Communications, Inc., producers of *Mister Roger's Neighborhood*; the National Council of Juvenile and Family Court Judges; and the Family Violence Prevention Fund. Ms. Groves received her master's degree from Boston University School of Social Work and her undergraduate degree from the College of William and Mary.

Chapter 6

Irwin Redlener

Children in a
Post-9/11 World

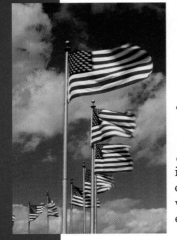

R aising children is always about nurturing their potential and meeting challenges. In fact, it can be said that some families may even grow and thrive through adversity. And sometimes the very process of meeting difficult challenges can strengthen resolve and teach life-changing lessons about solving problems in ways that have positive emotional and personal consequences for individuals. It can also be said that at almost every stage of history there has been, somewhere, crises, catastrophes, and struggles that pose enormous challenges to families. This is particularly true for children who must develop physically, emotionally, and cognitively, irrespective of the larger social, political, or economic context of their world, even if the context is the specter of terrorism in America.

There is a special set of concerns with respect to children in a post-9/11 world. With the enormous national effort being made to prevent terrorism and particularly to enhance response capacity to unconventional weapons of terror, the special needs of children must be accounted for in preparedness planning at all levels. The important principle is that children are not "little adults" in terms of how they might respond to many potential chemical or biological weapons.

The events of September 11, 2001, and beyond have created a unique set of circumstances for children in the United States. On 9/11, the nation was stunned by the brazen hijackings of four commercial jetliners that were used as missiles to attack highly visible targets in New York City and Washington, DC. One of the planes, undoubtedly diverted by the actions of passengers onboard, crashed into a relatively unpopulated area of Pennsylvania. The sheer extent and complexity of successfully planned and implemented acts of horrific violence, the destruction of seemingly invulnerable landmarks, and the ability to reach the Pentagon, a strong symbol of American power, were all important factors in understanding why Americans were so deeply affected by these terrible assaults. But there was more to it than the trauma of a single, infamous day.

Since 9/11, American children are growing up in a society that is in the process of adapting to new realities.

The fact is that 9/11 was but the first in a series of traumatic national events. Within weeks, a passenger jet filled with passengers en route to the Dominican Republic crashed into a middle-class residential neighborhood of New York City. Almost simultaneously, the nation was consumed with the possibility of wide-scale bioterror when cases of anthrax began appearing in Florida, Washington, DC, and New York City. Five lives were lost, and by the end of 2003, neither the motive nor the perpetrator had been discovered.

In the summer of 2002, concerned that terrorists might have "weaponized" smallpox, the government announced a plan to vaccinate 500,000 Americans against this deadly disease. A year later, the plan was aborted because participation was far below expectation. And on

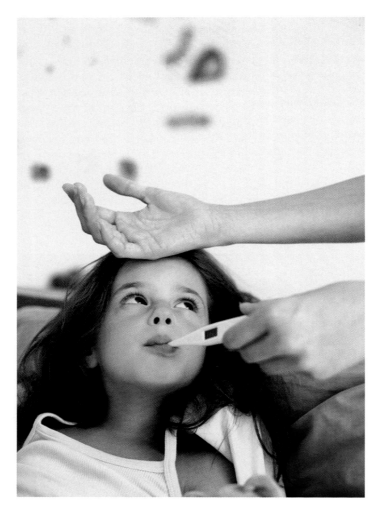

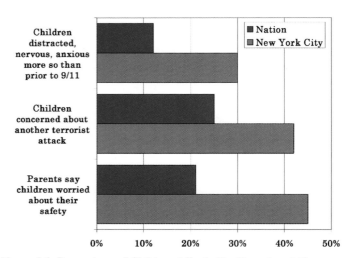

Figure 6.1: Percentage of Children Affected by Terrorism 1 Year after 9/11 by Location, 2002

Source: Children's Health Fund/Marist 2002

the international front, since 9/11, the United States has found itself embroiled in major conflicts in Afghanistan and Iraq while terrorist acts continue around the world.

In the immediate aftermath of 9/11, numerous studies demonstrated that a majority of Americans, including children, experienced stress reactions ranging from headaches, stomachaches, and the like to serious anxieties.[1-3] Reactions in New York City were highest, as expected, but by no means limited to the children whose parents or loved ones were among the 3,000-plus people who died on 9/11,[4] the 5,000 children who lived near the site of the World Trade Center attack,[5] or the more than 9,000 children who attended public schools near there.[6] Why is this so?

Before the first tower collapsed in lower Manhattan, the nonstop coverage of terrorism in America had begun and would continue without letup for months. The intensity of the coverage was virtually unavoidable, even for children. On television, for instance, film clips of hijacked planes crashing into the Twin Towers were shown repeatedly. Many experts cautioned that young children would find it difficult or impossible to distinguish repeated broadcast of the initial attacks from the possibility that attacks were continuing. Media exposure has not been established as a cause of posttraumatic stress disorder, but repeated exposure to graphic violent images has emerged as a risk factor.[7,8]

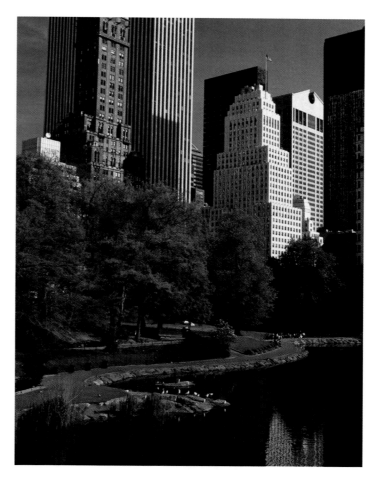

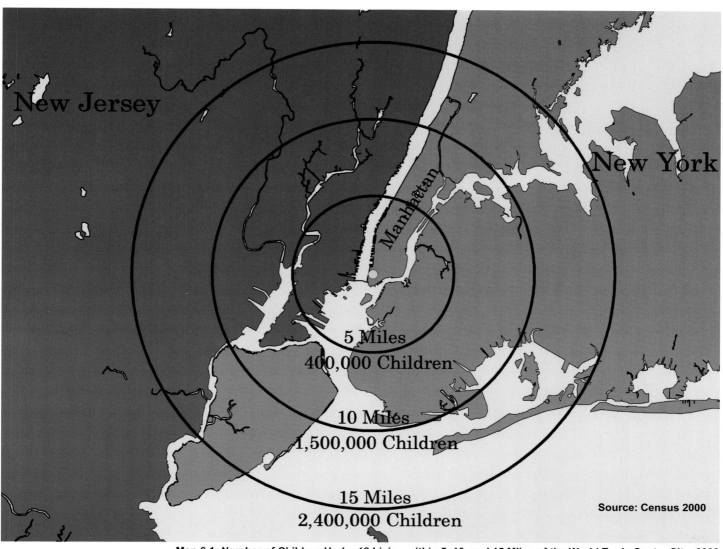

Map 6.1: Number of Children Under 18 Living within 5, 10, and 15 Miles of the World Trade Center Site, 2000

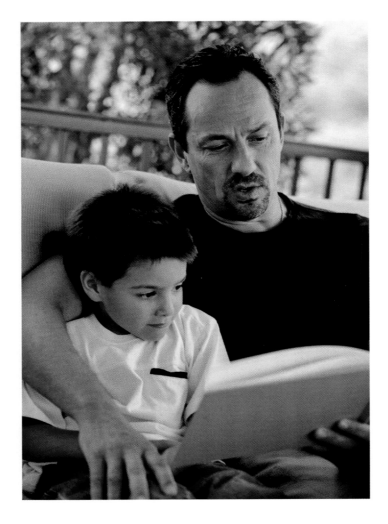

Several studies have shed light on how children have been faring since 9/11. In August 2003, the Children's Health Fund and the Marist Institute for Public Opinion conducted two concurrent surveys. One was national in scope; the other involved parents who lived in New York City. Among the more important insights from the two surveys were the following:

- There has been a persistent concern among parents and their children about the possibility of additional terrorism in the United States. Nearly 2 years after 9/11, 76% of Americans continued to believe that additional attacks were likely.

- Forty-two percent of parents and their children were concerned about their own safety and the safety of their families. Twenty-three percent of parents reported that, 2 years following 9/11, their children were still having multiple behavioral or psychological symptoms that seemed to be related to those events.

- Most affected were racial-ethnic minority children, especially Hispanics, and children in low-income families. Results from the New York City survey indicated that 32% of Hispanic, 22% of Black, and 15% of White children suffered from multiple symptoms. Parents of 18% of Hispanic children, 11% of Black children, and 7% of White children continued to report that their child(ren) showed feelings of depression and sadness. This finding is consistent with the results of a survey of the impact of 9/11 on New York City public school children that was conducted just 6 months after 9/11.[9]

This information does not suggest that children are necessarily experiencing clinical depression or posttraumatic stress disorder. A large number of children, however, are having concerns and problems that fall below the threshold of a psychiatric diagnosis but clearly reflect a level of anxiety and concern. These are the children who continue to have sleep disorders, difficulty in school, or more general evidence of anxiety—perhaps being extremely uncomfortable if their parent must fly out of town for a business meeting.

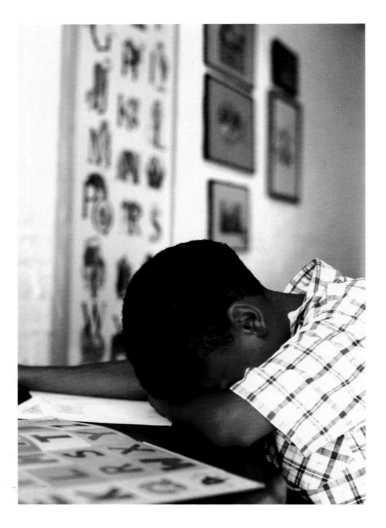

This new problem requires innovative solutions. Child health experts, physicians, and teachers must stand ready to address these problems. Efforts are already underway to ensure that emergency planning for bioterrorism in the United States includes essential information provided by child health experts. Children are more vulnerable to many of the chemical or biological agents that could be used by terrorists, and the treatments required for those who are exposed often differ markedly from protocols that would apply to adults.[10] Doctors, emergency workers, teachers, and others who may be first responders in the event of a terrorist attack need to know what to expect and what to do should the need arise. Pediatricians and family doctors are often the first people called by concerned parents who may want clarification of something they read or heard. It is essential that these professionals

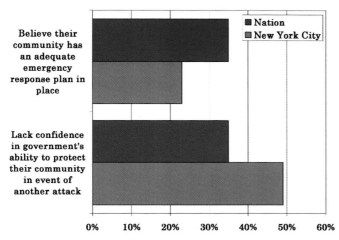

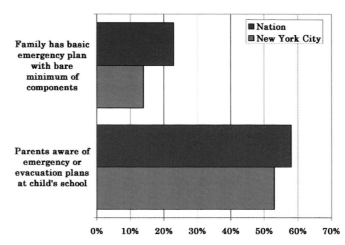

Figure 6.2: Respondents' Opinions on Community Preparedness and Their Own Confidence Levels by Location, 2003

Source: National Center for Disaster Preparedness/Marist 2003

Figure 6.3: Parents' Responses to Family and School Preparedness Questions by Location, 2003

Source: National Center for Disaster Preparedness/Marist 2003

have access to accurate information and are comfortable in responding to inquiries from parents or others.[11,12]

Parents, caregivers, and a child's surrounding community should educate themselves about the potential of future terrorist threats and the need for preparedness. Parents and caregivers should be alert to changes in a child's behavior as early indicators of distress. These will vary according to the child's age and developmental stage as well as preexisting psychological conditions. Preschool children may not say that they are worried about something specific; rather, there may be changes in play activities, certain themes expressed in drawings, or aggressive interactions with peers. Older children may be withdrawn or excessively aggressive in school or with siblings and friends. They may have disturbed sleep patterns and unusual or unexplainable physical symptoms such as abdominal pains. Young children may seem to require more attention, nonverbal contact, and reassurance. Most importantly, for all children, there should be severe limits on amount of exposure to distressing news or images on television.

Families should reinforce positive routines, such as gathering as a family at mealtimes, reading at bedtime, and engaging in weekend leisure activities. Stability and predictability in such activities help reassure that

> **Doctors, emergency workers, teachers, and others who may be first responders in the event of a terrorist attack need to know what to expect and what to do should the need arise.**

life is in order and that parents have imposed a sense of control that is vital to a child's sense of security.

Developing basic emergency plans for the family, child care centers, and workplaces is an essential step and is applicable to any crisis. Involving the whole family and community in such planning is both reassuring and imminently practical if a disaster—natural, accidental, or terror related—were to occur. These and other details about planning for emergencies can be obtained from the federal government's Department of Homeland Security or agencies such as the American Red Cross.

Since 9/11, American children are growing up in a society that is in the process of adapting to new realities. New feelings of vulnerability and a rapidly changing relationship to the rest of the world have created an environment that can adversely affect children and their families. It is essential to take those steps that will best ensure that children are protected, physically and psychologically, in the event of any emergency, including terrorism. At the same time, it is equally important that the new reality not undermine the ability of every child to grow and learn without fear. In every age and through every crisis, sustaining and nurturing a sense of optimism and infinite possibility about the future are fundamental responsibilities of all parents and those who care for children.

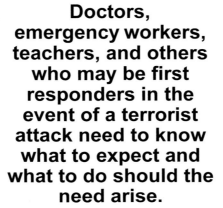

Irwin Redlener

Irwin Redlener, MD, a pediatrician and associate dean at the Joseph L. Mailman School of Public Health at Columbia University, is a nationally recognized expert on child health policy and disaster preparedness. He is also president and cofounder of the Children's Health Fund, a philanthropic initiative created to develop and support health care programs for medically underserved children. At Columbia, Dr. Redlener founded and directs the National Center for Disaster Preparedness, with a special focus on the needs of children in a post-9/11 world. The acclaimed New York Children's Health Project, the country's largest health care program for homeless children, was developed in 1987 by Dr. Redlener. It is the model for the Children's Health Fund network of innovative health care projects serving extremely disadvantaged children in 17 urban and rural communities across the country. In his role as pediatrician-child advocate, Dr. Redlener has published, spoken, and testified extensively on the subjects of health care for homeless and indigent children, terrorism preparedness, and national health policy.

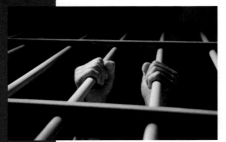

Chapter 7

Angie Vachio

Children of
Incarcerated Parents

The National Institute of Justice estimates there are 1.5 million of them; advocates estimate 5 million—no one knows for sure. We do know that they can be found in virtually every community, school, and state, but no one knows exactly who or where they are. They are children of incarcerated, or jailed, parents, and they are invisible in a system established to punish and isolate their parents from society.

Prisons are an old institution in our nation—in every nation. What has changed is that, since the 1980s, the United States has become the world's most aggressive jailer. Over the course of a generation, incarceration in our nation has increased by

500% with a current prison population of more than 2.2 million. With only 5% of the world's population, the United States holds more than 25% of all people imprisoned in the world.

Approximately 80% of our nation's prison population consists of parents with children of all ages. Their children are 7 times more likely to become involved in the juvenile and adult criminal justice systems than other children. Estimates suggest that 1 in 40 children in our nation today has a parent in prison. Our emphasis on imprisonment to fight crime may be helping to create the next generation of criminals. The link between generations is so strong that half of all juveniles in custody have a father, mother, or other close relative who has been in jail or prison. Yet, no system exists to identify these children, provide appropriate intervention and support, or recognize and respond to their unique needs.

According to the U.S. Bureau of Justice Statistics, most children of incarcerated parents are younger than age 10; the average age is 8. Additionally:

- African American children are 9 times more likely than White children to have a parent in prison. Hispanic children are 3 times more likely.

- Seventy-two percent of incarcerated parents were living with their children prior to arrest.

- Fifty-seven percent of imprisoned fathers and 54% of imprisoned mothers state that they have never had a personal visit with their children since entering prison.

- Seventy-nine percent of imprisoned mothers report that their children are living with grandparents or other relatives.

- Ninety percent of incarcerated fathers state that at least one of their children is living with their mother.

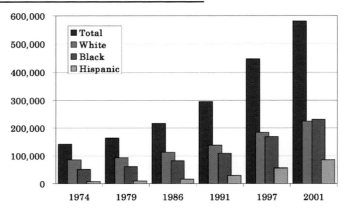

Figure 7.1: Estimated Number of Women *Ever* Incarcerated in a State or Federal Prison
Source: U.S. Department of Justice, Prevalence 2003

The fastest-growing segment of the prison population, which nearly tripled in the last decade, is women. Incarcerated women are predominantly nonviolent drug felons and are overwhelmingly mothers—mostly single mothers of dependent children. Eight percent to 10% are pregnant when they enter prison. On release, most will be rearrested, and one-third will be jailed or imprisoned again within 3 years, retraumatizing their children. Children of women offenders most often come from single-parent, low-income homes, headed by young women with little education, few job skills, and extensive histories of childhood victimization, domestic violence, and substance dependency. Yet, these women love their children. Most have appropriate parental attitudes and concerns, and no evidence exists that they are abusive or neglectful at greater rates than the general population. However, children of women offenders are at an extremely high risk for permanent separation from their mothers due to the requirements of the Adoption and Safe Families Act of 1997, which requires states

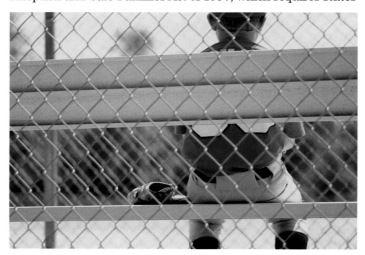

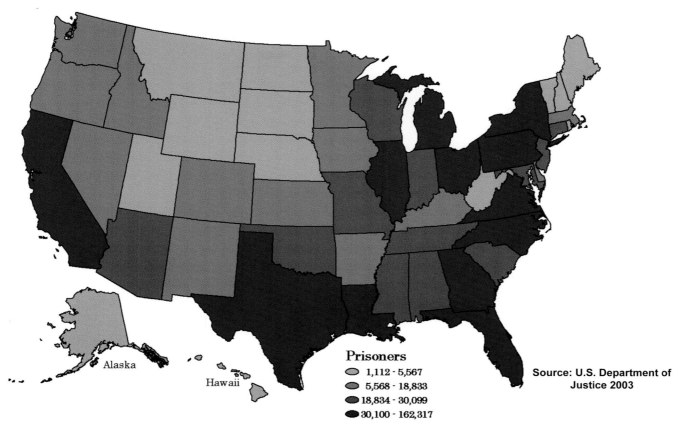

Prisoners
- 1,112 - 5,567
- 5,568 - 18,833
- 18,834 - 30,099
- 30,100 - 162,317

Source: U.S. Department of Justice 2003

Map 7.1: Prisoners Under the Jurisdiction of State or Federal Correctional Authorities, 2002

Approximately 80% of our nation's prison population consists of parents with children of all ages. Their children are 7 times more likely to become involved in the juvenile and adult criminal justice systems than other children.

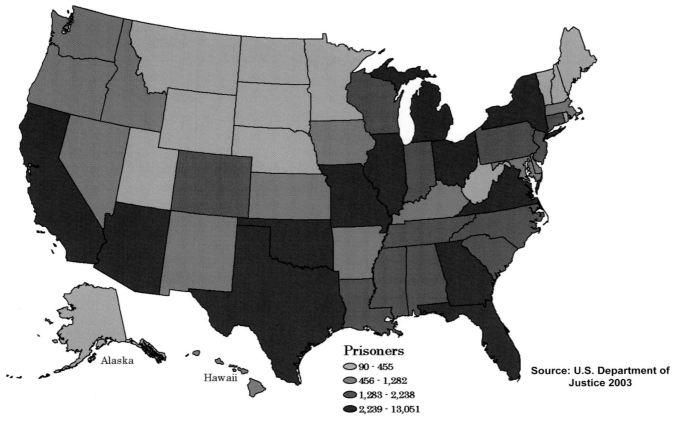

Prisoners
- 90 - 455
- 456 - 1,282
- 1,283 - 2,238
- 2,239 - 13,051

Source: U.S. Department of Justice 2003

Map 7.2: Women Under the Jurisdiction of State or Federal Correctional Authorities, 2002

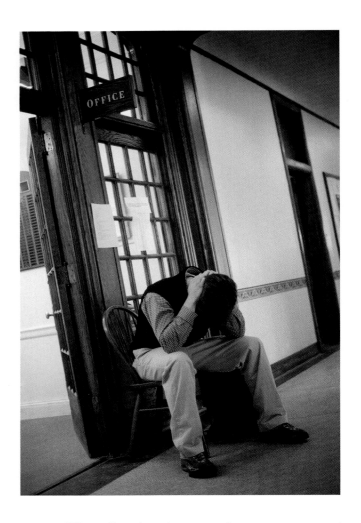 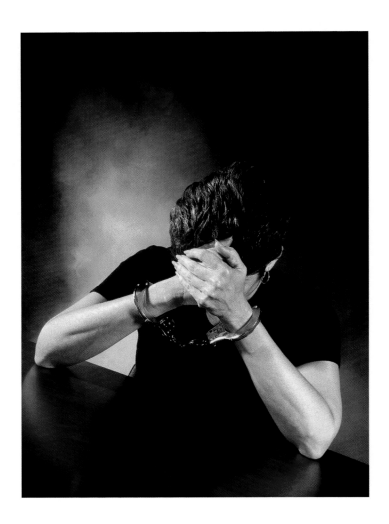

The fastest-growing segment of the prison population, which nearly tripled in the last decade, is women. Incarcerated women are predominantly nonviolent drug felons and are overwhelmingly mothers—mostly single mothers of dependent children.

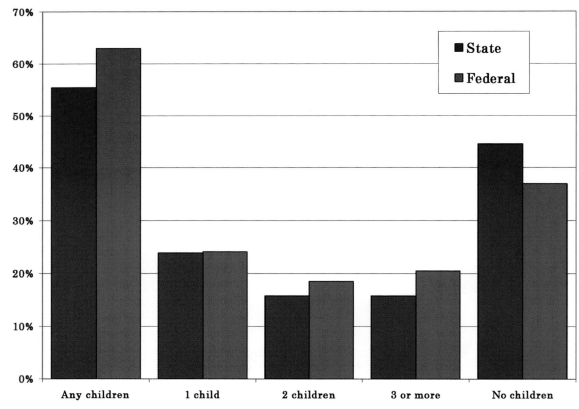

Figure 7.2: Percentage of Prisoners with Minor Children by Institution Type, 1997

Source: U.S. Department of Justice, Incarcerated Parents 2000

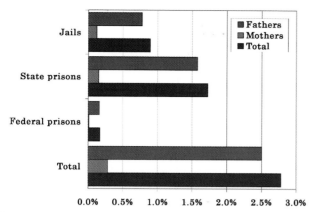

Figure 7.3: Percentage of All Children Under 18 with an Incarcerated Parent, 1997

Source: U.S. Department of Justice, Women Offenders 1999

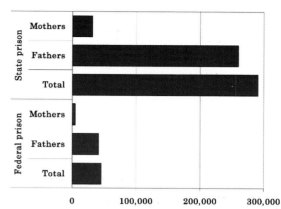

Figure 7.4: Estimated Number of Households with Minor Children Affected by the Incarceration of a Resident Parent, 1999

Source: U.S. Department of Justice, Incarcerated Parents 2000

to seek termination of parental rights when a child has been in foster care 15 out of 22 months. In addition, systems to promote healthy parenting relationships between inmate parents and their children are sparse.

The loss of a parent to incarceration has a profound impact on children, particularly when the parent-child relationship was strong prior to incarceration. Emotionally, children may experience trauma and feelings of anxiety, shame, guilt, and fear. Often, they feel anger toward their parents for what they may perceive as abandonment. Behaviorally, they may exhibit school-related problems, early pregnancy, gang involvement, drug use, and delinquency. Almost all sink further into poverty.

Across our nation, when an arrest is made and a judge passes sentence, no one asks whether the offender has children, if they are safe, or how they can be helped. Children with a parent in prison often face instability and uncertainty as to where they will live and who will care for them. Disproportionately, they have grown up in distressed communities with high poverty, high crime rates, poor schools, low parental literacy, and an absence of positive male role models. These conditions escalate the children's sense of abandonment and hopelessness. The children themselves often take on parental roles, worrying about their parents' safety and well-being. The children fear for their own futures and fear following in their parents' footsteps. They are stigmatized by having a parent in prison. They may suffer low

With only 5% of the world's population, the United States holds more than 25% of all people imprisoned in the world.

self-esteem and significant depression and sadness. Also disconcerting is that they frequently form relationships with others that are equally troubled since they often don't have parents or supportive adults to nurture them through these difficulties. These reactions will differ by gender, age, and the point in their childhood at which the separation from their parent occurred.

For the estimated 26% to 32% of children who witness the arrest of their parent, the event can be extremely traumatic. They see their parent as disempowered, leaving the child feeling exposed and vulnerable. Children, consequently, often feel embittered and contemptuous toward law enforcement. Once the arrest is made, if the children are not taken into custody, they again become invisible.

Children with parents in prison are a vulnerable and growing population, and it is imperative that we view the period of incarceration as an opportunity for intervention. By identifying these children and developing creative service responses, we can significantly lessen the trauma and begin to build on their strengths and their incredible capacity for resilience. Some possible services include providing support for guardians, keeping children in routine physical and verbal contact with their incarcerated parent, linking children to supportive services and people, and providing carefully planned community and reentry support for parents during both the incarceration and reintegration periods.

Angie Vachio

Angie Vachio, cofounder of the Peanut Butter and Jelly Preschools, and executive director of PB&J Family Services, Inc., headquartered in Albuquerque, NM, has dedicated her life to protecting children at risk of abuse and neglect. PB&J's ImPACT program operates in four New Mexico correctional facilities to reunify children with their incarcerated parents and reestablish the family unit once the incarcerated parent is released. In addition, PB&J has also founded the KidPACT program that provides support groups and other services for school-age children who have a parent in prison or come from a family with a history of criminality.

Vachio grew up in New York City and received her bachelor's degree from Adelphi University. She has a master's in special education from the University of New Mexico, and in 2002, Vachio received an honorary Doctor of Humane Letters from the University of New Mexico in recognition of her achievements in serving children and families. She was honored with being selected recipient of the U.S. Department of Health and Human Services' 2003 Commissioner Award for her outstanding contributions to the field of child protection.

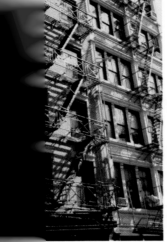

Chapter 8

Urban Housing

Henry Cisneros

I n the United States today, about 14.4 million American families have critical housing needs. This means that one in every seven households pays more than half of its income for housing or lives in substandard conditions. Housing experts tell us that a family that pays more than 30% of its household budget for shelter simply will not have enough money to address the other necessities of life such as food, medical care, transportation, children's clothing, and the other essentials.

The families with critical housing needs are most likely to be those who have incomes below 50% of the area median income and are more likely to be minority households. It is also true that about half of low- to moderate-income working families with critical housing needs have children, and the number of these families with more than three children per household is growing. Among those Americans with the most

severe housing needs—the homeless—the fastest growing segment is women with children. Even among working families, those with the most critical housing needs are likely to be female-headed households with children.

The implications for children living in substandard and over-crowded housing are profound. There are predictable health effects of living in places with poor ventilation, water leaks, drafts, and rampant communicable diseases. Among the most severe and persistent health problems that confront children in older and deteriorating housing are those associated with lead poisoning, which damages cognitive development. There are many well-documented

About 14.4 million American families have critical housing needs. One in every seven households pays more than half of its income for housing or lives in substandard conditions.

cases of toddlers who suffer lifelong learning disorders from eating paint chips found in older housing.

Beyond the overt health morbidities are the emotional effects of poor school performance, which stem from living in overcrowded conditions where it is difficult to establish the stability required for study and homework. Another category of housing-related effects are threats to the safety of children living in ill-secured apartment complexes and deteriorated public housing, where the sur-roundings may be characterized by gang activity, drug transactions, and physical abuse. It is not accidental that author Alex Kotlowitz titled his book about public housing *There Are No Children Here: The Story of Two Boys Growing Up in the Other America.* He

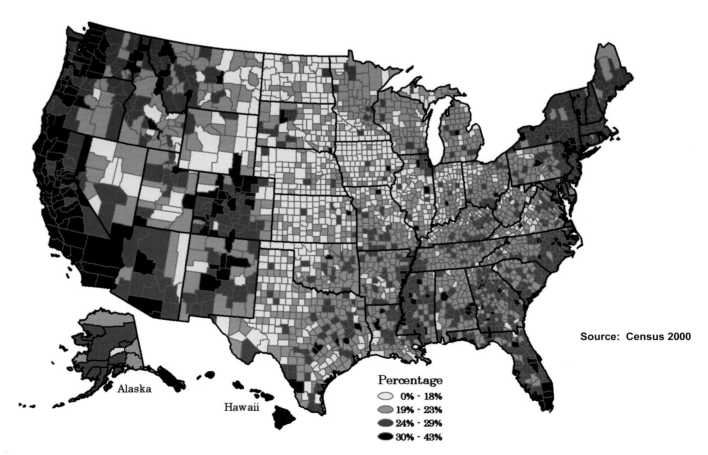

Source: Census 2000

Alaska

Hawaii

Percentage
- 0% - 18%
- 19% - 23%
- 24% - 29%
- 30% - 43%

Map 8.1: Percentage of Households Paying 30% or More of Their Income on Housing Costs

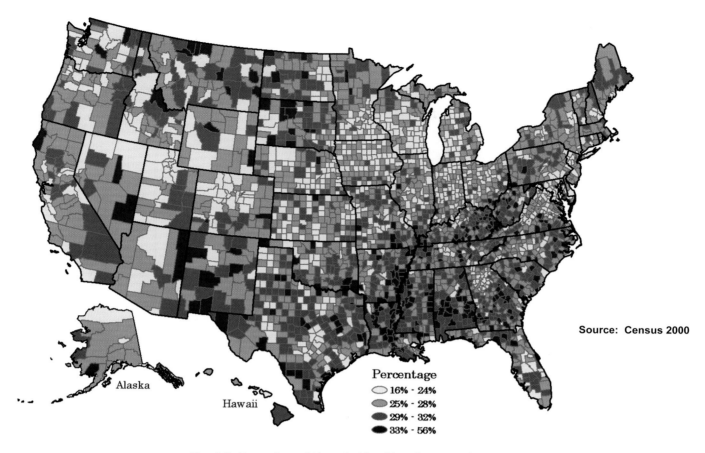

Source: Census 2000

Percentage
◯ 16% - 24%
◯ 25% - 28%
◯ 29% - 32%
⬤ 33% - 56%

Map 8.2: Percentage of Households with an Income 50% or Less of the Median Household Income

was describing conditions so intimidating in some urban public housing developments that children never get to enjoy childhood experiences and are forced to learn the survival skills that make them worldly and even dangerous before adolescence.

But the effects for children of poor housing conditions derive from more than the physical structures of individual residences. The importance of healthy environments extends to neighborhoods and communities. Among the aspects of designing communities with children in mind are such matters as careful planning of traffic flows to reduce the physical dangers to children. For example, when communities are built without sidewalks, children are forced to play in the streets, including riding bicycles or skating amidst traffic. Traffic considerations should include designing safe routes to schools and to neighborhood recreation amenities, with proper attention to street crossings and the slowing of traffic through areas with high concentrations of children.

Other children's issues that planners could address in the design of communities are those related to exercise and recreation. The lack of physical activity that results from such decisions as locating schools on distant sites can lead to obesity and unhealthy physical development. A report produced by the National Trust for Historic Preservation notes that only 13% of our nation's students walk to school, a result of spread-out neighborhoods, distant amenities, and communities dominated by cars.

Other children's health concerns related to homes and neighborhoods include those caused by environmental pollution. For example, many poor children live in neighborhoods with compromised air quality that leads to respiratory illnesses. One of the fastest-growing health challenges confronting children in our country today is asthma, which seems to be more prevalent in urban areas where homes have been located either adjacent to busy arterial streets—forcing children to breathe automobile emissions—or in industrial zones where smokestack emissions are at dangerous levels.

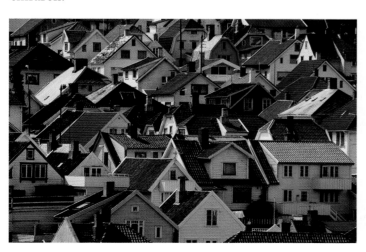

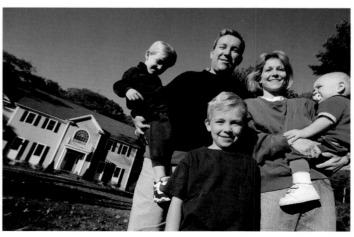

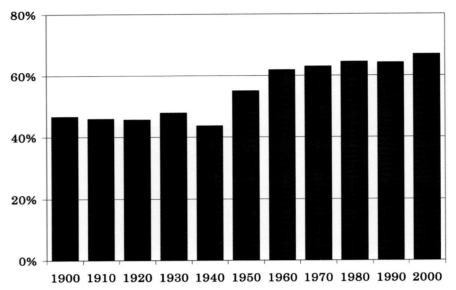

Figure 8.1: Home Ownership Rates in the United States, 1900-2000

Source: U.S. Census Bureau Housing 2002

At every step of "the continuum of housing," which identifies the major types of housing in our country, national and local officials, as well as private sector leaders, must be attentive to the importance of living conditions for children. This continuum makes it possible to focus on the role of each type of housing in the lives of children:

Emergency Shelters for the Homeless—The fastest-growing segment of the homeless population is women with children. While homeless shelters are simply no place for children to grow up, it is urgent to bring children off the streets. More shelter spaces are needed, and special accommodations must be made in homeless shelters for the special needs of children.

Transitional Housing—One way to move children beyond homeless shelters is to provide sufficient units of transitional housing, which is designed to enable families to receive supportive services such as job training, medical care, substance abuse treatment, counseling, and remedial education. Transitional units typically provide greater stability for children and are a longer-term housing resource. Many more units of transitional housing are urgently needed.

Housing conditions and health effects converge to raise issues of environmental justice. Over the years, many poor neighborhoods have been located near industrial plants, salvage yards, municipal dumps, and polluted waterways. All pose health dangers for the children who live in those neighborhoods.

A related policy challenge for community builders is to address housing patterns of racial segregation. When children live in racially segregated neighborhoods characterized by concentrated poverty, the outcomes are frequently poor school performance, arrested social development, and reduced economic opportunities.

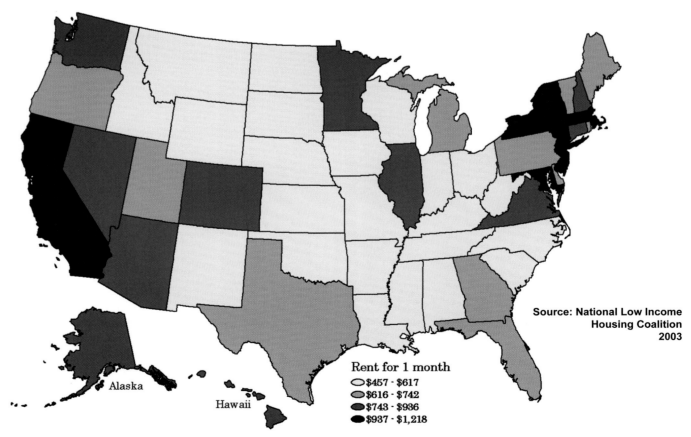

Source: National Low Income
Housing Coalition
2003

Rent for 1 month

○ $457 - $617
● $616 - $742
● $743 - $936
● $937 - $1,218

Map 8.3: HUD Proposed Fair Market Rent Levels for Two Bedrooms, 2004

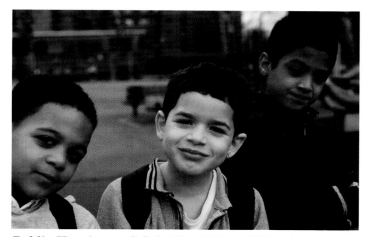

Public Housing and Subsidized Rental Housing—Many public housing developments and subsidized rental apartments have slipped into disrepair and are poorly managed. The result is that children live in chaos and frequently in danger. Efforts to transform the physical design of public housing through such national programs as Hope VI, which allows for the replacement of the worst of the overcrowded public housing with lower density and more secure homes, are important and must continue. The stock of subsidized rental units must be preserved and expanded.

Affordable Rental Units—A family with one full-time worker earning the minimum wage cannot afford the local fair market rent for a two-bedroom apartment in any major city in the country. That means multiple families with children must crowd into single units in many parts of the nation. The supply of multifamily developments must be increased.

Affordable Home Ownership—One of the greatest opportunities for stability for families is to become owners of their homes. Home ownership affords families not only the dignity of their own space, but also starts families on the ladder to economic mobility by allowing them to build equity that can be used to meet other family needs. Many studies have demonstrated that children who live in family-

owned homes have improved chances for advancements in life.

Quality Communities—Creating quality neighborhoods and communities supports the ultimate goal of providing safe and decent homes for families. Careful attention must be given to create the amenities, site designs, transportation patterns, and other dimensions of community building that are conducive to children living safely and growing up with prospects for achieving their potential.

A home in our society is many things. At the most obvious level, it is a place to live. But when we probe beyond the obvious and examine what that means, we understand that a home is where a family creates stability, relishes moments of peace together, enjoys nutrition in the form of home-cooked food, finds nurturing in time of sickness, feels safe and secure, safeguards its possessions, studies and pursues learning, plays, and hosts gatherings of extended family and friends. All of these activities and more are dimensions of the complete lives of children. Adults frequently refer to a home as the "American dream"; for children it can be a place to dream. Homes should be places where children can put their heads on their pillows at night, recalling the exploits and enjoyments of the day, far from the tumult of the outside world, dreaming of the future and their own place in it.

> **Homes should be places where children can put their heads on their pillows at night, recalling the exploits and enjoyments of the day, far from the tumult of the outside world, dreaming of the future and their own place in it.**

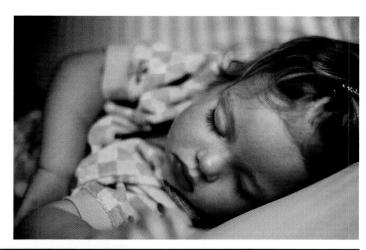

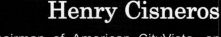

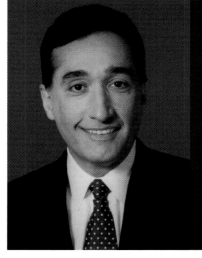

Henry Cisneros

Henry Cisneros, PhD, is the founder and chairman of American CityVista, an organization with the focus of building "villages within the city" in major metropolitan areas. Previously, Cisneros was president and chief operating officer of Univision Communications. From 1993 to 1997, Cisneros served as the secretary of the U.S. Department of Housing and Urban Development. Prior to joining the Cabinet, he was chairman of Cisneros Asset Management Company. In 1981, Cisneros became the first Hispanic American mayor of a major U.S. city—San Antonio. Mr. Cisneros served as president of the National League of Cities, chairman of the National Civic League, deputy chair of the Federal Reserve Bank of Dallas, and board member of the Rockefeller Foundation. He presently serves as chairman of the San Antonio Hispanic Chamber of Commerce and board member of KB HOME, Countrywide Mortgage, The Enterprise Foundation, the New America Alliance, and the American Film Institute. He holds a bachelor's and master's degree from Texas A&M University, a master's degree from Harvard, and a doctorate from George Washington University.

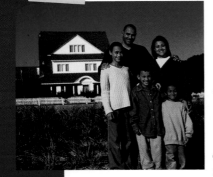

Chapter 9

Irwin Redlener

Homelessness
and Its Consequences

When a person or family is described as homeless, we think of people in despair. Yet, the very concept of "homelessness" transcends the simple reflection of difficult economic circumstances. It evokes a more unsettling description of people living in a state of disconnect from society itself. Having a home, a stable place of residence—even if the conditions are far less than may be desired—is a fundamental and almost universal goal of people in most human societies.

Most of us in the United States take our housing for granted. Whether luxurious or modest, and even if poorly maintained or literally run down, the vast majority of Americans grow up experiencing the notion of living somewhere specific. Children "go home" after school; parents "come home from work." The security of family, even when it is limited or consumed with other difficult issues, is closely tied to a stable place of being.

For homeless children and families in America, there is an altogether different reality. Understanding the implications and meaningful details of homelessness helps to clarify the health care challenges that homeless people and the service providers who care for them face on a daily basis. This is not just a matter of very disadvantaged children who need medical care and a food pantry; it is also about families who live in a state of social isolation and excessive risk physically and emotionally.

Having a home, a stable place of residence—even if the conditions are far less than may be desired—is a fundamental and almost universal goal of people in most human societies.

As is often the case in attempting to quantify social conditions, counting homeless people, especially children, is difficult. The first challenge is defining what we mean by "homeless." A straightforward approach might be to simply count the number of men, women, and children staying in official homeless shelters across the nation on any given day. In the late 1980s in New York City, for instance, the number of homeless children in the city's family shelter system comprised some 10,000

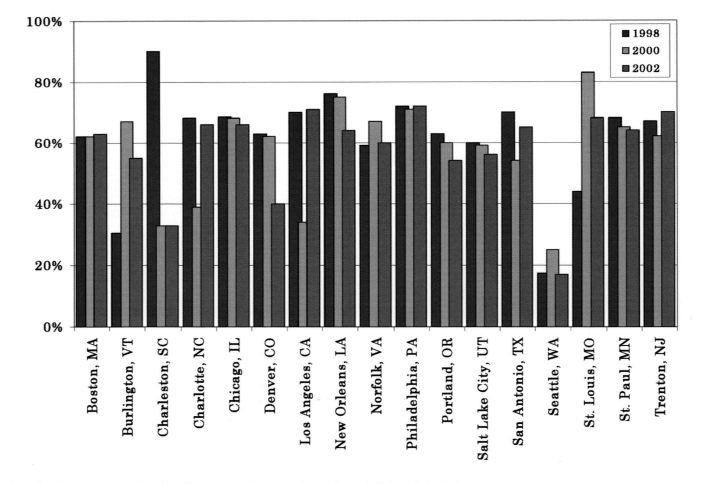

Figure 9.1: Percentage of Homeless Family Members Who Are Children in Select Major Cities

Source: U.S. Conference of Mayors 1998-2002

About Children

young people under the age of 20. By the summer of 2003, this number had risen to nearly 20,000.[1]

The problem is that these are just "snapshot" accounts taken at any moment in time. In reality, families move in and out of the shelter system over the course of a year, so that the actual number of children in the shelter each year might be 50% to 75% higher than reflected by the one-time count. Using the criterion of being homeless for some part of the year, a 2001 study by the Urban Institute suggested that as many as 1.4 million children, or about 10% of the children living in poverty, were homeless in the United States.[2]

Family homelessness is increasing. Homelessness in America is surveyed each year by the U.S. Conference of Mayors. Their most recent report issued in December 2003 found that 80% of the cities surveyed had needs for more emergency shelters than in the previous year, and they expected the number of families requesting shelter would increase during 2004. Currently, families with children comprise 40% of the homeless population compared to single homeless men who make up 41% of that population.[3] This is a starkly different face of homelessness than is generally expected.

Children in the family shelter system have been termed "attached" homeless children if they are living in a shelter with at least one parent or guardian. In large urban areas, there is another category of attached homeless children. These are children living with parents in temporary and transient conditions. For the most part, their families occupy squalid apartments, sometimes doubled and tripled up with other families. Often they do

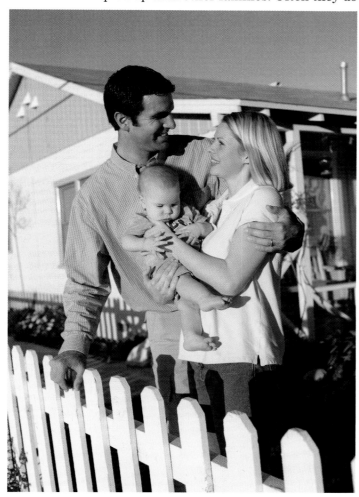

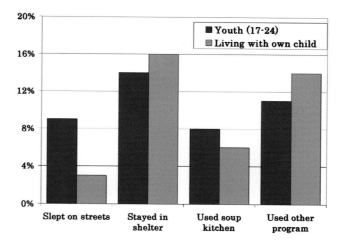

Figure 9.2: Percentage of Homeless Having Adverse Experiences Before Reaching Age 18 by Group Type, 1996

Source: Interagency Council on the Homeless 1999

not have legal tenancy rights, making their housing situation unstable. This is precisely the situation, for instance, with many indigent or near-indigent immigrant families who stay with a relative or friend in already overcrowded apartments or houses throughout the United States.

Severe overcrowding is a major problem in many inner-city and rural neighborhoods where such conditions lead to greater opportunity for the spread of infectious diseases as well as significant psychological stress for occupants. In New York City alone, it has been estimated that some 137,000 families with approximately 200,000 to 250,000 children are living in such situations.[4] The point is that they are both homeless and invisible to the authorities.

There are also "unattached" homeless children and youth, including thousands of children in the nation's foster care programs who are considered to be difficult to place or to adopt. These children may age out of the system and are simply released to the streets when they turn 18.

Youth who are living on the streets, including those who run away from home as well as those who are forced out by parents or guardians, are also classified as unattached homeless children. In fact, more than a million young people run away from home each year,[5] many becoming

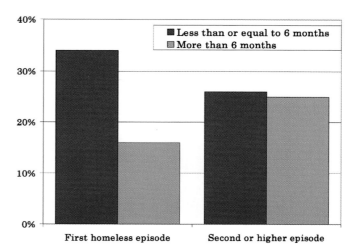

Figure 9.3: Percentage of Homeless by Length of Episode, 1996

Source: Interagency Council on the Homeless 1999

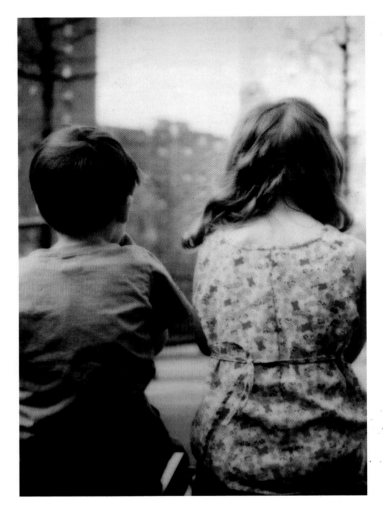

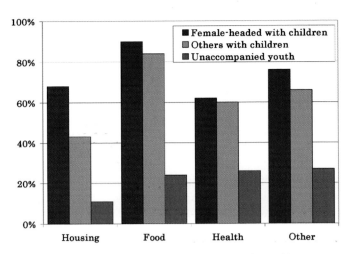

Figure 9.4: Percentage of Homeless Households Served by Homeless Assistance Programs by Service Type, 1996
Source: Interagency Council on the Homeless 1999

part of the 200,000 youth and young adults living on the streets at any given time. Young people living in extremely adverse home environments and some children with behavioral or emotional problems are particularly vulnerable to being forced out of their homes or even voluntarily leaving them. Cities such as New York, Miami, Phoenix, and Los Angeles may have the highest populations of such high-risk young people. Overall, "street youth" comprise at least 5% of America's homeless population.[3]

Finally, it should be pointed out that even if a family is legally housed, there can be distressing inadequacies in the qualitative aspects of the structure or infrastructure of the family's dwelling. It is not uncommon, for instance, to see families in urban neighborhoods living in buildings with significant and persistent housing code violations, including serious problems with plumbing and electrical service, nonworking elevators, and the like. Similarly, in many poor rural areas throughout the United States, there are countless houses obviously in terrible physical condition that are serving as homes for economically disadvantaged families.

Are such families and children housed or homeless? Clearly, they have shelter and may well have legal tenancy rights. On the other hand, severely substandard

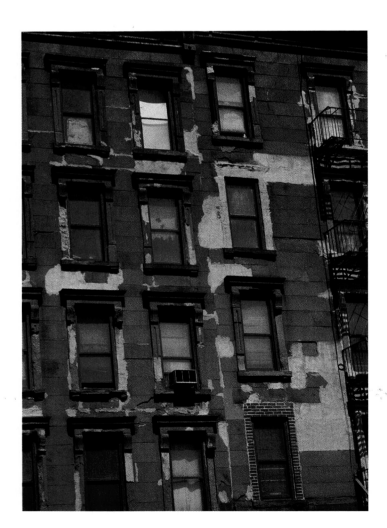

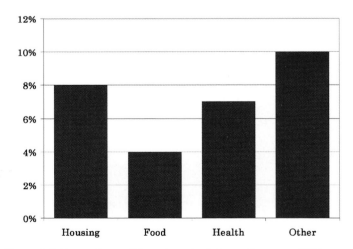

Figure 9.5: Percentage of Homeless Assistance Programs With Services for Runaway Youths, 1996
Source: Interagency Council on the Homeless 1999

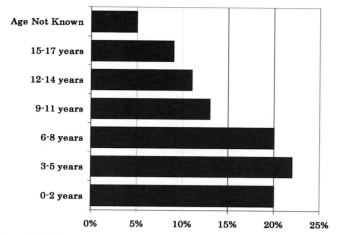

Figure 9.6: Percentage of Children Living with Homeless Parents by Age Group, 1996

Source: Interagency Council on the Homeless 1999

housing too frequently subjects the occupants, adults and children, to unacceptable risk of injury or illness. These families are living in the "gray zone," somewhere between literally without shelter and adequately housed.

Few things are more unsettling to children and adolescents than being homeless or living in severely inadequate housing. The very reality of losing one's home and being crowded into a neighbor's or relative's apartment or, far worse, being moved into an official homeless shelter is terribly distressing for most children. Generally speaking, such moves do not allow the children to take more than their most minimal possessions with them. The family, almost akin to the circumstances of refugees in war-torn areas, is suddenly thrust into unfamiliar environments which may well be perceived as threatening and overwhelming. Such circumstances certainly create stress and anxiety in children. A similar response in the parents or caregivers, who often feel a terrible loss of self-esteem and control, exacerbates the children's reactions.

In addition, homeless children are frequently cut off from previously stable relationships with friends, school, and social connections that existed in their original

> **Few things are more unsettling to children and adolescents than being homeless or living in severely inadequate housing.**

neighborhoods. Among the more important disconnections associated with homelessness for children is the loss of access to the usual source of health care. In fact, typically seen among homeless children is a significant deterioration of health status. Levels of immunization against childhood diseases, control of chronic conditions such as asthma and diabetes, and the ability to get timely care for acute illnesses all may suffer substantially when children are homeless for extended periods.

Studies around the country have consistently shown that homeless children experience more acute and chronic health conditions and developmental problems than poor, but housed, children. A 1991 study of children in Philadelphia shelters indicated that homeless children also had more accidents and injuries than their peers.[6] A New York City study on the impact of homelessness on preschool children—done in 1990 at the Martinique Hotel—showed that 75% of children in child care there showed speech-language delay and/or hyperactivity.[7] This is consistent with the 1994 finding that 78% of school-age children in Los Angeles County shelters were depressed, had behavior problems, or had severe academic delays.[8] Similar studies indicated that 72% of homeless mothers showed signs of depression or other psychiatric disturbance. Barely half of the homeless children eligible for special education services received them, and only 15% of homeless mothers in need of mental health services got any help.[9,10] More recently, an alarming rate of asthma (40%) was found among children entering the New York City shelter system,[11] a situation that the city is addressing through a variety of strategies to improve shelter conditions for homeless children with asthma.

Homelessness in the United States has become a seemingly intractable condition for millions of Americans. This means that children caught in the trap of poverty and homelessness will continue to face adversity and conditions that, if not abated, will affect their long-term ability to achieve their full potential and well-being as contributing members of society. Concerted, persistent efforts by advocates and policymakers will be essential in meeting this most difficult of domestic challenges.

Irwin Redlener

Irwin Redlener, MD, a pediatrician and associate dean at the Joseph L. Mailman School of Public Health at Columbia University, is a nationally recognized expert on child health policy and disaster preparedness. He is also president and cofounder of the Children's Health Fund, a philanthropic initiative created to develop and support health care programs for medically underserved children. At Columbia, Dr. Redlener founded and directs the National Center for Disaster Preparedness, with a special focus on the needs of children in a post-9/11 world. The acclaimed New York Children's Health Project, the country's largest health care program for homeless children, was developed in 1987 by Dr. Redlener. It is the model for the Children's Health Fund network of innovative health care projects serving extremely disadvantaged children in 17 urban and rural communities across the country. In his role as pediatrician-child advocate, Dr. Redlener has published, spoken, and testified extensively on the subjects of health care for homeless and indigent children, terrorism preparedness, and national health policy.

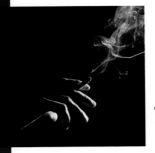

Chapter 10

*Michael Weitzman
and Megan Kavanaugh*

Tobacco and Health

Millions of children and adolescents are exposed every day to the harmful effects of tobacco through exposure to secondhand smoke or by smoking directly. While knowledge of the negative health effects of cigarettes and cigarette smoke dates back nearly a half-century,[1-4] it is primarily in the past 25 years that information has emerged regarding the adverse effects of secondhand smoke exposure on children. Passive smoking, also known as secondhand smoke or environmental tobacco smoke exposure, is linked to a broad spectrum of childhood health problems. In addition, cigarette smoking is a powerful addiction that begins most commonly before adulthood. While steps have been made to combat these problems, including laws banning smoking in public places and anti-smoking advertisement campaigns targeting youth, tobacco use remains the leading preventable cause of death in our country. Much work is needed before children can be considered safe from tobacco and tobacco smoke.

Smoking during pregnancy is the largest known risk factor for low birth weight,[5] which is considered to be less than 2,500 grams, or approximately 5½ pounds. The risk of sudden infant death syndrome (SIDS) doubles among infants whose mothers smoke.[6,7] Other than placing a baby on its back, abstaining from smoking is the most important thing a mother can do to prevent SIDS in her baby.[8]

Rates of pneumonia increase more than 50% among infants exposed to second-hand smoke.[9] Passive smoking also is linked to increases in asthma,[7] ear infections,[7,9] and even dental caries.[10] Children of smoking mothers are twice as likely to develop asthma as children of nonsmoking mothers.[11] Asthma is the most common chronic illness of childhood, a cause of more than 14 million days of missed school per year,[12] as well as a leading cause of children's hospitalizations. Ear infections are the leading reason children are given prescription antibiotics.[13,14] Reducing children's exposure to tobacco smoke would greatly decrease both of these common childhood problems.

Research also has increasingly examined the effects of prenatal and early passive exposure to cigarettes on children's intellectual functioning and behavior. Tobacco exposure is associated with alterations in newborn irritability, increased rates of behavior problems at all ages, attention deficit hyperactivity disorder behavior, and conduct disorder. Cognitively, tobacco exposure has been linked with decreased language development, small but significant decreases in IQ, and early school failure.[15]

The myriad negative health effects of tobacco smoke exposure come at a significant cost. For children, increased school absences bring social and academic consequences.[16] For parents, there is the financial cost of work days lost to care for a sick child along with the emotional cost of having a child with a chronic illness such as asthma. Nationwide, the direct cost of childhood medical expenditures alone due to environmental tobacco smoke exposure has been calculated to be a staggering $4.6 billion per year.[17]

It is estimated that over 15 million children in the United States are exposed to cigarette smoke in their homes.[18] Although a small decrease in the U.S. adult smoking rate

> **Each day in the United States, almost 5,000 adolescents smoke for the first time, and nearly 2,000 become established smokers.**

Figure 10.1: Percentage of U.S. High School Students Who Reported Smoking 1 or More Cigarettes During the Previous 30 Days

Source: Centers for Disease Control and Prevention 2002

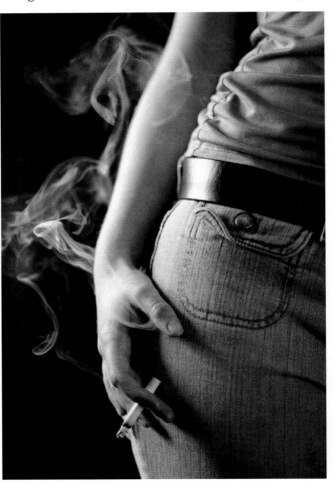

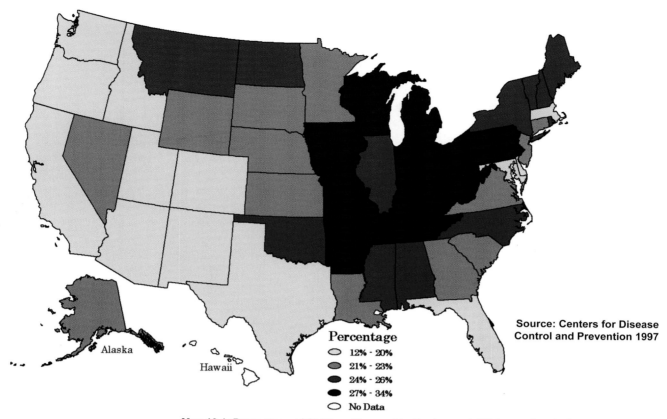

Percentage
○ 12% - 20%
○ 21% - 23%
○ 24% - 26%
○ 27% - 34%
○ No Data

Source: Centers for Disease
Control and Prevention 1997

Map 10.1: Percentage of Children Exposed to Enviromental Tobacco Smoke in the Home, 1996

has occurred in the past decade, nearly a quarter of adults are still smoking.[19] Approximately 40% of children live in homes with a smoker,[20] and 70% of parents who do smoke report that smoking is allowed within their homes.[18] While home exposure is a child's most common source of secondhand smoke,[21] children also are exposed in cars, in restaurants, and wherever they are near someone who is

smoking. Even though recent national data indicate a very significant 33% decline in smoking during pregnancy, 12.3% of pregnant women still smoke,[22] thereby exposing their children to the hazards of tobacco even before birth. The weight of evidence suggests a role of both prenatal and childhood tobacco exposure in contributing to behavior problems and cognitive deficits, as well as SIDS, asthma, and middle ear infections.[23]

In the United States, the rate of smoking among pregnant women with 9 to 11 years of education is 29% compared to a rate of 9.4% among women with 13 to 15 years of education, and only 2.1% among those with 16 or more years of education.[22] Adult smoking rates overall are significantly higher among certain minority groups, the less educated, and the poor.[19] For example, American Indians and Alaskan Natives have the highest percentage of smokers at 32.7% compared to the national average of 22.8%. These disparities also occur among children exposed

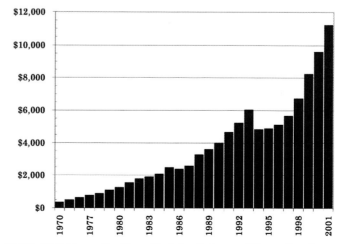

Figure 10.2: Domestic Cigarette Advertising and Promotional Expenditures (in Millions of Dollars)
Source: Federal Trade Commission 2003

47

to secondhand smoke, with children of poor and less-educated families disproportionately exposed.

These socioeconomic differences also exist when children themselves smoke.[24] This is particularly disconcerting given the large number of youth who continue to smoke. Twenty-nine percent of high school students have smoked within the past month,[25] down from peak rates of 36% in 1997,[26] but still almost double the U.S. Department of Health and Human Services' Healthy People 2010 goal of 16%.[5] Eleven percent of middle school students are current cigarette smokers, and 7% to 8% of children say they smoked a cigarette before the age of 11 years.[27] Each day in the United States, almost 5,000 adolescents smoke for the first time, and nearly 2,000 become established smokers.[28] In addition to cigarettes, children and teens are using other forms of tobacco. Among high school students, 15% have smoked a cigar in the past month, and 6.6% have used smokeless tobacco in the past month. Bidis, a type of Indian cigarette, and kreteks, or clove cigarettes, are also being smoked by more than 5% of high school students.[29]

Many factors influence whether children and adolescents begin to smoke. These include social influences of parental smoking, smoking status of friends, tobacco industry advertising campaigns,[30] and the depiction of smoking in movies.[31] The tobacco industry spends more than $11 billion each year on advertising and marketing to promote tobacco use.[32] Nearly one in three high school students and one in four middle school students have seen advertising for tobacco products on the Internet, and almost one-half of high school age tobacco users have bought or received items with a tobacco company name or picture on it.[27] Evidence suggests that these advertising methods are very effective.[33] The mounting evidence that viewing cigarette smoking in movies dramatically increases rates of youth initiation of smoking has led to a national movement in support of restricting smoking in the movies to R-rated movies.[31] Supporters of this restriction include the American Academy of Pediatrics, the American Medical

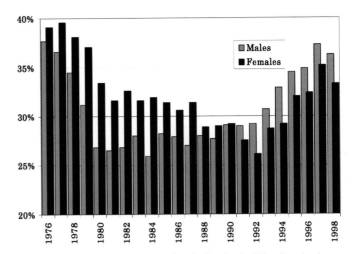

Figure 10.3: Percentage of 12th-Grade Students Who Smoked During the Previous 30 Days

Source: Monitoring the Future 1976-1998

Association, the World Health Organization, and attorneys general from 24 states.[34]

Among youth who try cigarettes even just once, approximately one in three will become regular smokers.[35] The lifetime habit of smoking undeniably has its roots in childhood, with 89% of adult smokers having tried a cigarette before age 18 and 71% becoming daily smokers by that age.[36] Nicotine is as addictive as cocaine and heroin,[37] and in a recent study, symptoms of nicotine dependence developed when young teens smoked an average of just two cigarettes 1 day a week.[38] Approximately 75% have tried to quit and have failed.[39]

Protecting children from the harmful effects of tobacco will require limiting, if not eliminating, exposure to environmental tobacco smoke, decreasing rates of smoking initiation, and increasing quit rates among youth who already smoke. Several groups strongly recommend smoking bans and restrictions to decrease such exposure.[40,41] Such bans exist in

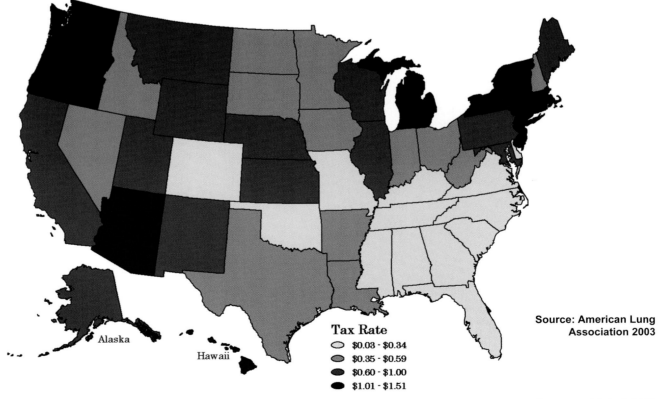

Source: American Lung Association 2003

Tax Rate
- ○ $0.03 - $0.34
- ○ $0.35 - $0.59
- ● $0.60 - $1.00
- ● $1.01 - $1.51

Map 10.2: State Cigarette Excise Taxes as of July 1, 2003

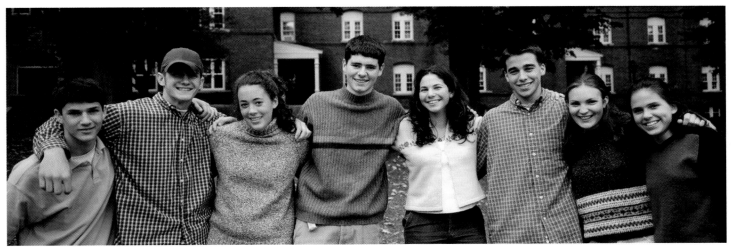

various degrees in the majority of states; however, the scope of the bans varies widely.[42] A slowly growing number of states, including California, Delaware, and New York, have banned smoking in almost all workplaces.[43] Multiple authorities, including the U.S. Public Health Service[44] and the American Academy of Pediatrics,[45] recommend that children's doctors offer advice about smoking cessation along with suggestions for limiting secondhand smoke exposure. Since children, and by extension their parents, see physicians often,[46] this approach seems wise. Among adults, brief advice from a physician has been shown to generate quit rates of 5% to 10% a year, and more intensive behavioral counseling and pharmacotherapy have resulted in quit rates of 20% to 25% per year.[40] Unfortunately, parental tobacco counseling is infrequent in the offices of children's doctors today.[47, 48]

To decrease smoking initiation by youth, the U.S. Surgeon General and others strongly recommend increasing the price of tobacco products and using youth-oriented anti-tobacco media campaigns in coordination with other efforts.[40,41] Each 10% price increase in cigarettes results in a 7% to 12% reduction in youth smoking and an approximate 4% overall decrease in adult smoking.[5] Accordingly, one Healthy People 2010 target is for the average state and federal taxes to be at least $2.00 per pack of cigarettes,[5] nearly double the current amount.[43,49] In accordance with federal law, all states have laws banning the sale of tobacco products to minors[50] but, unfortunately, these regulations often are not adequately enforced. More than half of high school students are not "carded" when buying cigarettes.[27]

For youth who have already developed an addiction to smoking, it is important to advise them to quit and to provide them with assistance when they wish to stop smoking. The U.S. Public Health Service recommendations are for clinicians to identify tobacco users, give a strong recommendation to quit smoking, and then provide cessation counseling for persons interested in quitting. Teenagers with nicotine dependence and a desire to quit can be given a prescription for at least one form of pharmacotherapy,[44] even though not one has been approved by the Federal Drug Administration for this age group.

To date, most of our nation's efforts to educate the public, and therefore curtail smoking, have focused on tobacco use as an adult problem. Indeed these commitments must be maintained. However, tobacco smoke exposure of children still remains an extremely prevalent problem. Every day, pregnant women smoke, endangering the lives of their future children, children "light up" for the first time, and parents expose their children to secondhand smoke. Raising the price of tobacco products, counseling parents about the dangers of smoking, and increasing restrictions on smoking in public areas are just three ways to address what remains our nation's number one substance abuse and environmental health problem.

Among youth who try cigarettes even just once, approximately one in three will become regular smokers.

Michael Weitzman and Megan Kavanaugh

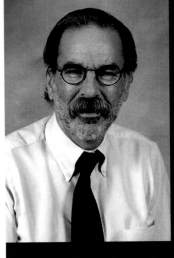

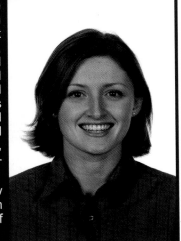

Michael Weitzman, MD, currently is executive director of the American Academy of Pediatrics' Center for Child Health Research and professor and associate chairman of pediatrics at the University of Rochester School of Medicine and Dentistry, where he was formerly director of the Division of General Pediatrics and pediatrician-in-chief at Rochester General Hospital. Prior to that, he was director of maternal and child health for the City of Boston and director of general pediatrics and the fellowship training program in academic general pediatrics at Boston City Hospital and Boston University School of Medicine. He has published over 150 original articles, chapters, books, and abstracts of scholarly work, and he is co-editor of two pediatric textbooks.

Megan Kavanaugh, BS, is a medical student research fellow at the Center for Child Health Research. She holds a BS from Duke University, and will receive her MD from the University of Rochester School of Medicine and Dentistry in 2005.

Chapter 11

Alan I. Leshner

Substance Abuse

Every major study of parental concerns shows children's potential substance abuse at or near the very top of the list. It is widely known that children's substance use can lead to a wide array of negative developmental outcomes, including school failure, delinquency, and, in the extreme, a seriously diminished and even shortened life.

Although the exact levels have varied a bit over time, about 50% of American youth will have tried an illegal substance by the time they graduate from high school. Most of that illegal drug use is of marijuana. In addition, when asked, 30% of 12th-grade youth stated they had smoked cigarettes in the past month. Fifty percent had used alcohol in the last month, and over 30% had been drunk in the last month.[1]

Not all children who try an abusable substance go on to become addicted or to develop other substance-related life problems, but the more often and the earlier they use drugs, the greater the likelihood they will develop problems. Conversely, if young people have not used marijuana, tobacco, or alcohol by the time they reach age 21, they are highly unlikely ever to become addicted. Moreover, there are dozens of known environmental and biological risk factors that increase the probability of initiating and continuing drug use. These factors are present at the level of the individual, the family, the community, and society as a whole.[2,3]

The relationship between substance use and youth development is not simple. Some effects result from direct exposure to drugs, whereas others relate to exposure to drug-using environments and their correlates. Exposure to abusable substances and "drug environments" can occur in at least three major, interrelated ways. These include passive exposure to abusable substances during gestation, exposure in drug-using households and communities, and substance use by children and youth themselves.

These are not independent relationships. Women who use drugs during pregnancy typically do not stop after the baby is born. Therefore, that same prenatally exposed child is likely to grow up in a substance-abusing household. Moreover, both prenatal exposure and living among drug users are powerful risk factors for later drug use by the child.

By itself, prenatal drug exposure can have significant effects on a child's developmental course. Perhaps the

> **About 50% of American youth will have tried an illegal substance by the time they graduate from high school.**

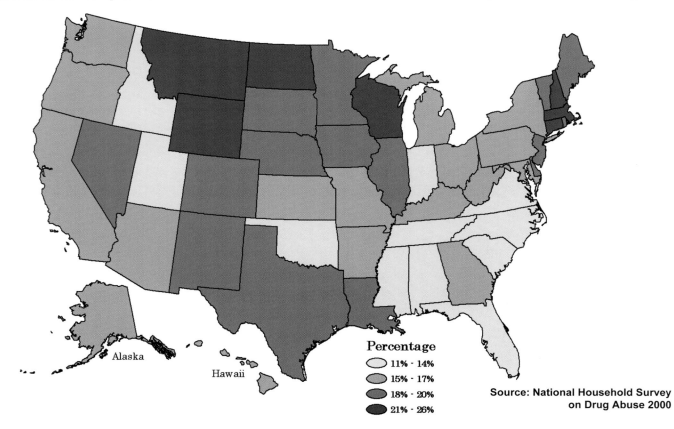

Percentage
- 11% - 14%
- 15% - 17%
- 18% - 20%
- 21% - 26%

Source: National Household Survey on Drug Abuse 2000

Map 11.1: Percentage of Youth Under 18 Using Alcohol in Last 30 Days

most dramatic prenatal drug effect is fetal alcohol syndrome. This disorder results from maternal alcohol use during pregnancy, and, in its most extreme forms, is expressed in severe developmental delays and cognitive disabilities. It is not clear just how much alcohol exposure is needed for fetal alcohol syndrome, but the fetus can be especially affected by the mother's drinking in the first months of pregnancy.[4]

Prenatal exposure to cocaine became a topic of great concern when the phenomenon of so-called "crack babies" was seen to accompany the crack epidemic that began in the mid-1980s. Although dramatic at birth, many differences dissipate over time, and the effects of prenatal cocaine exposure on later development and performance can often be quite subtle. This has led some people to conclude that there is no problem after all. However, studies of almost a dozen separate cohorts

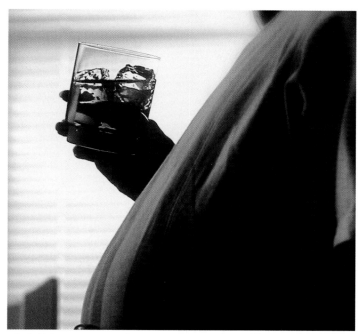

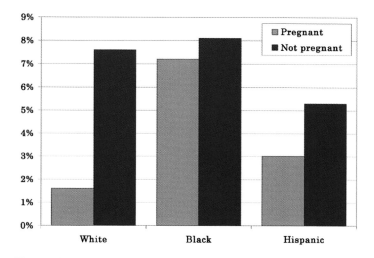

Figure 11.1: Percentage of Women Reporting Illicit Drug Use in Past Month by Pregnancy Status
Source: Substance Abuse and Mental Health Services 2001

of children exposed to cocaine prenatally conducted in the 1990s have shown that some children, though not all, do appear to experience subtle attentional, cognitive, and emotional deficits that can make them less successful in school and life in general.[5]

Recent observations that maternal drug use does result in cocaine binding to the fetal brain is greatly advancing our understanding of prenatal cocaine effects. This means that prenatal cocaine effects likely result from direct actions of the drug on the developing fetus, rather than from more indirect effects, like those from constrictions of maternal placental blood flow, as was originally thought. However, it is important that overlaying all direct effects of prenatal cocaine exposure is the fact that drug-using mothers typically also live in

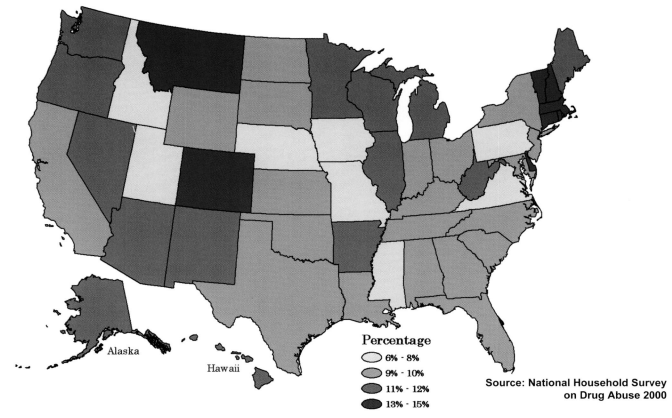

Percentage
- 6% - 8%
- 9% - 10%
- 11% - 12%
- 13% - 15%

Source: National Household Survey on Drug Abuse 2000

Map 11.2: Percentage of Youth Under 18 Using Illicit Drugs in Last 30 Days

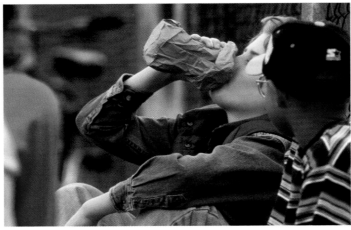

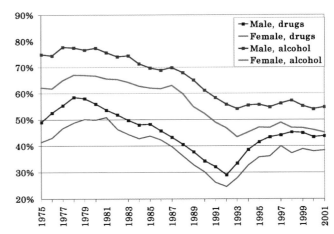

Figure 11.3: Percentage of 12th Graders Reporting Substance Abuse in Last 30 Days

Source: National Institute on Drug Abuse 2003

poverty, and the combination of poverty and living in a drug-using environment has a far more potent effect on later development than has any direct drug effect on the fetus.[6]

The effects of prenatal exposure to other drugs of abuse, including nicotine and marijuana, are not yet clear. Some studies suggest negative consequences and others suggest only transient effects.

As mentioned before, there are many risk factors that can increase the probability that someone will use drugs. The most widely known is low socioeconomic status, although it is difficult to know in any single case whether low socioeconomic status is a cause or a result of drug use. Other risk factors include substance use by parents and peers and poor family bonding.

There also is an array of what are called "protective factors" which help keep a child with many risk factors from going on to use drugs and develop substance-related problems. It is important to note that the majority of children with a large number of risk factors actually do not go on to use or develop problems with abusable substances. One of the most powerful protective factors is family involvement in the life of the child. Others include religious affiliation and group bonding. A full description of risk and protective factors can be found on the Web sites of the National Institute of Alcoholism and Alcohol Abuse (www.niaaa.nih.gov) and the National Institute on Drug Abuse (www.drugabuse.gov).

Among those who do try drugs, it is impossible to predict who will go on to develop more serious drug problems. We know that vulnerability to becoming addicted is determined by an interaction between hereditary and environmental factors, and they interact in complex ways. Genetic factors control well over 50% of the variability among individuals in the susceptibility to becoming addicted. Even though a genetic predisposition does not doom one to become an addict, the genetic contribution is pervasive enough to prompt many in the field to argue that individuals who come from families with extensive histories of addiction should consider avoiding all contact with substances of abuse. It also is important that, at least so far, most people cannot really know their genetic heritage in enough detail to know how biologically vulnerable they may be.

Environmental factors also play a tremendously important role in determining the progression from occasional use to addiction. Many of the same risk factors that make one more vulnerable to initial use are those that affect progression to addiction, although there are some differences.[2,3] A major risk factor for later addiction is growing up in a drug-using household–perhaps because of the intersection of the contributions to vulnerability of hereditary and environmental factors. Regular exposure of the child to drug-using behavior tends to normalize it.

Low socioeconomic status is another very powerful risk factor for addiction, as it is for initial drug use, although a common saying in the field is that "addiction is an equal opportunity destroyer." Like hereditary risk factors, environmental risk factors do not doom one to become an addict, but, by definition, they do increase the probability that one will have trouble with drug use.

Why does youth drug use lead to so many problems? The most obvious answer is that repeated drug use often leads to addiction, which is in so many ways an overwhelmingly maladaptive way of life. For addicted individuals, securing and using the drug become the most powerful motivators, lowering the relative priorities of such things as family integrity and

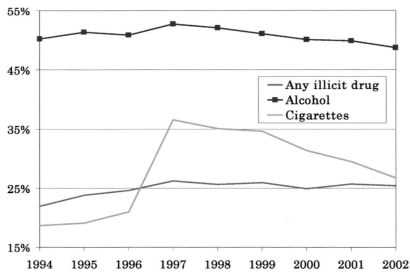

Figure 11.2: Percentage of 12th Graders Reporting Substance Abuse in Last 30 Days by Gender

Source: National Institute on Drug Abuse 2003

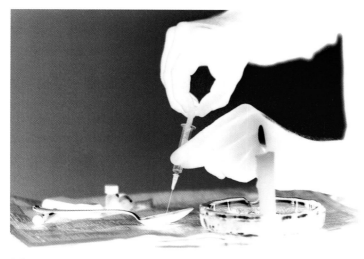

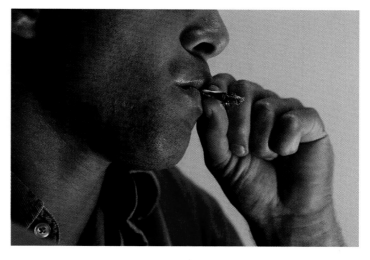

job success to the point that the individual's life comes apart.

But, statistically, relatively few young persons who try drugs go on to become addicted, so why such concern? Many studies suggest that even those who do not progress to very high levels of drug use can be negatively affected by drug use. Most obviously, drugs of abuse are intoxicating and therefore can interfere both with cognitive functioning and aspects of motor control, like the skills necessary to drive a car. Moreover, many drugs of abuse, like marijuana, interfere with short-term memory processes and can reduce school performance by residual memory loss that can last up to 48 hours after using the drug. Finally, youth substance use is correlated with many other negative behaviors during adolescence, including truancy and school failure, youth crime, and premarital pregnancy.

If young people have not used marijuana, tobacco, or alcohol by the time they reach age 21, they are highly unlikely ever to become addicted.

It is unlikely that this confluence of negative behaviors results from substance use alone. However, there is no question that both direct and indirect effects of youth substance use can have extremely negative consequences in the short and the long term. All of the exact mechanisms through which abusable substances exert their negative consequences are not yet known, but research is revealing more and more possibilities to explain them. For example, we now know that the adolescent brain is not fully formed but continues to develop.[7] It may well be that substance use actually alters the course or pace of brain development in ways that can lead to the kinds of negative outcomes that are seen after adolescent drug use.

Can youth drug use be prevented? It is a voluntary behavior, after all. But youth drug use levels have remained relatively stable and high for decades in spite of major efforts to curtail them. There is a science of drug use prevention, and principles of effective drug use prevention programming have been developed and published.[8] However, those principles are too infrequently incorporated into actual prevention programs, and, even when applied, these approaches seem insufficiently powerful to influence more than a small portion of the young people exposed to them. More research into youth motivation and behavioral self-control will be needed before we see the kinds of powerful prevention approaches that truly will be effective. In the interim, concerned parents are best served by becoming fully involved in the lives of their children and working to enhance protective factors like maintaining strong and positive family bonds, monitoring their children's activities and peers, and setting clear rules of conduct that are consistently enforced and followed by all members of the family.

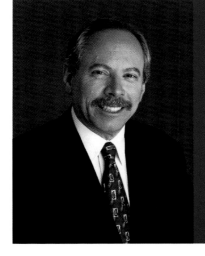

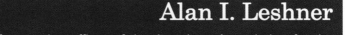

Alan I. Leshner

Alan I. Leshner, PhD, is chief executive officer of the American Association for the Advancement of Science and publisher of *Science*. Dr. Leshner formerly was director of the National Institute on Drug Abuse. He also has held senior positions at the National Institute of Mental Health and the National Science Foundation (NSF). Dr. Leshner went to NSF from Bucknell University, where he was professor of psychology. While on the faculty of Bucknell, he also held long-term appointments at the Postgraduate Medical School in Budapest, Hungary; at the Wisconsin Regional Primate Research Center; and as a Fulbright Scholar at the Weizmann Institute of Science in Israel. He is the author of numerous book chapters and papers in professional journals. He also wrote a major textbook on the relationship between hormones and behavior. Dr. Leshner received his undergraduate degree in psychology from Franklin and Marshall College and his MS and PhD degrees in physiological psychology from Rutgers University. In 1996, he received the Presidential Distinguished Executive Rank Award, the highest award in federal service.

Part Two: About Their Family Life and Well-being

Families nurture, protect, encourage, and support children. During recent decades, single-parent families, families led by grandparents, and foster family settings have come to share dominance with the nuclear family consisting of mother, father, and children. Parents and other providers must negotiate the necessities of working life, the requirements of change, the blending of families, and sometimes the struggles of living in poverty. The conclusions presented in the following chapters express different views on these issues; however, the problems that are approached represent some of the primary struggles facing children as families change. Supporting families represents a critically important and ongoing task of all societies. Learning how our society is providing requisite underpinnings to families is an urgent task and responsibility.

Chapter 12

Kristin Anderson Moore
and Sharon Vandivere

Turbulence:
The Effects of Change

Adjusting to a major change—such as the divorce or remarriage of a parent, a new school, or a residential move—can be difficult for children. Sometimes, change occurs repeatedly during the course of a year in an important area of a child's life. Alternatively, changes may occur in multiple contexts. Sometimes change occurs throughout a child's life. Children in these circumstances are said to experience a high level of *turbulence*, and they tend to have poorer developmental outcomes than children with less turbulent lives.

While change can be positive for children, such as moving to a better neighborhood, even positive changes can be stressful. For example, a move to a better neighborhood might mean loss of friends and a challenging school transition. Furthermore, many types of change can undermine children's development. Extreme examples include horrific experiences, such as war, while more commonplace examples include experiencing frequent turnover in doctors[1] or being in a classroom where fellow students and teachers change frequently. In this chapter, however, we focus on turbulence that is directly and uniquely experienced by the child and his or her family, rather than on general societal disruptions, such as war or measures of instability in services and in the lives of others.

Thus far, research has explored how turbulence within particular contexts affects children. Researchers have

Researchers have repeatedly found that multiple changes are related to poorer development and outcomes for children.

repeatedly found that multiple changes are related to poorer development and outcomes for children. For example, studies of residential mobility have shown that children whose families move frequently do not develop as well as children whose families stay in a consistent family home over time. A review of multiple studies found that moving is linked with poorer academic performance, grade retention, and high school drop-out rates.[2]

Research on education has shown that children who change schools repeatedly have poorer academic performance and more behavior problems in school.[3] Similarly, research on child care has found that having a large number of child care providers or frequent changes in providers is associated with poorer development for young children.[4] Turnover in day care teachers has been linked with poorer social development among preschool-age children.[5]

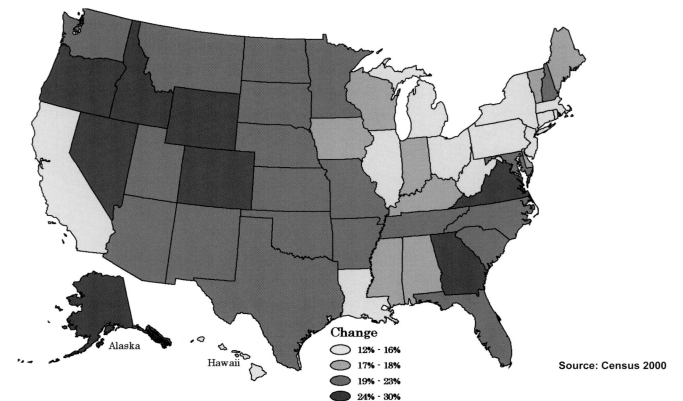

Change
- 12% - 16%
- 17% - 18%
- 19% - 23%
- 24% - 30%

Source: Census 2000

Map 12.1: Percentage of Population Over Age 5 Living in Different County in 2000 Than in 1995

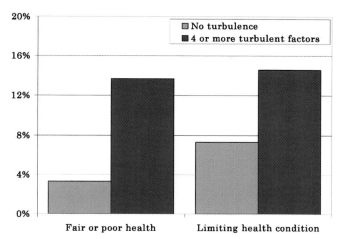

Figure 12.1: Percentage of Children Under 18 with Health Problems by Level of Turbulence, 1997

Source: Moore, Vandivere, and Redd 2004

Demographers have found that changes in family structure can undermine children's development. Children of divorced parents are more likely than other children to have problems in socioemotional development, school achievement, and high school completion.[6,7] Several studies have shown that the level of behavior problems among children in stepfamilies and among those living with single parents is higher than for children in families with two biological parents.[8] In fact, it may be that any change in family composition—rather than a specific type of change, such as a divorce—may be turbulent for children.[9] The lives of children with cohabiting parents may be particularly turbulent.[10]

While further work is warranted to develop brief, reliable, and valid measures of turbulence, work to date indicates that turbulence can be measured, varies across families, and is related to children's outcomes.[11,12] Among children under age 18, analyses of the combined 1997 and 1999 waves of the National Survey of America's Families indicate that 3% had moved from state to state during the past year, 7% had changed residences in the past 6 months, 2% had moved in with other people at some point during the prior year due to financial difficulties of the family, 8% had a parent who had begun a new job within the past 3 months, and 1% had a change in their or a parent's health for the worse in the past year. Among 6- to 17-year-olds, 3% had changed schools twice or more in the past year. Overall, 19% of children experienced one turbulent event in the prior year, and 4% experienced two or more turbulent events.

Many types of turbulence are interrelated. A divorce may trigger changes in neighborhood and school. While some children experiencing the disruption of their parents' marriage are able to stay in their home and school, others experience a cascade of disruptive events. The turbulence concept can capture and measure the accumulation of these disruptive events. Distinguishing among children with greater and lesser degrees of

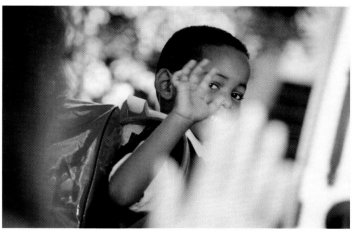

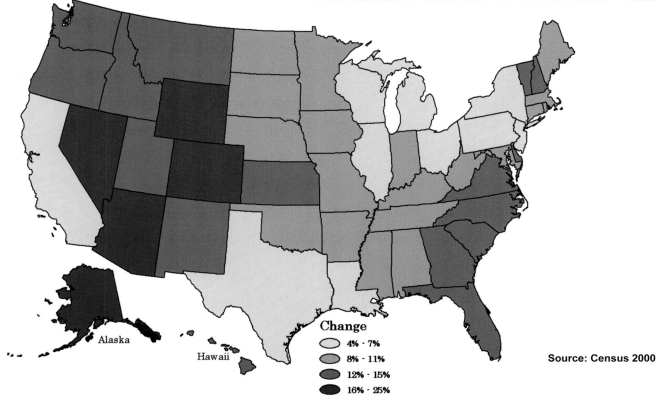

Change
4% - 7%
8% - 11%
12% - 15%
16% - 25%

Source: Census 2000

Map 12.2: Percentage of Population Over Age 5 Living in Different State in 2000 Than in 1995

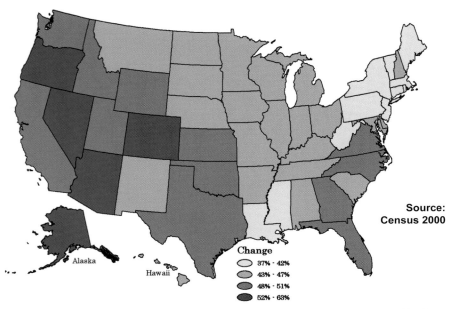

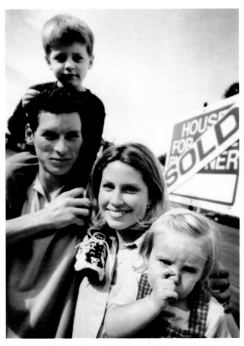

Source: Census 2000

Change
○ 37% - 42%
◔ 43% - 47%
◑ 48% - 51%
● 52% - 63%

Map 12.3: Percentage of Population Over Age 5 Living in Different House in 2000 Than in 1995

turbulence is important, since turbulence is conceptualized as having an additive (or possibly multiplicative) effect on children's development. That is, a child experiencing only a divorce in the family but no other major changes is more likely than a child experiencing no turbulence to have problems, while a child experiencing a divorce and a move to a new neighborhood has an increased probability of experiencing problems. A child experiencing even more turbulence—for example, a divorce accompanied by a move to a new neighborhood and a school change—is likely to be at even greater risk for developmental problems.

Indeed, cumulative turbulence is consistently related to poorer development among children. Defining high turbulence as experiencing four or more changes in the past year, 32% of 6- to 11-year-olds and 53% of 12- to 17-year-olds in high turbulence families experienced a high level of behavioral and emotional problems, 46% of 6- to 17-year-olds experienced a low level of engagement in school, and 39% of 12- to 17-year-olds had been suspended or expelled.[12] These

percentages are more than double—and sometimes triple—the percentages for children who have not experienced high levels of turbulence.

Families experiencing high levels of turbulence are likely to be having other kinds of problems, so it is difficult to know for certain whether turbulence causes poor outcomes among children or whether the negative outcomes are due to other circumstances that occur simultaneously with turbulence. For example, children of teen mothers are likely to experience multiple changes in living arrangements and in child care arrangements.[13] Additionally, disruptive changes are more frequent among children in low-income families. Despite, or because of, the link between turbulence and other challenges and difficulties that families face, turbulence represents an important concept for researchers and policy analysts.

The concept of turbulence has a number of uses. It can serve as a social indicator to identify a group of children at risk for poor developmental outcomes. It can also be used to monitor how the proportion of

Change in marital status — 5.2%
Other family reason — 20.2%
New job or job transfer — 10.6%
To look for work or lost job — 1.8%
Other job-related reason — 4.0%
Housing-related reason — 54.6%
Other reason — 3.7%

0%   20%   40%   60%

Figure 12.2: Type of Location Change for Children Under 18 Experiencing Move, 1998-2002

Source: Geographic Mobility/Migration 2003

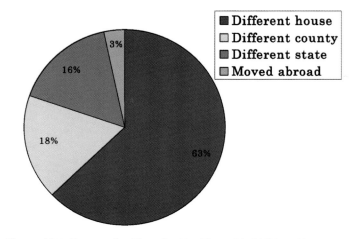

■ Different house
□ Different county
■ Different state
▨ Moved abroad

3%
16%
18%
63%

Figure 12.3: Reason for Move for Families with Children Under Age 16, March 2001-March 2002

Source: Geographic Mobility/Migration 2003

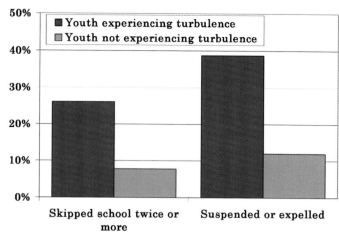

Figure 12.4: Problems at School for Children Ages 12 to 17 by Level of Turbulence

Source: Moore, Vandivere, and Redd 2004

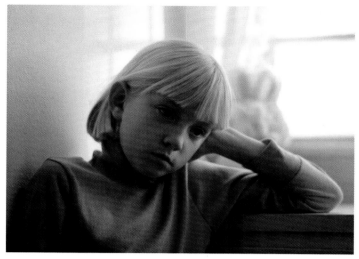

children experiencing high levels of disturbance differs across important subpopulations or changes over time. For example, rising levels of turbulence following a policy change or an economic downturn would signal problems for children. Analysts can also use turbulence as an outcome measure in studies of program and policy effectiveness. If a job training or parenting education program has a goal of promoting stable environments for families, evaluators can compare the levels of turbulence of the program group with a control group.

Basic research studies can use turbulence to take a "whole child" approach to children's development. Thus, instead of focusing only on specific types of change in children's lives, such as changes in the schools that children attend, researchers might explore whether other

While change can be positive for children, such as moving to a better neighborhood, even positive changes can be stressful.

changes are also occurring in the lives of children. Controlling for a variety of individual turbulent experiences might lead researchers to identify root causes of poor development. For example, it might be changes in family composition or instability in early child care that are causing problems as much as, or more than, changes in school. On the other hand, if the negative effects of changes build on each other in a multiplicative way, then examining cumulative changes across domains might be a more powerful predictor of child outcomes than changes in any single domain.

In sum, while further measurement work and research are needed, turbulence represents a useful integrating concept that helps us see children's lives as a whole. Assessing turbulence in children's lives can provide important information about what their lives are like and how they are faring.

Kristin Anderson Moore and Sharon Vandivere

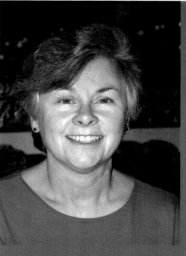

Kristin Anderson Moore, PhD, is a social psychologist and the president of Child Trends. In addition, she serves on the advisory group for the National Survey of Family Growth, the Packard Foundation's Advisory Board for the Future of Children, the technical review panel of the Early Childhood Longitudinal Study Birth Cohort, and the Advisory Council for the National Institute for Child Health and Development. Dr. Moore was a founding member of the Task Force on Effective Programs and Research at the National Campaign to Prevent Teen Pregnancy and served as a member of the bipartisan federal Advisory on Welfare Indicators. In 1999, Dr. Moore was awarded the Foundation for Child Development's Centennial Award for her achievements on behalf of children. She was also designated the 2002 Society for Adolescent Medicine Visiting Scholar. Dr. Moore obtained her PhD in sociology from the University of Michigan.

Sharon Vandivere, MPP, is a senior research analyst at Child Trends with a background in psychology and public policy. She has worked on projects involving indicators of children's well-being. Ms. Vandivere currently manages Child Trends' participation in the Assessing the New Federalism project. Assessing the New Federalism is a multiyear, joint research project with the Urban Institute to analyze the devolution of responsibility for social programs from the federal government to the states. She has coauthored research policy briefs focusing on child and family well-being published through Child Trends and the Urban Institute.

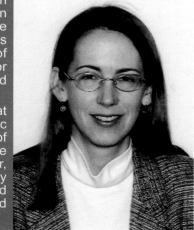

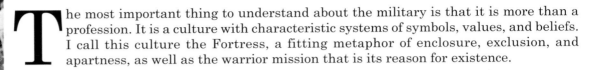

Chapter 13

Mary Edwards Wertsch

Children of the Fortress:
America's Most Invisible Culture

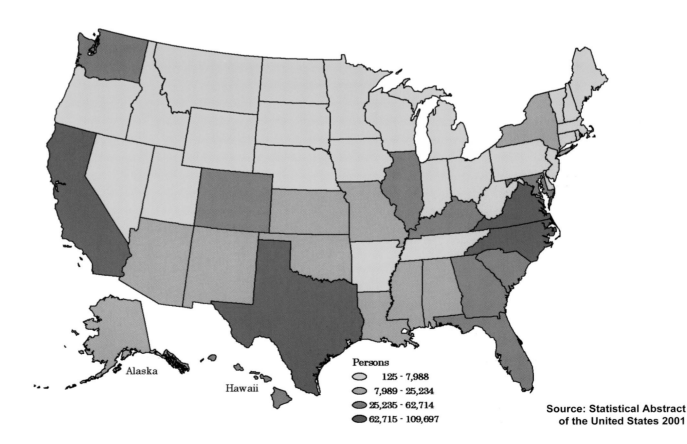

The most important thing to understand about the military is that it is more than a profession. It is a culture with characteristic systems of symbols, values, and beliefs. I call this culture the Fortress, a fitting metaphor of enclosure, exclusion, and apartness, as well as the warrior mission that is its reason for existence.

The Fortress is most unusual as cultures go. It cannot be defined racially, ethnically, religiously, geographically, linguistically, or in any of the other ways cultures are typically described. Furthermore, the majority of its uniformed members were not themselves Fortress-born. Instead they elected to immerse themselves in it temporarily, perhaps for a few years, perhaps for a career—but always with the idea of eventually leaving the Fortress for civilian life. Inside the Fortress, there are no old people. In a certain sense, it is the concept and material resources of the Fortress that stay and the people who merely move in and out, like a long-running play with a continuously changing cast.

But that is the Fortress as experienced by adults. It is different for the children. For them, the Fortress is not a choice, but a given. Its values and beliefs are acquired, not through training, but by a kind of cultural osmosis. Its rhythms of moving, settling in, and moving again are not aberrations from a hometown norm, but the norm itself.

> **For military children . . . the Fortress is a mother culture as intense, defining, and powerfully shaping as any culture on earth.**

For military children, who have no hometowns and may barely know their extended families, the Fortress is a mother culture as intense, defining, and powerfully shaping as any culture on earth. The cultural antecedents of today's military children, in this country and all around the world, were the youngsters whose mothers were camp followers, dragging the children along in the dust of armies on the march, or whose mothers hung about ports. These mothers were laundresses, seamstresses, cooks, wives, or prostitutes of the soldiers and sailors. The exceptions primarily would have been the children of officers who grew up in proper houses on military installations. But even if children were growing up inside the protective confines of a military base, they were definitely not on the Fortress radar screen. Even as our military expanded, building more bases, housing, and

Persons
- 125 - 7,988
- 7,989 - 25,234
- 25,235 - 62,714
- 62,715 - 109,697

Alaska

Hawaii

Source: Statistical Abstract of the United States 2001

Map 13.1: State Populations of Military and Civilian Personnel in U.S. Military Installations, 1999

schools, the military-as-institution did little to research or support the needs of wives and children.

Even after World War II, when global responsibilities led to tremendous expansion of the peacetime military, wives and children were often treated as bothersome complications and potential threats to readiness. Enlisted men of lowest rank were forbidden to marry by the military that controlled every aspect of their lives. Higher-ranking personnel could have families, but the military provided little to ease the difficulties of Fortress life for them. A very telling saying entered military banter everywhere: "If the Army/Navy/Air Force/Marine Corps had wanted you to have a family, it would have issued you one."

With the end of the draft and the creation of the All Volunteer Force in 1973, however, it became clear that families would become a bigger part of the picture.

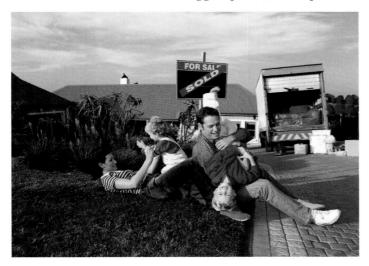

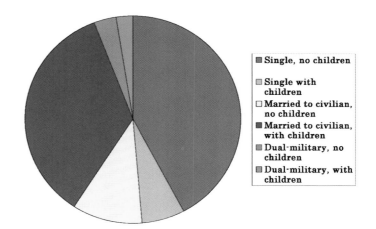

- ■ Single, no children
- ■ Single with children
- □ Married to civilian, no children
- ■ Married to civilian, with children
- ■ Dual-military, no children
- ■ Dual-military, with children

Figure 13.1: Family Types Among Active Duty Military Personnel, 2001

Source: Military Family Resource Center 2002

Restrictions on marriage of junior enlisted personnel were dropped. The first Family Support Center was opened by the Navy in 1979, and Army Community Centers followed suit. Now, 30 years into the All Volunteer Force, a military once overwhelmingly composed of single men has been transformed into one in which uniformed personnel are significantly outnumbered by dependents. According to the 2001 Demographics Report of the Department of Defense, there were nearly 1.4 million active duty service members and nearly 1.9 million family members.[1]

So it is that families, once barely visible to the military-as-institution, are now one of the prime forces shaping it. There is no doubt that families are absolutely essential to an all-volunteer military, and the morale and readiness of the force can be strongly impacted by family issues. Studies have shown that family discontent is one of the

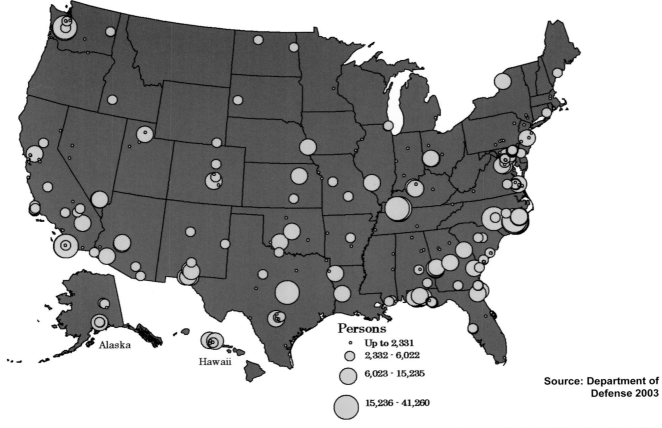

Persons

- ○ Up to 2,331
- ○ 2,332 - 6,022
- ● 6,023 - 15,235
- ● 15,236 - 41,260

Source: Department of Defense 2003

Map 13.2: Number of U.S. Military Personnel by Installation Location, 2003

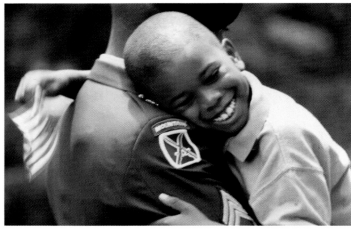

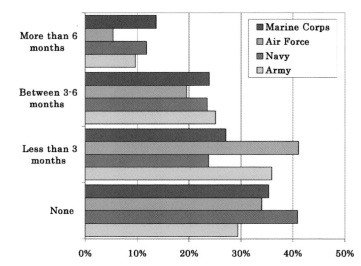

Figure 13.3: Military Youth, 10 to 18 Years Old, Experiencing
Family Separations, 1999
Source: Military Family Resource Center 1999

principal reasons service members choose to leave the service early.[2] When one considers that it costs more than $6 million to train a single pilot,[3] it becomes clear that the Department of Defense has good reason to devote resources to understanding and addressing the issues of military families.

It is important to understand that life inside the Fortress is radically different from life in civilian America. It is the particular combination of traits that makes it unique. The Fortress is characterized by:

- fierce idealism, born of devotion to the military mission,

- rigid authoritarianism, essential for a command structure,

- a strict class system, marked by the great divide between enlisted and officer, as well as many gradations of rank,

- a great deal of absence from family life by the parent(s) in uniform,

- extreme mobility,

- separateness, and often alienation, from the civilian community, and

- constant preparation for war.

These traits are endemic to the Fortress and always have been. They were as true of the Roman Legion as they are of today's U.S. armed forces.

These traits translate into the following challenges for today's 1.2 million American military children under the age of 18:

Loss is the principal psychological challenge of every military childhood. First, the mobility of the military means that every child will be uprooted numerous times, losing everyone in his or her world other than family members. Military families move, on average, every 2.9 years.[4] This is enough to ensure that a typical military child will attend five to seven schools in 12 years. Second is the threat of loss of a parent in the line of duty. This is exacerbated in wartime, particularly in the 6% of military families with single parents and in the 6% with dual-military parents.[1]

Some military children must deal with parental alcohol abuse. The 1998 Department of Defense Survey of personnel found that military men are more likely to drink and drink heavily than their civilian counterparts. The rate of heavy drinking among military men ages 18 to 25 was 1.8 times the rate for young civilian men.[5]

There is insufficient child care capacity for military children. The Department of Defense has made significant improvements in its child care facilities and programs in the past 20 years,

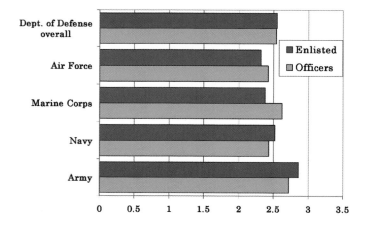

Figure 13.2: Average Number of Dependents per Family, 1998
Source: Department of Defense 1998

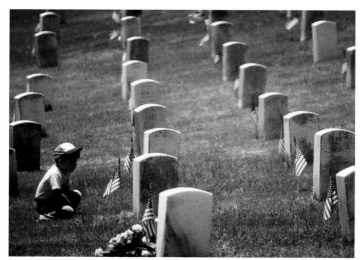

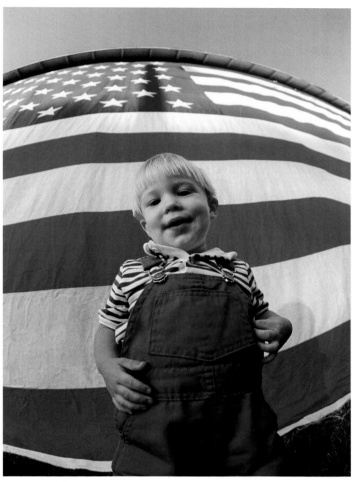

Financial stress is a major problem for many military families. Military pay is still about 6% below civilian pay for comparable work.[7] There is still a shortage of base housing, and more than 60% of what does exist is considered substandard by the Department of Defense.[8] Finding affordable housing may put the family too far from the base to avail itself of the support services there. Financial stress can contribute to family breakdown and ranks as one of the principal quality-of-life reasons members elect to leave the service.

Military behavior is often mirrored inside the family. The authoritarian nature of the military is frequently echoed inside military families and can contribute to stress, family violence, and insecurity in children.

Military children may not have an easy life inside the Fortress, but they often emerge from it with qualities that serve them extraordinarily well for the rest of their lives.

The Department of Defense deserves credit for instituting programs in recent years that have improved life for military children and should be supported and encouraged to do more. Congress must also seriously address the pay gap and other issues that subject military personnel and their families to unreasonable stress even as they risk catastrophic loss for the sake of their country. In the meantime, military children will continue to cope as they always have, doing the best they can to adapt to what the Fortress requires of them.

Military children may not have an easy life inside the Fortress, but they often emerge from it with qualities that serve them extraordinarily well for the rest of their lives. One is resilience in the face of change. Another is an anti-racist attitude that is strongly encouraged by the diversity and values of the Fortress itself. But the most powerful of all is the bedrock idealism implicit in every aspect of Fortress life. Military children who absorb this understand that there are more important things than money and that meaning in life derives from serving a cause larger than one's self.

working to meet accreditation standards, increasing the pay of child care workers, and expanding the number of child spaces. Still, there is more work to do. By 2000, the Department of Defense had met 58% of its child care need; the plan is to meet 80% by 2005.[6]

Some military families are reluctant to use available resources. Most bases now have centers that provide advice, counseling, and education for military parents and children. However, they are used almost exclusively by enlisted and lower-ranking officer families and not by career officers. This is because the ethos of the Fortress still makes it a career risk for an officer or any of his or her dependents to admit to any kind of problem.

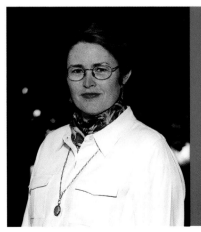

Mary Edwards Wertsch

Mary Edwards Wertsch, BA, is the author of the nonfiction book, *Military Brats: Legacies of Childhood Inside the Fortress* (Harmony Books, 1991; Aletheia Publications, 1996), which examines the military as a home culture for children and sets out the positive and negative psychological legacies of that life. As the daughter of a career Army infantry officer, she lived in 20 houses and attended 12 schools by the age of 18. She has given talks on the subject of military culture in the United States and abroad. Her professional background is in journalism, and she lives in St. Louis, Missouri, with her husband and two sons. She currently is working on a companion guide to her book for use by discussion groups. She also is compiling an anthology of fiction, nonfiction, and poetry about military childhood by established writers who are military brats.

Chapter 14

Judith Wallerstein

The Consequences of
Divorce

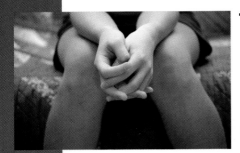

Growing up in America has changed. Divorce began to rise steeply in the early 1970s. Since 1972, over a million children each year have experienced their parents' divorce. By the beginning of the 21st century, a quarter of adults in their 20s and 30s had spent important childhood years in divorced or remarried families, or both. Although the statistics vary somewhat from year to year, partly because of the decrease in marriage and the increase in cohabiting couples with children, the incidence of divorce has hovered around the 45% mark for first marriages and 60% for second marriages for two decades. Divorce has risen throughout Europe, South America, and Asia during these same decades, but the United States continues to lead the world. Rising concern about high divorce rates in this country has led to a nationwide increase in premarital counseling, largely under church auspices, and to an increase in educational

programs by governmental entities, churches, and colleges. The aim of these activities is to promote marital quality and stability.

Research has grown since the early 1970s from almost no studies at all to enough projects to create a substantial library of findings. We have learned that the breakup is almost always profoundly upsetting to children. We have become increasingly aware of long-term effects that become visible many years later in the difficulties that adult children of divorce encounter in establishing lasting relationships in love and marriage. The course and quality of their growing-up years in the post-divorce family—including their frequently lowered socioeconomic status; the diminished availability of parents, especially fathers; the dwindling financial support during college years; and even their playtime and friendships, which are curtailed due to the time they devote to traveling back and forth to be with each parent in separate homes—are different from that of the child in the reasonably functioning, intact family. Indeed, because half of children of divorce are 6 years old

Since 1972, over a million children each year have experienced their parents' divorce.

or younger at the time of the divorce, their knowledge of life within the two-parent family is limited. Their expectations of relationships between men and women are influenced by the marital breakup and post-divorce relationship of their parents and by the success or failure of the remarriage of one or both parents.

Most of the psychological research on divorce has reflected the middle-class Caucasian child's experience. Studies have shown a post-divorce descent into poverty, with its attendant hazards, of many mother-headed families, especially families that previously were middle class. Only a trickle of studies has reported on children in Non-Caucasian or poverty-level populations; few have considered ethnic or racial groups in which the extended family is the dominant family structure, a structure that might provide greater security to the child after the divorce.

Divorce is a different experience for adults than for children. To the adult, divorce is a necessary and valid remedy for a seriously troubled relationship. Although

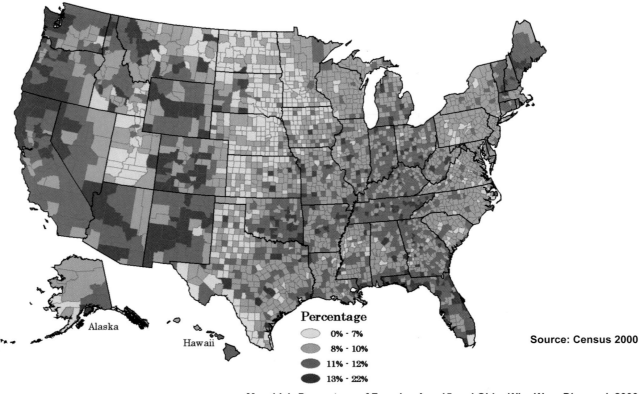

Alaska

Hawaii

Percentage
0% - 7%
8% - 10%
11% - 12%
13% - 22%

Source: Census 2000

Map 14.1: Percentage of Females Age 15 and Older Who Were Divorced, 2000

parents worry about their children, they expect that the children will understand their decision and that they will adjust quickly to new family circumstances. Parents rarely realize how little the children understand and how much help the children need to accept the changes. Further, parents certainly cannot anticipate how hard it will be to provide that help during the stressful years ahead as each parent struggles to rebuild a separate social, economic, and sexual life.

Splitting up the family to solve the parents' problems makes no sense to children. Few children are aware of their parents' growing dissatisfaction during the marriage, and they are rarely prepared for the breakup of their family. In most families, there is no overt conflict between the unhappy parents during the marriage that could prepare the children. Not surprisingly, children who have little inkling of what is to happen are more troubled than those in chronic high-conflict families where divorce can surely bring relief to parent and child, unless the conflict continues or even rises during the post-divorce years.

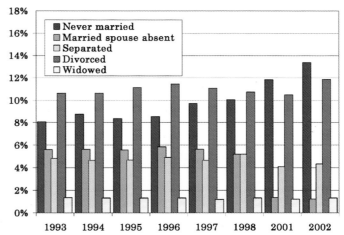

Figure 14.1: Marital Status of Single-parent Householder with Own Children Present (Under Age 18)

Source: U.S Census Bureau 2004

The early responses of children and adolescents are governed by their age and developmental stage at the time of the breakup. Having seen one parent leave the household, preschool children fear that they, too, will be abandoned. Their frequent sleeplessness, crankiness, regressions, and phobias express these acute fears, and they are very much in need of extra time and comforting from parents.

Young school-age children often develop learning problems and display aggression on the playground. In their worry about their parents and their fear that calm and order in the family will never be restored, many forfeit a year of school progress. Preadolescents are often very angry at their parents for divorcing. Underlying their anger is their fear that they will lose the stability of the family that enables them to pursue their crowded developmental agenda of school, peers, and activities. Compassion for the troubled parents also develops at this time, especially among school-age and young adolescent girls. Children sometimes sacrifice school and friends to care for a needy parent.

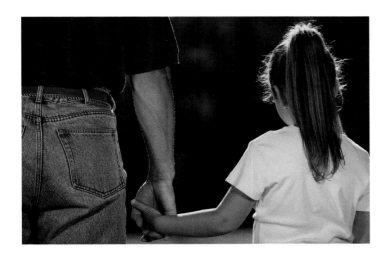

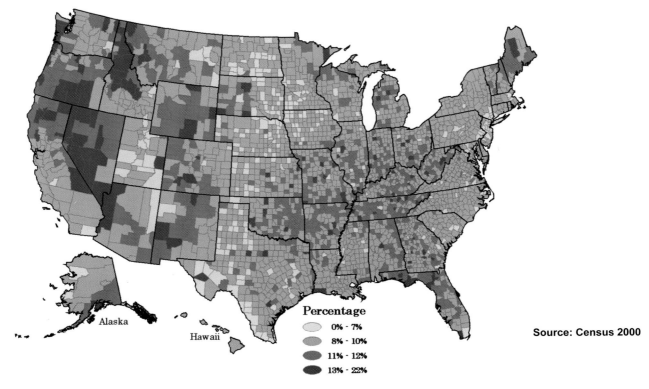

Source: Census 2000

Percentage
- 0% - 7%
- 8% - 10%
- 11% - 12%
- 13% - 22%

Alaska

Hawaii

Map 14.2: Percentage of Males Age 15 and Older Who Were Divorced, 2000

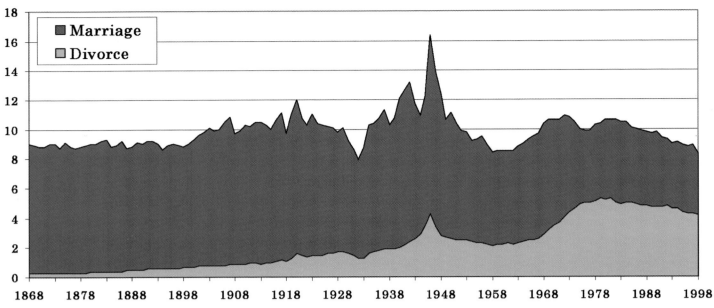

Figure 14.2: Marriage Rate and Divorce Rate Per 1000 Persons

Source: National Center for Health Statistics 1973, 1989, Statistical Abstract of the United States 2000

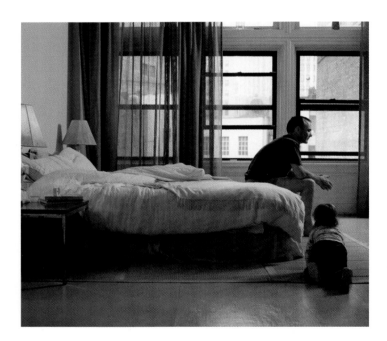

Adolescents, who often take charge of running the household after the breakup, worry about their future: Will my relationships fail as well? Who will pay for my college? Will my parents recover from this crisis? Who will take care of me, and who will take care of them? Teens are often closely tied to a troubled parent by compassion compounded by anger at the parent they blame for the divorce.

As they enter late adolescence and young adulthood, many children of divorce fear heartbreak and loss in their adult relationships. They are haunted by memories of their parents' unhappiness and complain of being unprepared for marriage. Many decide that the way to avoid divorce is to avoid marriage. Census figures show a lower incidence of marriage and a higher incidence of divorce in this population as compared with adults raised in intact marriages. Many eventually overcome their anxieties by the time they reach their 30s and go on to create stable, loving families. Others continue to suffer with sorrow and loneliness. Approximately 20% to 25% are likely to be maladjusted in their adult lives, according

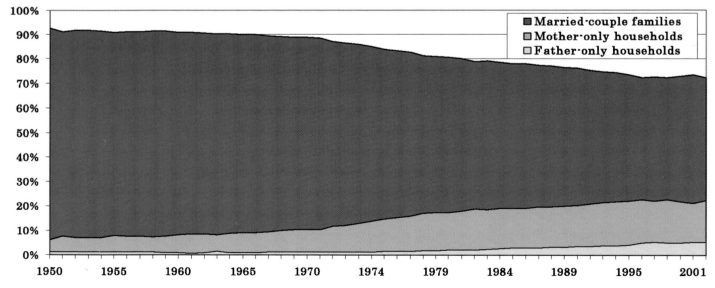

Figure 14.3: Family Type for Families with Children Under 18

Source: U.S. Census Bureau 2003

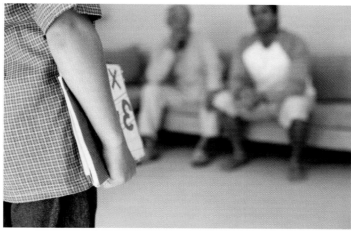

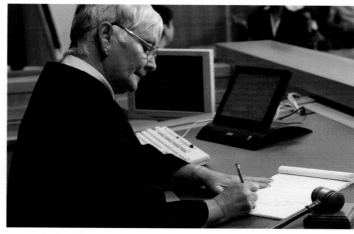

to one recent long-term study. On the other hand, one of the good outcomes of divorce is that, as adults, many children of divorce are highly competent in the workplace. They learn early to take responsibility for themselves and for others.

The central arena of public policy for children of divorce has been the courts and, secondarily, the legislature. Since family law and courts vary widely from state to state, divorce policies and practices have been a patchwork quilt. There is growing recognition that the adversarial stance of the court is ill-suited to promote much needed post-divorce cooperation between parents. As a result, mediation of the differences between the parents by trained media-tors has been introduced in a growing number of courts to protect children from parental conflict. However, courts and mediators have been criticized for tilting toward the legal rights of parents since few take the opportunity to hear the expressed wishes of the child. Court orders for custody or visitation rarely include the flexibility that allows for the expectable changing needs of the developing child.

Divorce has risen throughout Europe, South America, and Asia during these same decades, but the United States continues to lead the world.

Traditionally, the courts and the community have regarded the mother-custody family as the heir to the two-parent family. However, there has been increased recognition of the importance of both parents to the development of children. Although most children still remain in the sole custody of their mothers, the courts and society have shown increasing interest in greater participation of fathers in the post-divorce family. Joint custody has become more common to ensure that growing children have two supportive parents. There are many instances in which this arrangement works well for children and parents, but, by and large, a good outcome only occurs when the parents cooperate in their post-divorce parenting and respect each other's contribution.

In recent years, the collection of child support has been more rigorously enforced, and children have benefited from greater economic security. However, many women and children continue to experience a serious drop in economic protection. Recently, courts throughout the United States have established brief educational programs to help parents explain the divorce to their children and to avoid continued conflict. In a few places, children's groups parallel the parent groups and are designed to help the children understand and accept the many changes in their families. With the exception of these court-sponsored educational programs, counseling serv-ices for divorcing parents or their children have been rare. A major problem has been that attorneys, mental health professionals, pediatricians, nursery school teachers, and educators are not well informed about the consequences of divorce for children. Most are unfamiliar with ways to help parents select the appropriate custody plan. Although there is widespread community recognition that a divorce is a crisis for children, as well as their parents, our society still is inadequately prepared to provide divorced parents the advice and support they need, for themselves or for their children.

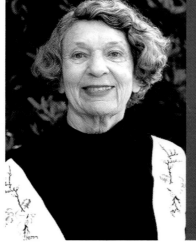

Judith Wallerstein

Judith Wallerstein, PhD, is an authority on the effects of divorce on children and their families. She is senior lecturer emerita at the University of California at Berkeley and founder of the Judith Wallerstein Center for the Family in Transition in California, a major center for research, education, and counseling for families in separation, divorce, and remarriage. Findings from her groundbreaking investigations have been widely published in scientific journals and lay publications and presented worldwide to community groups and meetings of medical, legal, and mental health professionals. Her books include *Surviving the Breakup: How Children and Parents Cope with Divorce*, written with Joan B. Kelly. Subsequent bestsellers include *Second Chances: Men, Women and Children a Decade After Divorce*, written with Sandra Blakeslee, and *The Unexpected Legacy of Divorce: A 25-Year Landmark Study*, written with Julia Lewis and Sandra Blakeslee. Her latest work, a guide for divorcing parents, is *What About the Kids? Raising Children Before, During and After Divorce*, written with Sandra Blakeslee. She has received numerous awards from national medical, psychological, and legal groups and from legislative bodies.

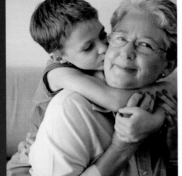

Chapter 15

Grandparents
Raising Grandchildren

Donna M. Butts and Jaia Peterson

Since the beginning of time, family members have stepped up to raise children when parents were no longer able or willing to do so. Relatives, primarily grandparents, have been the silent thread offering children stability, roots, and unconditional love. Yet until recently, these family caregivers—who are often referred to as kinship caregivers—were rarely recognized or rewarded for their sacrifices. Although the unexpected responsibility of raising children later in life can have dramatic consequences, the number of children raised by grandparents increased from 2.2 million in 1970 to 4.5 million in 2000. This alone has helped to force the issue from the fringes to mainstream attention.

Today, 6 million children, or 1 out of every 12, live in households headed by a grandparent or other relative. Over 2 million children live in grandparent-headed households without a parent present. Most experts agree substance abuse by a parent has been the number one reason for the significant increase in kinship caregiving, but other issues such as poverty, death, incarceration, military deployment, and HIV/AIDS all play a part in creating skipped-generation households.

Kinship care families are as diverse as other families in the United States, and their needs and strengths are just as complex. For the first time, the U.S. Census Bureau began collecting data on these families through the 2000 decennial census. Mandated through welfare reform, the census now asks three questions about grandparents raising grandchildren. The results were released in the fall of 2003 by the Census Bureau and pointed to the stark reality that 19% of grandparents raising grandchildren had incomes below the poverty line. Census data

also revealed that while relatives cared for 6% of all White children, 17% of African American children were in the care of relatives. These families lived in all states, but the southern and southwestern states had a higher prevalence of kinship care families.

Often the families find themselves living together after little or no time to prepare for a new resident. Caregivers recount how their worlds suddenly changed with a middle-of-the-night knock on the door by a protective services worker dropping off a related child for safe placement. This leads to a dramatically different lifestyle for the child and caregiver. The time in life many older adults refer to as "my time" disappears. Given that 39% care for the children for 5 or more years, many kinship caregivers will never see "my time" again.

Many kinship caregivers believe this new family configuration will be temporary and only last for a few

> **Today, 6 million children, or 1 out of every 12, live in households headed by a grandparent or other relative.**

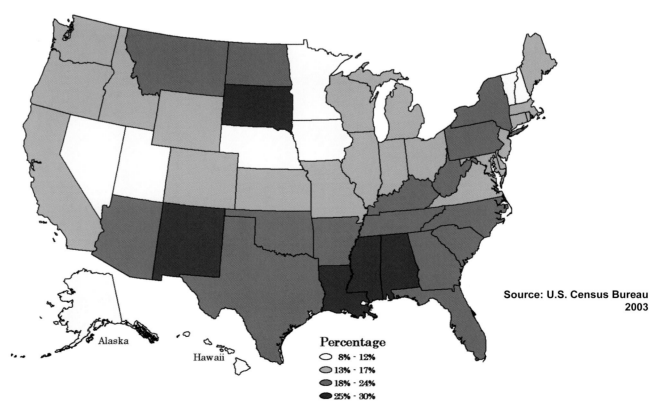

Source: U.S. Census Bureau
2003

Percentage
- 8% - 12%
- 13% - 17%
- 18% - 24%
- 25% - 30%

Map 15.1: Percentage of Households in Poverty with Grandparents Responsible for Grandchildren, 1999

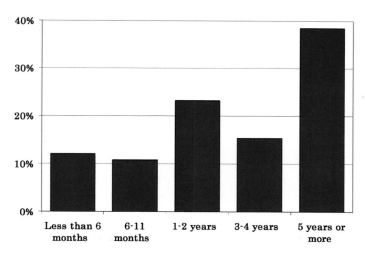

Figure 15.1: Percentage of Grandparents Responsible for Grandchildren Living with Them by Stay Length, 2000

Source: U.S. Census Bureau 2003

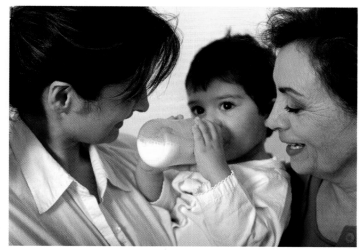

months. They hope that eventually the biological parent will be able to resume parental responsibility, and they are concerned that legal action to obtain guardianship would sever or jeopardize delicate family relationships. This means most of the children live in informal arrangements with their relatives without a formal legal relationship. Pursuing legal guardianship, custody, or adoption can be costly and time consuming. For some kinship caregivers, it is simply too expensive to retain legal counsel, and they do not have access to free or affordable legal services. Others find that in order to gain legal standing, the state must first take custody of the child. They fear losing the child to a system they do not understand or, even worse, believe they will face public scrutiny and questioning about their parenting abilities. Whatever the reason, these caregivers are providing a tremendous service to their families and to the country. If even half of the children who are not currently in the system were to enter formal foster care, conservative estimates indicate it would cost taxpayers more than $6.5 billion each year while overwhelming a foster care system that is already bulging at the seams.

Kinship care families face a wide range of challenges and barriers that vary significantly depending on their legal relationships and needs. In a recent survey of grandparent and other relative caregivers conducted by the Children's Defense Fund, respondents reported that

what they needed most was accurate information about existing programs and services that were available to their families. Others needed assistance in accessing things such as counseling, financial assistance, affordable housing, health insurance, education for the children, and respite care. The lack of a legal relationship can lead to children being denied any of these services and programs. This is of particular concern because children in the care of relatives are more likely to have special educational, medical, and mental health needs often created by the conditions that led to their alternative living arrangement. The caregivers and children are also more likely to experience depression, guilt, attachment disorders, and anxiety. They share a sense of social isolation, believing that they are different from others in their peer groups. Support groups, along with respite care, can play an important role in helping to alleviate stress. In addition to providing accurate information and access to services, support groups help the families understand that they are not alone.

The median age of a grandparent raising a grandchild is 57. Because of this, many caregivers are working outside the home and need to be able to access employer-sponsored benefits designed for families, such as child-related leave and child care. Relative caregivers need to be able to include the children they are raising as dependents on their employer-sponsored health insurance policies. A survey of 51 major companies across the United States revealed that none of the companies allowed relative caregivers who were raising children without legal custody, guardianship, or adoption to include these children as eligible beneficiaries on their employer-provided health insurance. Few companies

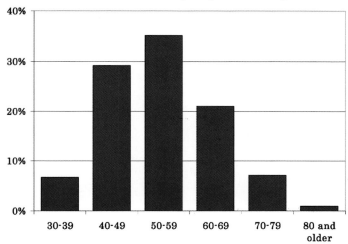

Figure 15.2: Percentage of Grandparents by Age Who Are Responsible for Grandchildren Living with Them, 2000

Source: U.S. Census Bureau 2003

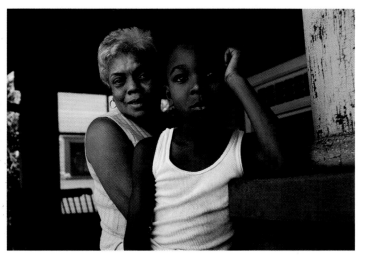

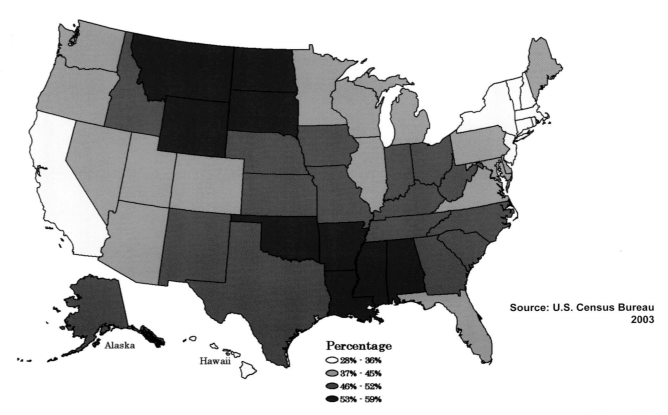

Source: U.S. Census Bureau
2003

Percentage
- 28% - 36%
- 37% - 45%
- 46% - 52%
- 53% - 59%

Alaska

Hawaii

Map 15.2: Percentage of Grandparents Who Are Responsible for Grandchildren Living with Them, 2000

allowed their relative caregiver employees who were informal caregivers to access the companies' child care services. Only half of the corporations allowed employees to take leave to stay home with sick children, and in most cases, they were required to use vacation or sick leave. Nearly all companies surveyed offered employee assistance and counseling programs that are accessible to all employees; however, none of them offered specific programs for relative caregivers.

Beyond the workplace, there are many creative programs through public agencies and private nonprofits that support the needs of kinship caregivers. Local area agencies on aging across the United States may offer support groups, respite care, or information and referral services to assist older grandparents who are raising grandchildren. State and county child welfare agencies, which are responsible for responding to local child abuse, neglect, and other child welfare issues, often offer direct services or referral services to kinship caregivers. Furthermore, faith-based and community-based organizations across the United States such as Volunteers of America, Catholic Charities, and land grant university

extension services offer a variety of services ranging from support groups to legal assistance to respite care. At least two states, New Jersey and Ohio, offer kinship navigator programs that are hotlines or helpdesks that caregivers can call to help navigate the services available to them in their state.

Two recently enacted federal laws have set guidelines for programs to help kinship caregivers: the National Family Caregiver Support Program and the Living Equitably: Grandparents Aiding Children and Youth Act (LEGACY). The National Family Caregiver Support Program, which was enacted in 2000, allows 10% of its funding to be used to provide support services to grandparents over the age of 60 who are raising grandchildren. Services include information about available resources, assistance to caregivers in gaining access to the services, individual and family counseling, support groups, respite care, and other supplemental services. The LEGACY Act, which was signed into law in December 2003 as part of the American Dream Downpayment Act, calls for a national study of the housing needs of grandparents and other relatives raising children, training for local Department of Housing and

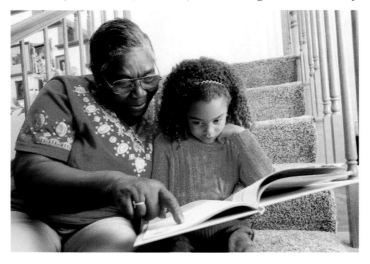

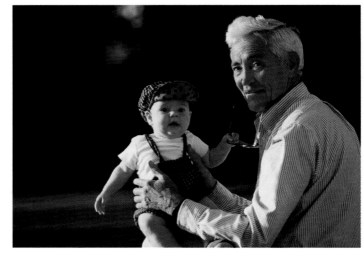

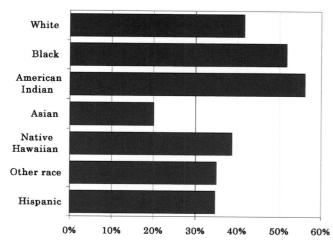

Figure 15.3: Percentage of Grandparents Living with Grandchildren Who Also Are Responsible for Their Grandchildren by Race, 2000

Source: U.S. Census Bureau 2003

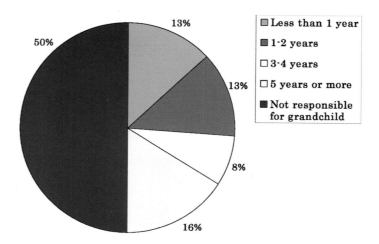

Figure 15.4: Duration of Responsibility for Grandchildren of Grandparents Age 30 to 59, 2000

Source: U.S. Census Bureau 2003

Urban Development officials on issues affecting grandparents raising grandchildren, and funds for two to four organizations across the country to develop housing specifically for grandparents raising grandchildren.

Several states have enacted varied legislation to assist grandparents in gaining educational and medical consent for children. Educational and medical consent laws, which vary by state, help grandparents and other relatives raising children to enroll children in school, participate in individual education plans, approve necessary medical procedures, and gain access to medical records.

There are several different types of state laws related to guardianship and legal custody other than adoption and foster care. They include *subsidized guardianship*, which allows relatives caring for a child in state custody to obtain guardianship and provide a permanent home for the child while receiving a monthly stipend to help provide for the needs of the child; *standby guardianship*, which provides an option for terminally ill parents to designate a standby guardian if parents become incapacitated or die; and *de*

facto custodian, which gives caregivers the same standing as parents in custody cases if they satisfy the definition of "de facto custodian," who is generally the primary caregiver of a child who has lived with that person for a certain period depending on the child's age.

Given that 39% care for the children for 5 or more years, many kinship caregivers will never see "my time" again.

Many children thrive when raised by grandparents and other relatives. Children living with relatives maintain connections to their family members, traditions, and identity. In many cases, kinship caregivers enable sibling groups to remain intact when otherwise they would be placed in different homes. The children are able, to a greater extent than foster children not in kinship care, to maintain relationships with their birth parents and other family members. They experience fewer placements leading to a more stable living situation and are likely to stay within the same community and school system. While grandparents and other relatives face many barriers, most are committed and willing to undertake the sacrifices necessary to raise another generation of children. Our country and our communities are stronger because of them.

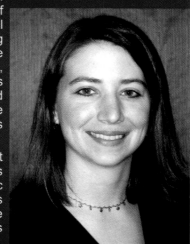

Donna M. Butts and Jaia Peterson

Since 1997, Donna M. Butts, BA, has served as the executive director of Generations United (GU), the only national membership organization focused solely on promoting intergenerational public policies, strategies, and programs. GU represents more than 100 organizations comprised of more than 70 million Americans and houses the National Center on Grandparents and Other Relatives Raising Children. She has more than 30 years of experience working with nonprofit organizations at the local, national, and international levels. A graduate of Stanford University's Executive Program for Nonprofit Leaders, Butts has served on the National Kinship Care Advisory Panel and the International Consortium of Intergenerational Programmes and is a respected author and speaker.

Jaia Peterson, MS, is the public policy director at Generations United. Her work includes advising Congress on intergenerational issues, coordinating the GU Public Policy Committee, and editing the GU newsletter, *Together*. Peterson received a masters degree in social work from Syracuse University and has worked in child protective services, refugee resettlement, and many other capacities with individuals and families from a variety of cultural backgrounds.

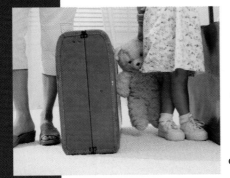

Chapter 16

Moira Szilagyi

Foster Care

Foster care is intended to be a temporary haven for children whose families are unable to meet their basic needs for health and safety. It is based on the premise that children do best when raised in family settings, although about 20% of foster care children (mostly adolescents) reside in group homes or residential treatment facilities. The average length of stay in foster care is 33 months and ranges from a few days to many years.

Seventy percent of children enter foster care as a result of a court-ordered placement due to child abuse and neglect. Nearly 30% of foster care children (almost all adolescents) enter care through a court-ordered process called Persons in Need of Supervision or through juvenile delinquency petitions. Less than 1% are placed voluntarily by

parents. Efforts to prevent foster care placement have resulted in increased numbers of children being placed with relatives, neighbors, or family friends over the last decade. *Kinship care* is an informal, unregulated system that is estimated to provide care for about one-third of children in out-of-home care.

The most recent information from the U.S. Department of Health and Human Services indicated that 542,000 children were in foster care as of March 2001, with about 250,000 entering and leaving the system each year. Just over half were male (52%), and they ranged in age from birth to 21 years, although most states still discharge youth at age 18. The vast majority of these children resided in large urban settings. In 2000, about 1% of the U.S. child population was in foster care. Utah had the overall lowest rate (0.25%) while Wisconsin and the District of Columbia had the highest at 2.7%. Minority children continue to be overrepresented in the foster care system; they also stay longer and are less likely to be adopted.

Children entering the foster care system have health needs in excess of children who are living in poverty with one or more parents. Multiple, cumulative adverse events and exposures that place children at risk for foster care also contribute to their overall poor health

status. Prenatal risk factors include exposure to toxins, maternal malnutrition, and infections transmitted from parents such as HIV, herpes, syphilis, and hepatitis B or C.

> **Children entering foster care beyond the neonatal period have lived in financially destitute, chaotic, emotionally deprived environments characterized by violence and inconsistent caregiving.**

Children entering foster care beyond the neonatal period have lived in financially destitute, chaotic, emotionally deprived environments characterized by violence and inconsistent caregiving. A recent study revealed that over 80% had experienced significant violent incidences prior to placement. Many had lived with multiple caregivers and had not benefited from exposure to the sustained, predictable nurturance necessary for normal emotional and psychological development. Seventy percent had experienced physical and/or sexual abuse, the rate of which is often underestimated at the time of placement.

Older youth entering foster care often have behavioral and emotional issues arising out of ongoing family discord or violence, abuse or neglect, or their own mental health issues. Many older youth have engaged in high-risk behaviors, including substance abuse, elopement, truancy, sexual activity, and criminal behavior. Rates of special education services, school absence, and school failure of children entering foster care exceed those of other children living in poverty.

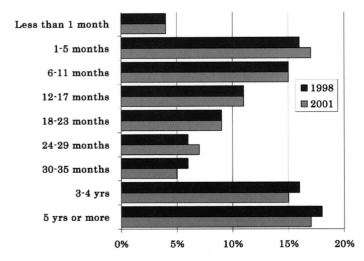

Figure 16.1: Estimated Number of Children in Foster Care

Source: U.S. Department of Health and Human Services 2003

Figure 16.2: Children's Length of Stay in Foster Care

Source: U.S. Department of Health and Human Services 2000, 2003

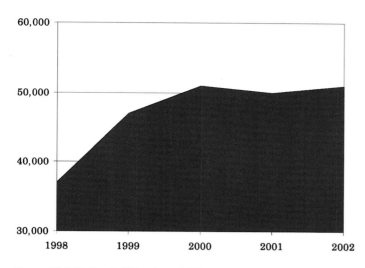

Figure 16.3: Estimated Number of Children Adopted

Source: U.S. Department of Health and Human Services 2003

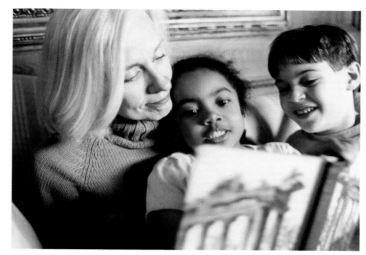

Entry to foster care is a traumatic event for all but the youngest child. Separation from parents or long-term caregivers and placement in a home with strangers are crises for the child. For reasons of health or safety, children are often removed suddenly, without planning, despite sometimes long involvement with child protective and preventive services. Because it preserves some semblance of family and familiarity, placement with kin is believed to be less traumatic, although studies show that kinship providers are often older, poorer, and less healthy than nonrelative foster parents. In addition, children living in kinship care often have less access to services despite equivalent needs. Most or all of the child's major relationships may be disrupted because of the inability to place siblings together or to find homes in the child's original community.

Fortunate children find themselves in homes with patient, nurturing, authoritative foster or kinship parents who gently, but consistently, offer affection, guidance, and support. In some communities, children spend variable amounts of time in a shelter until a foster home is identified, a suitable kin placement is found, or the child is reunified with a parent.

Children undergo a process of adjusting to foster care characterized most often by an initial period of shock, grief, and loss. A few children immediately display significant externalizing behavior, but most only begin to display significant behavior issues after the initial period of loss has passed.

Visitation, the single best predictor of reunification, is fraught with difficulty for the foster care child. It often occurs in sterile environments, gradually increasing in frequency and moving to the parent's home as the parent demonstrates an ability to keep the child safe. Inconsistent visitation or rejecting behavior by a birth

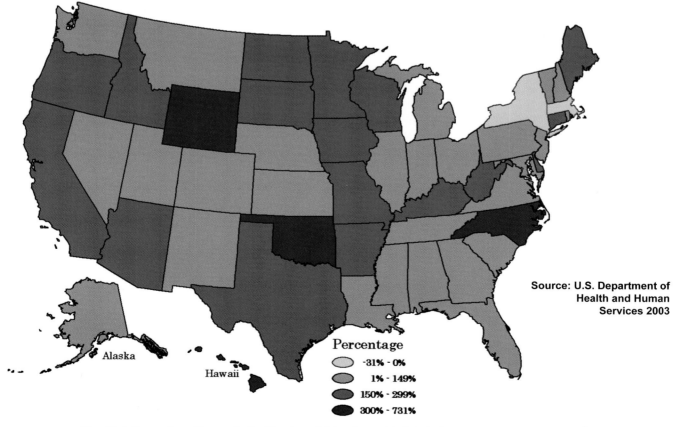

Source: U.S. Department of Health and Human Services 2003

Percentage
- -31% - 0%
- 1% - 149%
- 150% - 299%
- 300% - 731%

Map 16.1: Percentage Change in the Number of Adoptions with Public Child Welfare Agency Involvement, 1995-2002

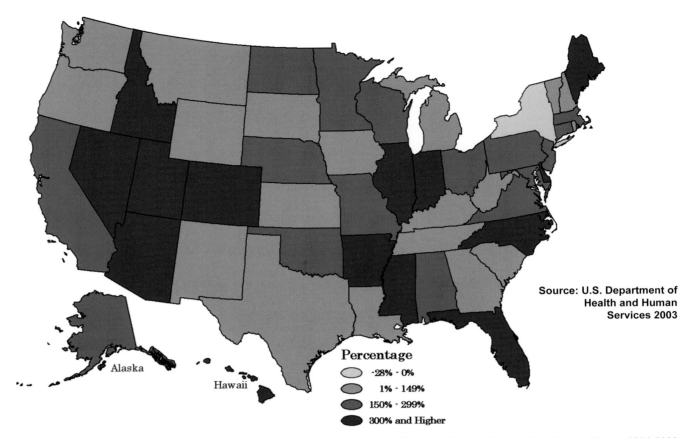

Source: U.S. Department of
Health and Human
Services 2003

Map 16.2: Change in Federal Foster Care Expenditures, 1991-1999

Percentage

○ -28% - 0%

○ 1% - 149%

○ 150% - 299%

● 300% and Higher

parent reinforces feelings of rejection. Separation at the end of visits can be traumatic, and there is a lack of therapeutic support during visitation.

Discord among foster and birth parents is particularly confusing for children. Most foster care children love their birth parents and worry about them. The separation or reunion of siblings; the illness or death of a parent (foster or birth); or the incarceration, unknown whereabouts, or admission to rehabilitation services of a birth parent can frighten a child. Changes in case-workers or therapists reinforce feelings of loss and a sense of impermanence. Children in foster care feel powerless, alienated, and humiliated by their peers or their circumstances. Removal from one's family, place-ment with strangers, and the uncertainty of foster care can overwhelm the limited life skills, coping skills, and adaptability of children.

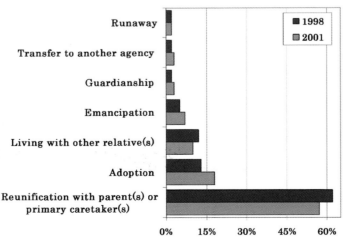

Figure 16.4: Outcomes for Children Exiting Foster Care

Source: U.S. Department of Health and Human Services 2000, 2003

According to 2001 U.S. Department of Health and Human Services' figures, 67% of foster care children were ultimately reunified with their parent, relative, or prior caregiver, while 18% were adopted, and 7% "aged out" of the system. Approximately 20% reentered foster care within 12 months after discharge. Fifty thousand children, an all-time high, were adopted out of foster care in 2001. Nationally, about 65% were adopted by their foster parent. Most were freed through a lengthy legal process called *termination of parental rights,* which by federal law may begin when a child has been in foster care for a minimum of 15 out of the prior 22 months; the average time from termination of parental rights to adoption was 16 months.

The overall health status of children in foster care is abysmal. They have very high rates of chronic medical, developmental, emotional, behavioral, and dental problems. An appropriate array of mental health services for foster care children and their families is their single greatest health need. Younger children in foster care suffer more from emotional disorders related to their circumstances, while older children have a higher incidence of true psychiatric illness. Unfortunately, failure to achieve a permanent home in a timely manner, the unpredictability and uncertainty of foster care, and cumulative adverse events erode their well-being over time. There is a dearth of funding for mental health, especially for newer approaches that may hold greater promise for these children and their families (therapeutic visitation, assessment in the child's environment(s), and foster/birth parent mentor-ing). Often children and families do not have access to mental health care services following their release from the foster care system. This is due to inadequate integration of health and permanency planning.

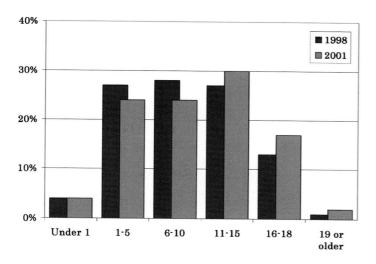

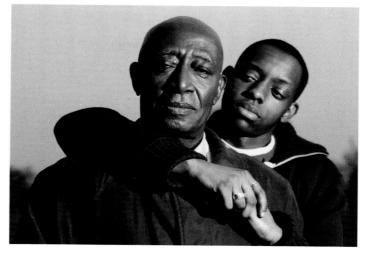

Figure 16.5: Ages in Years of Children Exiting Foster Care

Source: U.S. Department of Health and Human Services 2000, 2003

There are multiple barriers to providing for the health needs of this population, the most important of which are the high mobility of the population, the lack of care coordination through a medical home, the lack of appropriate mental health services, and the complexities of the foster care bureaucracy. Multiple changes in foster care placement result in fragmented health care. The diffusion of authority and responsibility among foster parents, birth parents, and child welfare staff compound the fragmentation. Legal guardianship remains with the family of origin unless the child is freed for adoption, and the unavailability of the birth parent to consent for health care can prevent sharing of health information and timely health services.

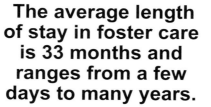

The average length of stay in foster care is 33 months and ranges from a few days to many years.

Health care financing issues that pose barriers to care include delays in Medicaid activation, the scarcity of health practitioners willing to accept Medicaid, and inadequate reimbursement of mental health, developmental, and dental services. Children in foster care are also under-immunized and behind in well-child care, and many children in foster care experience only sporadic crisis-oriented care from a variety of providers since most lack a medical home.

Despite our vast knowledge of what children need and how to support them through the process of foster care, the system continues to lack the resources to apply that knowledge in meaningful ways to benefit children and their families. In addition to needed resources, there are several fundamental changes that could improve the health outcomes, well-being, and permanency of children in the foster care system. They should have a medical home with practitioners willing to work collaboratively with the foster care system. There should be appropriate financing of an array of mental health services to meet the needs of the children living in foster care and their families. A centralized health care professional or team responsible to the foster care agency should offer health care management to enhance communication among health, child welfare, mental health, education, and legal professionals. This would promote the integration of the health plan into the permanency plan for our nation's foster care children.

Foster care should be a window of opportunity for healing, for both children and their families. Optimizing the health outcomes of foster care children enhances well-being, stability in foster care placements, and the achievement of permanency in a "forever family."

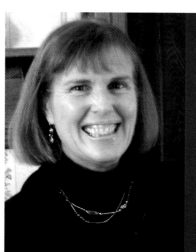

Moira Szilagyi

Moira Szilagyi, MD, PhD, is assistant professor of pediatrics at the University of Rochester School of Medicine and Dentistry and the medical director of foster care pediatrics for the Monroe County, New York State Department of Health. The editor of *Fostering Health: Health Care for Children in Foster Care*, Szilagyi has contributed to national efforts to improve health services and health outcomes for children in foster care and has served on the Committee on Early Childhood, Adoption, and Dependent Care at the American Academy of Pediatrics and its section on adoption and foster care. She has served as faculty for a breakthrough collaborative on foster care health care developed by the National Institute for Child Health Quality and has served in an advisory capacity to various local, state, and national groups interested in this area. She has written several articles and chapters on the health needs of this population and continues to educate doctors in training and her peers and colleagues about children in foster care.

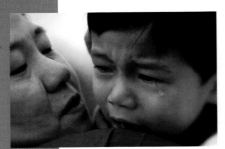

Chapter 17

Steven A. Camarota

Children of Immigrants

The United States is currently experiencing the largest sustained wave of immigration in its history. Data from the U.S. Census Bureau show that in March of 2003 the nation's total foreign-born population reached 33.5 million, an increase of almost 14 million since 1990 and triple the number in 1970. The Census Bureau defines the foreign-born as persons in the country who were not U.S. citizens at birth, including naturalized American citizens, legal permanent residents, and illegal immigrants. (For convenience the terms immigrant and foreign-born are used synonymously in this article.)

While the total foreign-born population has grown dramatically, only about 1 out of 10 immigrants was under age 18 in 2003, and immigrant children accounted for only about 4% of all children in the country. There are 3 million foreign-born children in the United States, and roughly one-third are thought to be illegally in the country. There are relatively few foreign-born children because the vast majority of immigrants come to the United States as adults. Although foreign-born children are modest in number, children born in the United States to immigrant parents represent a large and growing share of the nation's child population. Children born in this country, even those whose parents are illegal immigrants, are automatically U.S. citizens.

In 2003, there were 12.8 million children in immigrant-headed households, and they accounted for more than 17% of all children in the country. However, less than one-fourth of these children were immigrants themselves. In 1970, the 3.1 million children in immigrant households represented only about 4% of all children in the country. The share of children from immigrant backgrounds was higher if one considers all those with either a father or a mother born in another country. In 2003, 22% of children in the United States (16 million) had at least one parent born abroad. Again, only 3 million of these children were immigrants themselves; the rest were born in the United States.

In 2003, 22% of children in the United States (16 million) had at least one parent born abroad.

The economic and social experiences of children from immigrant households are directly linked, of course, to that of their parents and vary enormously depending on the parents' country of origin. The differences between groups are so great that it is often difficult to generalize about the condition of children from immigrant backgrounds. Some immigrants come to the United States very well educated, and, as a result, their children enjoy a very high standard of living. However, many immigrants have

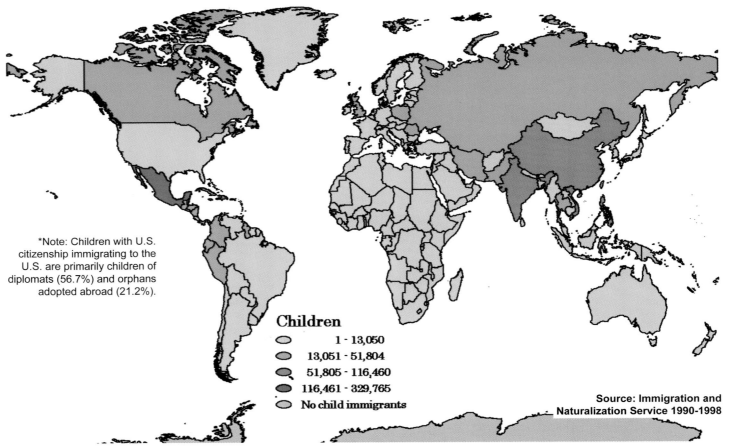

*Note: Children with U.S. citizenship immigrating to the U.S. are primarily children of diplomats (56.7%) and orphans adopted abroad (21.2%).

Children
- ⬭ 1 - 13,050
- ⬭ 13,051 - 51,804
- ⬭ 51,805 - 116,460
- ⬭ 116,461 - 329,765
- ⬭ No child immigrants

Source: Immigration and Naturalization Service 1990-1998

Map 17.1: Number of Countries' Immigrants to the U.S. That Were Under 18 Years Old, 1990-1998

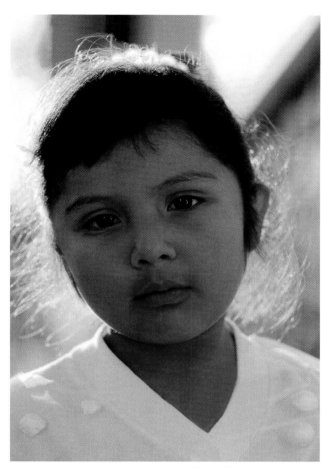

relatively few years of schooling. Their children often live in or near poverty, lack health insurance, have high dropout rates, and suffer from the problems that typically afflict children from low-income families.

Almost one in four children from immigrant households lives in poverty compared to one in seven children of natives. Although they accounted for only about 17% of all children in the United States, children in immigrant households accounted for 26% of those in poverty. Overall figures, however, obscure the very large differences that exist between groups. Children whose parents come from Canada, Europe, East and South Asia, and Sub-Saharan Africa tend to have poverty rates that are as low or, in some cases, significantly lower than that of natives. In contrast, children in households headed by persons from Mexico, the Caribbean, and the rest of Latin America have dramatically higher rates of poverty than natives. It must be remembered that children whose parents come from the Western Hemisphere tend to exert a very large impact on the overall figures because about two-thirds of children in immigrant households come from this part of the world.

Another significant problem for the children of immigrants is that many do not complete high school. This problem is most pronounced among children who arrive in the United States. as teenagers, but it is also common among the U.S.-born children of immigrants. About one-fourth of the children in immigrant households drop out of high school by age 18, although many eventually

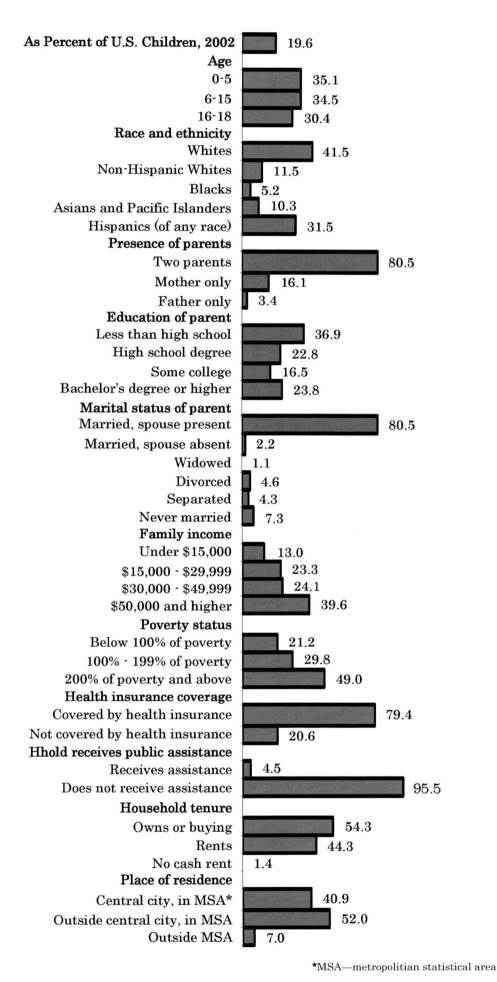

*MSA—metropolitian statistical area

Figure 17.1: Percentage of Children with at Least One Foreign-born Parent, 2002

Source: U.S. Census Bureau 2003

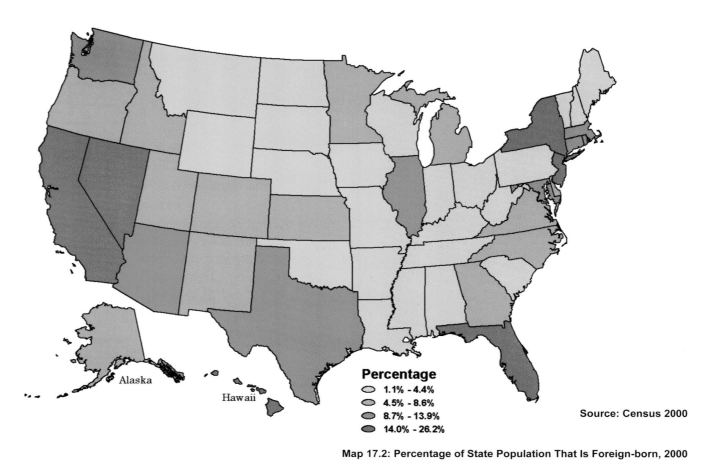

Percentage
- ◯ 1.1% - 4.4%
- ◯ 4.5% - 8.6%
- ◯ 8.7% - 13.9%
- ⬤ 14.0% - 26.2%

Alaska

Hawaii

Source: Census 2000

Map 17.2: Percentage of State Population That Is Foreign-born, 2000

Although they accounted for only about 17% of all children in the United States [in 2003], children in immigrant households accounted for 26% of those in poverty.

	In poverty	In or near poverty[1]	Without health insurance	Household head lacking high school education
Mexico	31.1%	70.1%	30.6%	63.4%
Central America	26.1%	59.4%	27.5%	52.3%
Caribbean	23.3%	53.1%	20.5%	32.4%
South America	21.6%	46.0%	21.9%	19.0%
Middle East	19.4%	39.5%	13.0%	9.4%
Sub-Saharan Africa	14.4%	37.1%	7.6%	5.9%
East Asia	13.0%	32.9%	11.6%	12.3%
Europe	11.6%	29.3%	11.2%	15.2%
South Asia	5.6%	24.0%	9.1%	4.0%
Canada	5.4%	18.7%	7.2%	13.1%
Children in immigrant households	24.3%	54.1%	22.5%	31.2%
Children in native households	14.9%	34.7%	9.3%	13.3%

[1]Near Poverty defined as less than 200% of poverty threshold.

Figure 17.2: Selected Socioeconomic Characteristics of Children Based on Country of Birth of Head of Household, 2003

Source: Center for Immigration Studies 2003

get their GED. For children whose parents come from Latin America, as many as one in three does not complete high school. These rates have significant negative implications for the social mobility of these children because there is no single better predictor of success in the modern American economy than educational attainment.

One of the most severe problems children of foreign-born parents face is a lack of health insurance. Nearly 23% of children in immigrant households lack health insurance, in comparison to 9% of those from native households. This is despite a successful effort in recent years by the federal government and states to provide coverage to low-income children, including those born to immigrants, under the State Children's Health Insurance Program. Again, enormous differences exist between immigrant groups, with those from the Western Hemisphere having the lowest rates of coverage. Although many immigrant children suffer

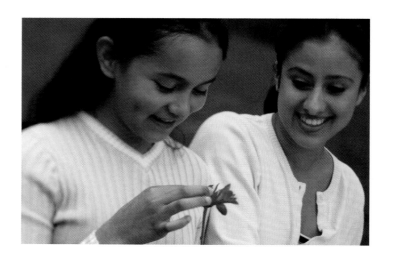

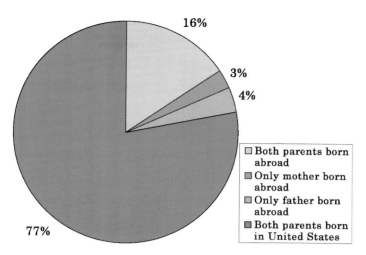

16%

3%

4%

77%

☐ Both parents born abroad
■ Only mother born abroad
☐ Only father born abroad
■ Both parents born in United States

Figure 17.3: Place of Birth for Parents of All Children in United States, 2003
Source: Center for Immigration Studies 2003

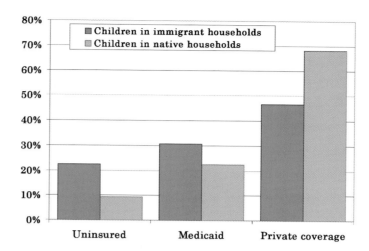

■ Children in immigrant households
☐ Children in native households

Uninsured   Medicaid   Private coverage

Figure 17.4: Health Insurance Coverage by Household Type, 2003
Source: Center for Immigration Studies 2003

from a lack of insurance, 30% of children in immigrant households do receive Medicaid.

Although many social indicators suggest that children from immigrant backgrounds often need access to social services or have special educational needs, there are a number of significant impediments. Limited education, language barriers, unfamiliarity with government services, and legal status sometimes work to prevent immigrant parents from accessing programs for their children, even though they might be eligible. Of course, it must be added that despite these barriers, legal immigrants use such programs as food stamps, Supplemental Security Income, public housing, and Temporary Assistance to Needy Families at somewhat higher rates than natives.

Politically, another factor complicates immigrants' access to social services. Many groups that advocate for immigrant rights lobby hard to make programs for people with low incomes available to immigrants. However, some conservative groups that support keeping immigration levels high do not support giving immigrant families access to these programs. One of the main arguments for immigration is that it creates benefits for the native-born population, but extensive use of social services by immigrants and their children tends to undermine this argument. As a result, many advocates of immigration are hesitant to call attention

to the needs of immigrant families or provide them with access to services. This was clearly the case in 1996 when Congress, as part of welfare reform, made newly arrived, legal immigrants ineligible for some programs. This inherent tension surrounding immigration likely will continue to play a major role in determining what access immigrants and their children have to the social safety net.

The current wave of immigration shows no signs of abating any time soon on its own. Absent a change in U.S. immigration policy, the number of children from immigrant backgrounds will continue to grow. How these children fare in this country has become critically important to the nation's future since they comprise an ever-increasing share of the nation's population.

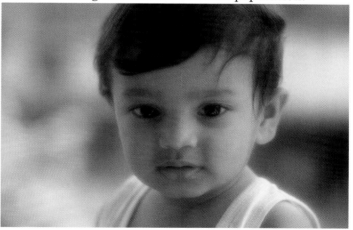

Steven A. Camarota

Steven A. Camarota, PhD, is director of research at the Center for Immigration Studies in Washington, DC. Dr. Camarota earned his PhD from the University of Virginia and a master's degree from the University of Pennsylvania. He has testified before Congress numerous times on immigration-related issues. His articles on the impact of immigration have appeared in academic journals and the popular press including *Social Science Quarterly*, *The Washington Post*, *The Chicago Tribune*, and *National Review*. He appears frequently on *CNN, MSNBC, Fox News Channel, NBC Nightly News*, and *ABC World News Tonight*. His most recent works, published by the Center for Immigration Studies, are *Where Immigrants Live: An Examination of State Residency of the Foreign Born* and *Back Where We Started: An Examination of Trends in Immigrant Welfare Use Since Welfare Reform*. Other recent work includes *The Open Door: How Militant Islamic Terrorists Entered and Remained in the United States, 1993-2001*. He is the lead researcher on a Census Bureau project that is examining the quality of data on the foreign-born in the American Community Survey.

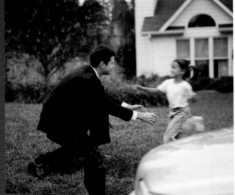

Chapter 18

*Deborah Belle
and Brenda Phillips*

Experiences in the
After-school Hours

The after-school hours present many U.S. parents and their children with dilemmas that are not easy to resolve. The school day is several hours shorter than the full-time workday, and the school year is interrupted by frequent holidays and early release days. U.S. workers now work more hours per year than workers in any other industrialized nation, and U.S. jobs increasingly require work in the evening and weekend hours when child care is particularly hard to arrange.[1] Not only are parents often away at work while their children are out of school, but grandparents, neighbors, and family friends are also likely to be employed and unavailable to supervise children. Close to half of all U.S. children spend at least part of their childhoods in single-parent

households,[2] further reducing the pool of adults available to care for children after school. Studies indicate there is twice as much demand for after-school care as available programs can meet.[3]

The United States has the highest poverty rate in the industrialized world,[4] making it difficult for many parents to purchase child care assistance. In 1998, the sole parent or both parents of 5.3 million low-income 6- to 12-year-olds were at work in the after-school hours.[5] Only 10% to 30% of these low-income children attended after-school programs, and low-income children were more likely than affluent children to be on their own for long periods.[5]

Children without adult supervision in the after-school hours have very different experiences. Some children are alone for many hours into the evening, others for

This is the peak time for violent juvenile crime, and the greatest danger is in the first hour after school.

much briefer periods. Some children are required to remain in their homes and are forbidden to invite friends to visit. Others spend the after-school hours "hanging out" with peers. For some children, the move to self-care is part of a larger move toward taking responsibility for running the household. Children may supervise younger siblings, do substantial housework, and prepare the family's evening meal during their after-school hours. To some children, unsupervised time means freedom from adult authority, to others it represents valued responsibilities, and to others it entails onerous restrictions. Often there is no clear demarcation between supervised and unsupervised time. Adults may be accessible when needed although physically absent, or they may be physically present but emotionally unavailable.[6]

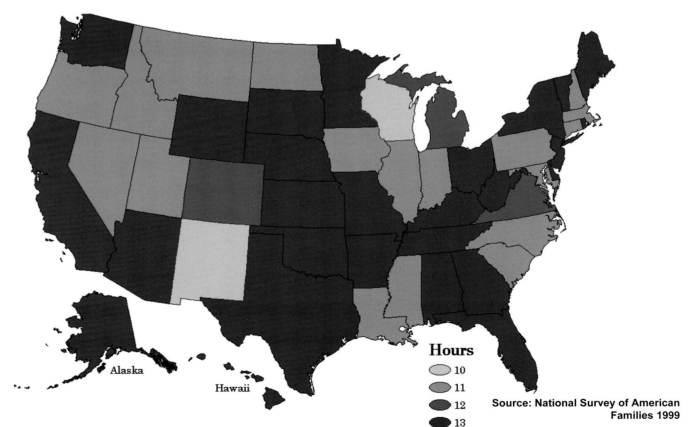

Hours
- 10
- 11
- 12
- 13

Source: National Survey of American Families 1999

Map 18.1: National Estimate of the Average Hours per Week Children Spend in Before- or After-school Programs

Low-income parents face particular difficulties in finding acceptable after-school arrangements for their children. Frequently, they cannot afford the activities their children desire or cannot arrange their children's transportation home from these programs. Neighborhoods are often dangerous, limiting children's options for outdoor play. Poor parents are disproportionately employed in evening and weekend work and in jobs offering no flexibility for attending to children's needs. Many parents cannot receive telephone calls at work alerting them to a problem at home.

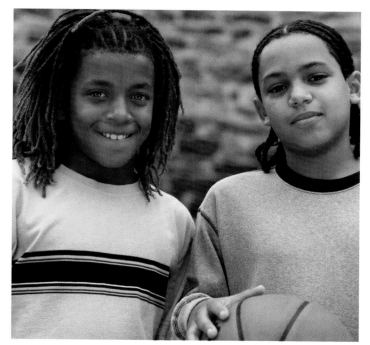

Much research documents the dangers young people face during the after-school hours. This is the peak time for violent juvenile crime, and the greatest danger is in the first hour after school is dismissed.[7] Drug use and risky sexual behavior may also be particularly likely when young people are unsupervised after school.[7] Spending unsupervised time with peers, particularly away from home, is associated with higher levels of delinquency, substance use, and susceptibility to peer

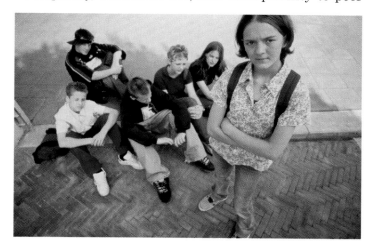

pressure.[8,9] Spending longer hours without adult supervision increases the risks to young people's well-being.[7] Conversely, parental monitoring, parental warmth, and a nonpermissive parenting style seem to protect unsupervised adolescents from many problem behaviors.[7,9,10] Not surprisingly, the risks of unsupervised time are greatest and the benefits of after-school programs are strongest for low-income young people and those in dangerous neighborhoods.[11–13]

Many after-school programs succeed beautifully in meeting the needs of young people. At the heart and soul of such programs are strong relationships between youth and staff in which staff view young people positively, rather than focus on possible deficits.[14] Staff

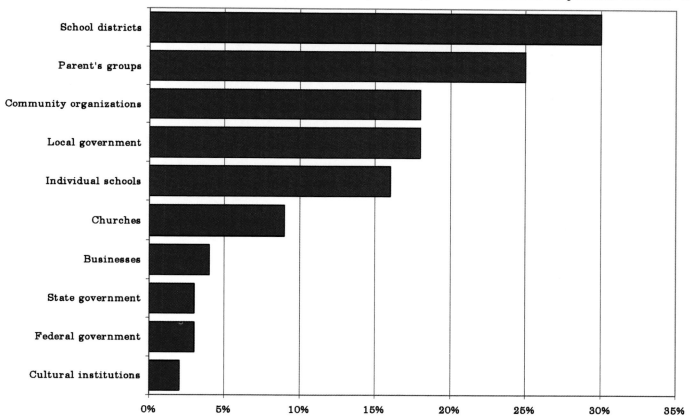

Figure 18.1: Types of Organizations/Agencies Responsible for Setting Up After-school Programs

Source: U.S. Department of Education 1999

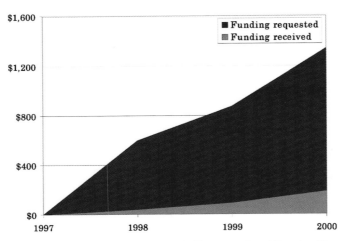

Figure 18.2: Total After-school Funds Requested and Received by Schools Across the Nation in Millions of Dollars
Source: Department of Education 2000

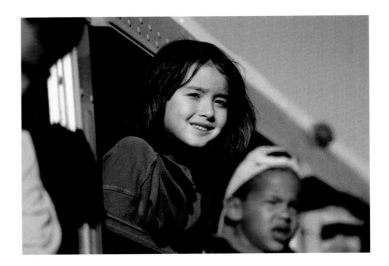

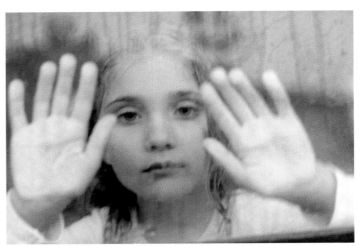

and youth have fun together, and staff help the young people make productive choices about their lives while fostering essential skills.

However, after-school programs today are often asked to fulfill multiple, conflicting agendas.[3,5] Some view their primary purpose to be a continuation of the work that schools carry out earlier in the day, educating students in academic subjects. From such a perspective, fun and unstructured time are suspect and may be derided as mere babysitting. A heavy focus on what should be learned can easily turn into a program oriented on deficits rather than one that accentuates assets of the children. The need to accomplish a fixed

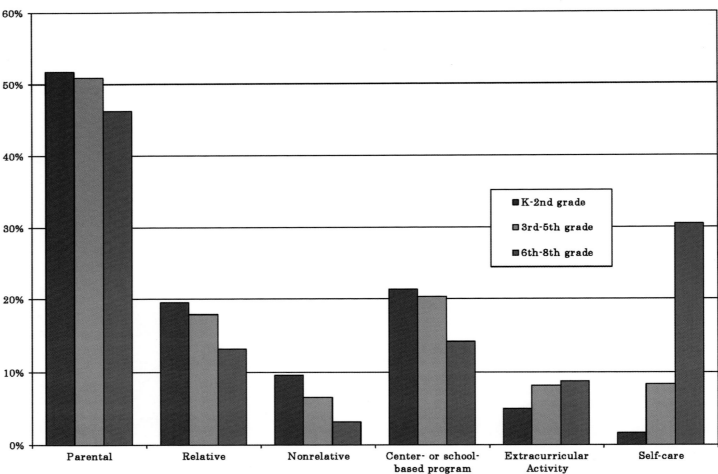

Figure 18.3: Percentage of Children by Type of After-school Care Arrangement and Grade Level, 2003

Source: U.S. Department of Education 2003

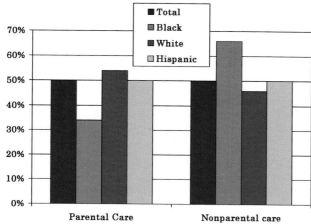

Figure 18.4: Percentage of Children (Kindergarten-8th Grade) Who Participated in After-school Care Arrangements

Source: U.S. Department of Education 2003

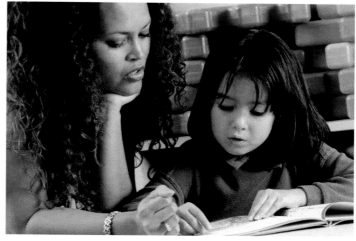

academic agenda also erodes the time and space needed to allow staff to bond closely with young people. Program evaluation and future funding are heavily dependent on demonstrations of improved academic performance on standardized tests. As Garey noted, such evaluation criteria do not assess "how happy the children are, how safe they are, how many friends they make, or how healthy and fit they are."[3]

Some after-school programs are fundamentally crime-prevention tools that contain young people and therefore prevent them from injuring themselves or others. Garey described one after-school program that did not allow parents to pick up their children until they had been at the program for three hours.[3] This conception of after-school care as containment conflicted with parents' needs and wishes to care for their own children.

Many U.S. children, particularly those from low-income families and those in dangerous neighborhoods, have a great need for thoughtfully designed after-school programs. Research has illuminated this need and the

> **The risks of unsupervised time are greatest and the benefits of after-school programs are strongest for low-income young people and those in dangerous neighborhoods.**

difference that programs can make in the lives of young people.

However, the immensity of the problem goes beyond the dearth of after-school programs. Many U.S. parents must work so many hours and often in such inflexible circumstances that they are not able to provide the parental care their children need. Employers should be challenged to find ways to allow the parents in their workforce to care for their children properly. Parents who can make and receive telephone calls at work, bring children to the workplace on occasion, and take time off from work to be with their children at home will do a better job of parenting and may actually be more productive at work as their anxiety about their children's safety lessens. Higher wages would allow some parents to leave a second job or to reduce hours at work, thus becoming more available to children. Government action, including raising the minimum wage, may be required to fulfill these goals. Children and parents in the United States face challenges that are unique in the industrialized world. Nowhere else do parents work such long hours and with such little support. Surely we can do better.

Deborah Belle and Brenda Phillips

Deborah Belle's, PhD, most recent book is *The After-School Lives of Children: Alone and with Others While Parents Work*. Earlier, she edited *Lives in Stress: Women and Depression and Children's Social Networks and Social Supports*. She has been a William T. Grant Foundation faculty scholar and a fellow at the Bunting Institute and at the Radcliffe Public Policy Center. She is a professor of psychology at Boston University, where her current research focuses on the emotional and physical health costs of economic inequality and on the ways in which individuals and families make sense of poverty and homelessness in a wealthy nation.

Brenda Phillips, MA, is a presidential fellow and doctoral candidate in Human Development at Boston University. She trained as a child psychotherapist at Saint Michael's College in Vermont and obtained a master's degree in clinical psychology. Ms. Phillips has also been a student research fellow at the Social Science Research Center at Saint Michael's, studying moral development in young children. She is currently conducting research with Dr. Deborah Belle on issues of economic inequality. Brenda is particularly interested in forces of social oppression and how they impact children's socioemotional development.

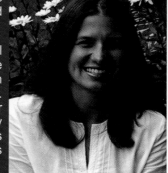

Chapter 19

Helen Blank

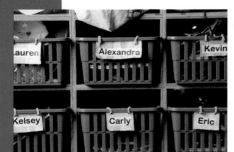

Challenges of
Child Care

Child care touches the lives of millions of American families. Each day, an estimated 12 million children less than 6 years old—including children whose mothers do not work outside the home—spend some or all of their day in the care of someone other than their parents.[1] These children may be in a variety of settings—with neighbors, with relatives, in child care centers, or in neighborhood family child care homes where providers care for a small number of children. Many are cared for in several different settings within a day or a week.

Child care makes it possible for parents to work and support their families, and it makes a sizable contribution to the national economy. According to a study sponsored by the National Child Care Association, Americans paid

approximately $38 billion for licensed care for their children in 2001.[2] The licensed child care sector employed 934,000 workers, which was slightly more than were employed as public secondary school teachers. The study further indicated that parents with children in these child care programs earned more than $100 billion in 2001, and those wages and salaries, when spent, generated almost $580 billion in income for others and $69 billion in tax revenues.

There is a growing recognition that the early years spent in child care are very important to a child's development. Studies have repeatedly shown that good-quality child care and early education help children develop, enter school ready to succeed, improve their skills, and stay safe while their parents work. A strong preschool experience that gives children the opportunity to build their language and literacy skills helps to ensure that

they can benefit from classroom instruction once they enter elementary school.

> **Children in high-quality care demonstrate greater mathematic ability, greater thinking and attention skills, and fewer behavioral problems.**

A National Center for Educational Statistics study showed that children who acquired particular skills—the ability to recognize shapes, letters, and basic numbers and the ability to understand the concept of relative size—before entering kindergarten had significantly higher overall reading and mathematics scores near the end of their kindergarten and first grade school years.[3] Other findings of the study revealed that children who had been read to at least three times a week, who had a positive attitude toward learning, and who were in very good to excellent health as they entered kindergarten also had higher scores. This study demonstrates the critical importance of the child care settings in which millions of preschool children spend large amounts of time.

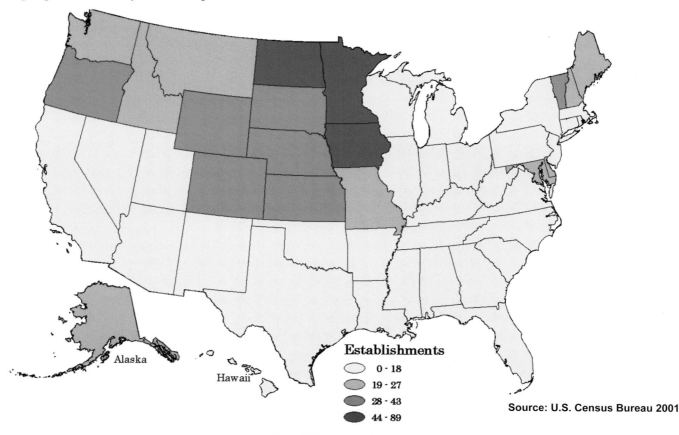

Establishments
- 0 - 18
- 19 - 27
- 28 - 43
- 44 - 89

Source: U.S. Census Bureau 2001

Map 19.1: Total Child Care Establishments per 1,000 Children Under Age 5, 1987

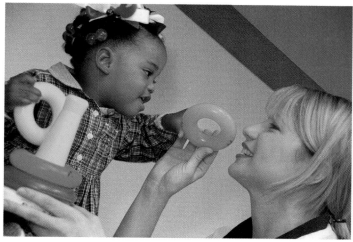

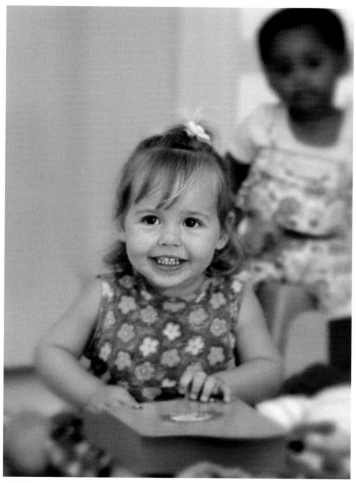

Children need comprehensive, high-quality early experiences that promote all aspects of development, including social, emotional, physical, and cognitive development. According to a report by the National Research Council, *Eager to Learn: Educating Our Preschoolers*, "Cognitive, social-emotional, and motor development are complementary, mutually supportive areas of growth all requiring active attention in the preschool years....All are therefore related to early learning and later academic achievement." A high-quality program must address each of these critical development areas to ensure that children are ready to learn.[4]

All children, particularly low-income children, reap benefits when they are exposed to quality child care environments. A four-state study has been following a group of children to compare high-quality child care with lower-quality child care.[5] So far, results from the study show the children's progress from age 3 through second grade. The most recent findings reveal that children in high-quality care demonstrate greater mathematic ability, greater thinking and attention skills, and fewer behavioral problems. These differences hold true for children from a variety of family backgrounds, with particularly significant effects for at-risk children. A number of longitudinal studies have shown that good programs can improve low-income children's futures in

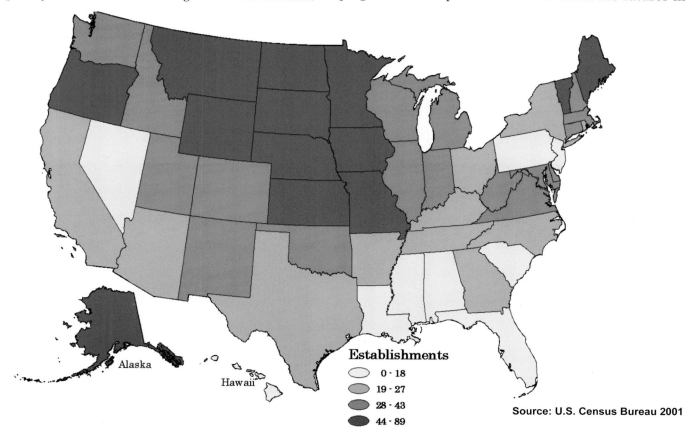

Establishments

- ⬭ 0 - 18
- ⬭ 19 - 27
- ⬭ 28 - 43
- ⬭ 44 - 89

Source: U.S. Census Bureau 2001

Map 19.2: Total Child Care Establishments per 1,000 Children Under Age 5, 1997

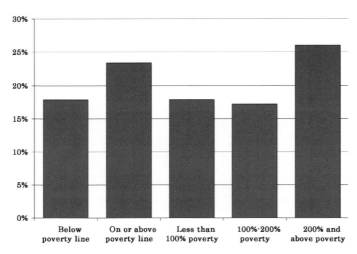

Figure 19.1: Percentage of Children in Organized Child Care by Poverty Status (Under Age 5), 1999

Source: U.S. Census Bureau 2003

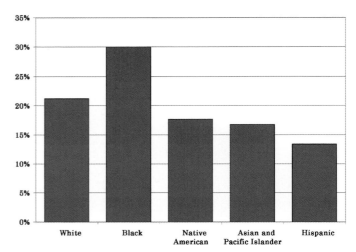

Figure 19.2: Percentage of Children in Organized Child Care by Race and Ethnicity (Under Age 5), 1999

Source: U.S. Census Bureau 2003

areas such as school achievement and higher-learning activities while decreasing their involvement with the criminal justice system.[6]

Although low-income children may have the greatest need for good-quality child care, limited assistance is available to help low-income families pay for child care. Available funds fall far short of meeting the need. Nationally, only one out of seven children eligible for child care assistance under federal law receives help.[7] Families pay approximately 60% of child care costs, government pays 39%, and private sector businesses and nonprofit organizations contribute less than 1%. In contrast, families pay only about 23% of the cost of a public college education, with government and the private sector paying the rest.[8] Yet, child care is expensive. According to the Children's Defense Fund, full-day child care can easily cost from $4,000 to $10,000 per year—at least as much as college tuition at a public university.[9] Yet, one out of four families with young children earns less than $25,000 a year.[10] Calculations show that if both parents hold full-time, minimum wage jobs, the family would have only $21,400 in pre-tax annual income.[9] The Children's Defense Fund analysis indicates that this family could not afford to pay even 10% ($2,140) of its income for child care, much less the higher amounts charged by many facilities. Low-income families often have to settle for cheaper and possibly inferior child care.[9] Case studies of low-income

families waiting for child care assistance in several communities highlight the multiple challenges that low-income parents face when they cannot get help to pay for child care.[11-16] These parents find it more difficult to work, are forced to place their children in potentially unsafe situations, and confront serious financial difficulties. A significant number have to leave their jobs and turn to welfare.

With millions of children from all income levels in child care, programs must have strong standards to help ensure quality, and programs should be monitored regularly. Parents must be the first line of defense in monitoring their children's care, but it is essential for government to play a supportive role as well. Studies have found that parents need help to monitor and evaluate the quality of care their children receive since some aspects of a child care program are difficult for them to observe.[17] For example, most parents are able to see a program only when they drop off and pick up their children. Periodic visits to child care programs by state licensing officials can result in identification of poor-quality programs, improvement of these programs, and protection of children when dangerous situations are found. In fact, state licensing officials rated such visits the most effective way to ensure compliance with state licensing requirements.[18] Yet, with inadequate state investments in child care

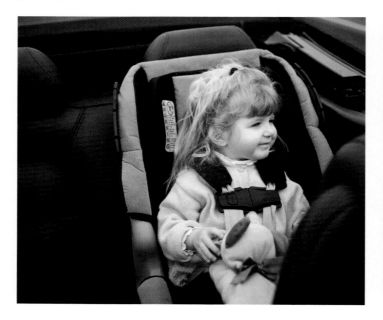

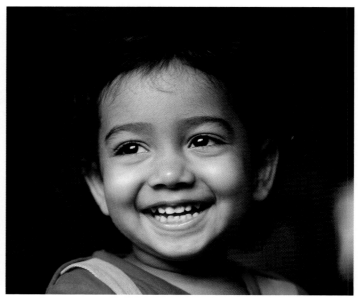

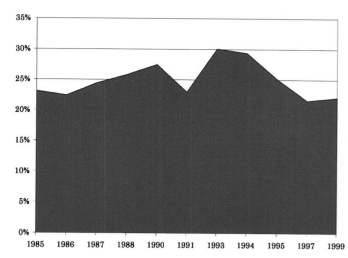

Figure 19.3: Trends in Organized Child Care for Children Under Age 5

Source: U.S. Census Bureau 2003

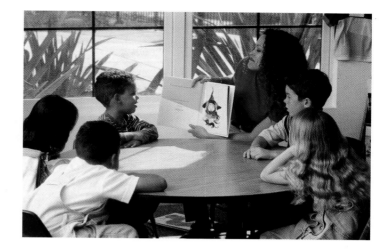

licensing staff, many states find it difficult to monitor child care programs thoroughly.

No uniform quality standards govern all child care and early education programs nationwide, and many programs are exempt from any regulation or licensing requirements. Family child care homes that care for small numbers of children are likely to be exempt from regulation unless they serve children who receive public funds. Strong state licensing requirements can help to ensure children's well-being. Licensing can help regulate specific aspects of quality of care such as low staff-to-child ratios and adequate training of providers. These standards improve the overall quality of caregiving and are linked to children's positive intellectual and social development.[19] Unfortunately, requirements in many states are too weak to protect children's health and safety adequately. For example, early childhood educators recommend that a single caregiver be responsible for no more than 3 or 4 infants, 4 or 5 toddlers, or 10 preschool-age children. Yet, only 10 states have licensing requirements to ensure that child care centers have these staff-to-child ratios.[20]

Research also shows that the staffs who care for children on a daily basis play an essential role in children's develop-

> **Many states do not require [child care] providers to have even a basic knowledge of child development issues, and many states require little or no training for providers.**

ment and experiences. Trained and educated teachers contribute to improved cognitive and other developmental outcomes. Better-trained staffs are more likely to create warm, caring environments that are responsive to the needs of children and help prepare children to succeed in school.[17,21-23] Yet, recruiting and retaining qualified staffs are challenging tasks. Child care providers earn an average salary of $16,980 a year with few benefits.[24,25]

Many states do not require providers to have even a basic knowledge of child development issues, and many states require little or no training for providers before they are allowed to work with children. While cosmetologists must attend as much as 2,000 hours of training before they can get a license,[26] 30 states allow teachers in child care centers to begin working with children before receiving any training in early childhood development. Thirty-two states allow family child care providers to begin caring for children before receiving any such training.[20]

Child care for children in the United States affects all Americans, not just parents. Preschool-age children who are cared for in nurturing and safe learning environments are more likely to succeed in school and, therefore, in life. Given the importance of affordable, quality child care to children's futures, their families' ability to work, and the strength of our current and future economy, child care is an issue that demands significant attention and investments from both the public and private sectors.

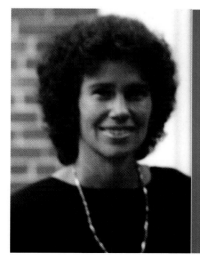

Helen Blank

Helen Blank, MUP, is a senior fellow at the National Women's Law Center. Ms. Blank served 24 years as the director of Child Care and Development at the Children's Defense Fund where she spearheaded efforts to expand funding for early care and education programs. She led the coalition that helped to enact the first comprehensive child care legislation and developed a guide for implementation of the legislation. In 1991, she led an effective campaign to ensure that regulations for the legislation allowed states to use new federal funds in the best interests of children. She was also a leader in efforts to increase child care funding in welfare reform. She has authored numerous major reports, articles, and papers on state child care and early education policies. Ms. Blank is a member of the advisory board of Corporate Voices for Working Families, the T.E.A.C.H.® Early Childhood advisory committee, the Easter Seals advisory committee, the Child Care Food Program Sponsors' Forum, and the advisory board for the Local Initiative Support Corporation. Ms. Blank has a bachelor's degree from the University of Michigan and a master's degree in urban planning from Hunter College of the City University of New York.

Chapter 20

Ellen Galinsky

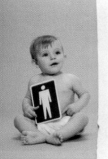
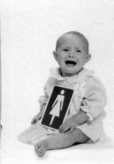

Gender Roles

While there is a great deal of research about how boys learn about being boys and girls learn about being girls, the public debates have focused on whether the differences that are found are large or small, whether they are genetic or forged by the way children are raised, and whether the cultural "myths" about masculinity and femininity are harmful.[1-4] What has not been included in most of the studies and popular books, other than anecdotally, are the voices of young people themselves. We have not known how young people see gender roles, especially gender roles for adults—that is, until recently. Two nationally representative studies that I have conducted are beginning to fill in the blanks on how young people see men and women in their major societal roles: working and caring for their families.

The first is a nationally representative study of boys and girls in the 3rd through 12th grades, which was conducted in 1998 and first published in 1999 in my book, *Ask the Children.*[5] The 1,023 children in the sample represent the diversity of children growing up today in the United States, including diversity in income level, racial and ethnic backgrounds, and family configurations. The study also included a nationally representative group of employed parents to enable comparison of the views of young people and adults.

Children were asked how strongly they agreed or disagreed with a number of statements, including "It is much better for everyone involved if the man earns the money and the woman takes care of the home and the children." More than two in five children (43%) strongly or somewhat agreed that the traditional gender division of labor was better for "everyone involved." However, there were big differences between older and younger children: more than twice as many 8- to 12-year-olds strongly agreed with this statement (22%) than did 13- to 18-year-olds (10%).

Equally striking were the differences between boys and girls in their feelings: almost twice as many boys (19%) strongly agreed with this statement as did girls (11%). The omnipresent polling in this country has made us aware that there is a gender gap in politics. Here we found a gender gap in children's views of the proper role of men and women, and it occurred at very young ages.

> **Forty-two percent of girls strongly agreed that it is acceptable if men and women do not follow traditional gender roles, but only 25% of boys strongly agreed.**

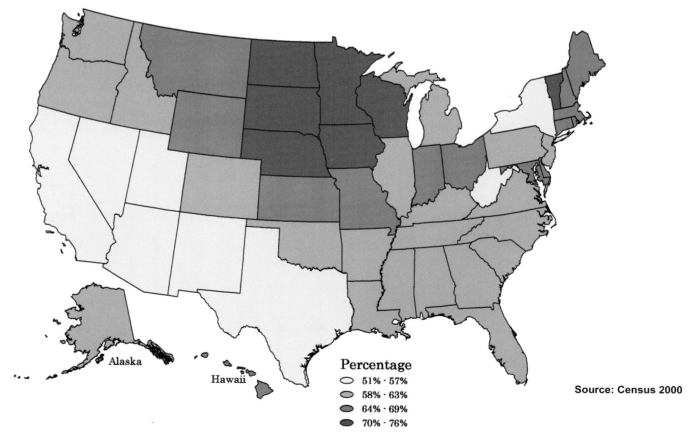

Alaska

Hawaii

Percentage
- 51% - 57%
- 58% - 63%
- 64% - 69%
- 70% - 76%

Source: Census 2000

Map 20.1: Percentage of Children Under 18 in Two-parent Families in Which Both Parents Work, 2000

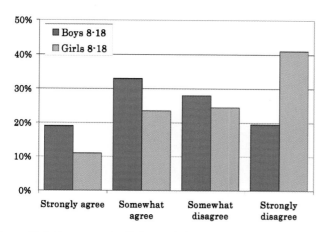

Figure 20.1: Response to: "It is much better for everyone involved if the man earns the money and the woman takes care of the home and the children."

Source: Galinsky 2000

Further analyses revealed that older girls were less traditional than were younger girls, but boys' attitudes did not change as they aged. Thus, the gap between the views of boys and girls was larger among older children than among younger children.

Not surprisingly, children's home lives affected their opinions. Children with an at-home mother were almost twice as likely to agree strongly that it is better if the man earns the money and the woman cares for the family (24%) than those with an employed mother (14%). It makes sense that children support the lifestyle choices of their parents and the culture they experience.

Do children differ from parents on how they see gender roles? I found that children's views were less traditional than parents' views. For example, 22% of employed parents strongly agreed with the statement "It is much better for everyone involved if the man earns the money and the woman takes care of the home and the children," while only 15% of children with employed parents strongly agreed.

Children in the 7th though 12th grades also were asked whether they agreed or disagreed that "A mother who works outside the home can have just as good a relationship with her children as a mother who does not work." More than 8 in 10 young people (82%) agreed with

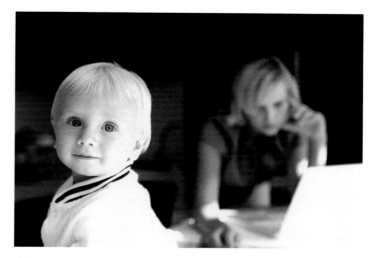

this statement, but as before, there were gender differences. Girls (89%) were more likely than boys (75%) to feel that a mother can have equally good relationships with her children regardless of whether she is employed or not.

The children also were asked to respond to the statement "Children do just as well if the mother has primary responsibility for earning the money and the father has primary responsibility for caring for the children." The majority of the children (70%) agreed with this statement, but again, there were gender differences. Forty-two percent of girls strongly agreed that it is acceptable if men and women do not follow traditional gender roles, but only 25% of boys strongly agreed.

Views of other work and family issues followed the same pattern; there were differences in the views of boys and girls regarding gender roles in the future. Girls were more likely than boys to disagree with the notion of traditional gender roles. Furthermore, while girls' attitudes became even less conventional as they grew up, boys' attitudes did not change. Subsequent analyses revealed that factors beyond their gender and age influenced children's views, including family structure, whether children thought their parents liked their jobs, and whether they thought their parents put family first or not.

The fact that girls' and boys' expectations of gender roles diverged has important implications for the adult relationships they will form in the future—when men's

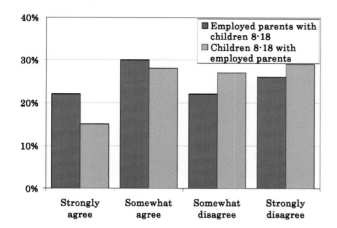

Figure 20.2: Response to: "It is much better for everyone involved if the man earns the money and the woman takes care of the home and the children."

Source: Galinsky 2000

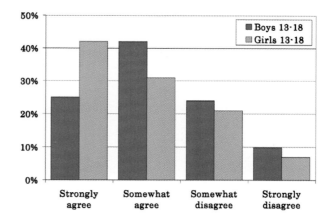

Figure 20.3: Response to: "Children do just as well if the mother has primary responsibility for earning money and the father has primary responsibility for caring for the children."

Source: Galinsky 2000

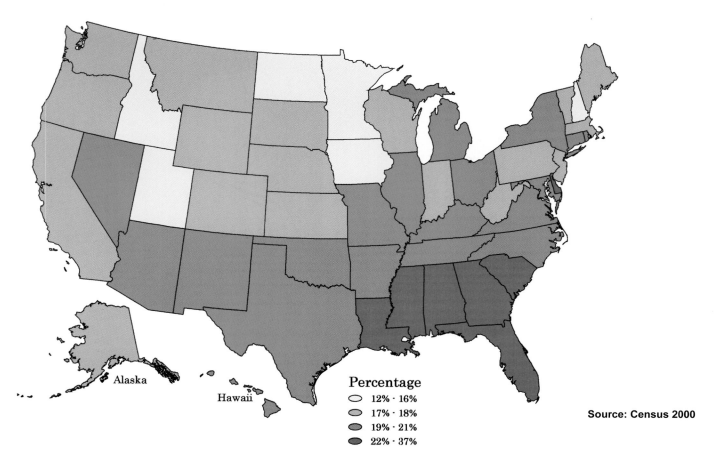

Percentage
○ 12% - 16%
○ 17% - 18%
● 19% - 21%
● 22% - 37%

Source: Census 2000

Map 20.2: Percentage of Children Under 18 in Two-parent or Single-mother Families in Which Only the Mother Works, 2000

and women's expectations of their roles and responsibilities could conceivably collide. As a mother interviewed for *Ask the Children* said, "If young men and women don't see eye-to-eye on their expectations, they will simply replay some of the conflict-ridden scripts our generation has been playing."

In the second study, *Youth and Employment: Today's Students, Tomorrow's Workforce*, we explored 10th, 11th, and 12th graders' expectations for their own futures.[6] This study of a nationally representative sample of 1,028 young people, which was part of the Families and Work Institute's *Ask the Children* series, showed that girls and boys differed in their expectations of how they will care for their children. (Ninety percent of students who planned to have a job also planned to have children.) For example, girls (81%) were more likely than boys (59%) to say they will reduce their work hours when they have

children. Boys (73%) were more likely than girls (28%) to expect their spouses to reduce their work hours when they have children. One of the most important findings was that while only 28% of girls expected their spouses to reduce their work hours, 59% of boys said they will reduce their work hours when they have children. Young women may not understand that young men want to be very involved in their families!

Will they do so? It is, of course, impossible to say, but there are signs that both men's and women's roles are changing at work and at home. According to a 1995 Families and Work Institute study, *Women: The New Providers*,[7] not only were more women employed, many had extended their role definitions of nurturing their families to include providing for their families economically. We also have found that men are increasingly involved in caring for their families. The

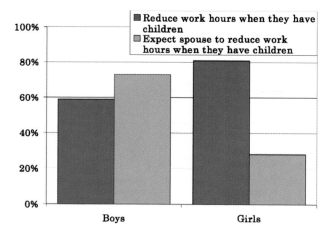

Figure 20.4: Child Care Responsibility Expectations of 10th, 11th, and 12th Graders

Source: Families and Work Institute 2001

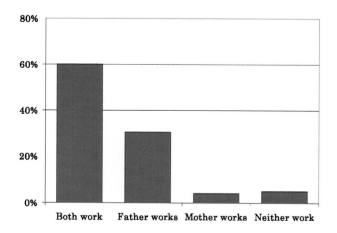

Figure 20.5: Percentage of Children Under 18 in Two-parent Families by Parents' Work Status, 2000

Source: Census 2000

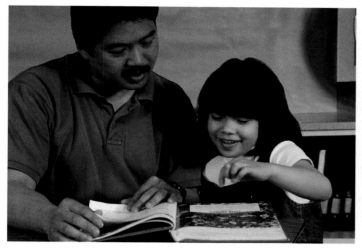

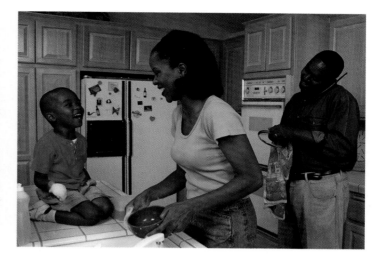

Families and Work Institute's nationally representative study of the U.S. workforce, the *2002 National Study of the Changing Workforce*,[8] indicates that 30% of women in dual-earner families reported that their husbands took equal or more responsibility for the care of their children, up from 24% 10 years ago. Fathers in dual-earner couples were also spending 48 minutes more doing household chores and taking care of their children on workdays than comparable fathers did 25 years ago. In fact, the gap between the amount of time that mothers and fathers in dual-

Most young people of both genders wanted to have the experiences of working and parenting, and boys expected to have an active role in caring for their children.

earner couples spent had narrowed from 88 minutes to 48 minutes per workday.

Taken together, these studies indicated there were differences in attitudes about gender roles between boys and girls and between young people and adults. Young people held less traditional views of gender roles than adults held, and there were differences between the views of boys and girls that began early and persisted. Additionally, girls' attitudes became less traditional as they grew up, while boys' attitudes did not change. However, most young people of both genders wanted to have the experiences of working and parenting, and boys expected to have an active role in caring for their children.

Roles are changing among today's adults, too, with more women providing for their families economically and men taking more responsibility for the care of their children. The convergence and divergence of gender roles and attitudes about them will continue to shape interactions between males and females. Discovering these similarities in roles and attitudes gives us a glimpse into the relationships of the future, where it seems that both males and females want to work and to care for their children. Thus, it is important that we move beyond cultural expectations of roles. It is important that we ask the children what they want in their futures and then truly listen to their responses.

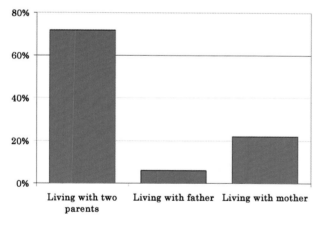

Figure 20.6: Percentage of Children Under 18 by Family Type, 2000

Source: Census 2000

Ellen Galinsky

Ellen Galinsky, MS, is the president and cofounder of Families and Work Institute (FWI), a Manhattan-based nonprofit organization that conducts research on the changing family, changing workforce, and changing community. She is the author of the book *Ask the Children: The Breakthrough Study That Reveals How to Succeed at Work and Parenting* and coauthor of Family and Work Institute's other *Ask the Children* studies, including ones on youth and employment and youth and learning. She is overseeing a 13-part television series on early learning. Ms. Galinsky coauthored the 1992, 1997, and 2002 *National Study of the Changing Workforce*, a nationally representative study of the U.S. workforce, and *The 1998 Business Work-Life Study*, a nationally representative survey of employers. She is a past president of the National Association for the Education of Young Children and serves on many boards, commissions, and task forces. Ms. Galinsky previously was on the faculty at the Bank Street College of Education. She is the author of numerous books, reports, and articles in academic journals and popular magazines.

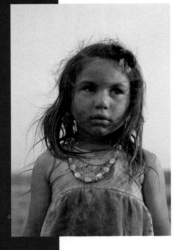

Chapter 21

Richard Wertheimer

Poverty

In 2001, there were 11.7 million children living in poverty in the United States.[1] This means that 16% of all children were living in families with incomes below the official poverty threshold, which was $17,960 for a family of four with two children and $14,269 for a family of three with two children.

All members of a family, including its children, are poor if the family's income is below the poverty threshold. The U.S. government bases the poverty threshold on the number of adults and children in the family. Noncash benefits such as food stamps or public housing are not included when measuring family income. The Earned Income Tax Credit also is not included. Every year, the government adjusts the poverty thresholds using the Consumer Price Index to reflect increases in the cost of living.[1]

Between 1970 and 2001, the percentage of children in poverty was cyclical with peaks occurring in the wake of recessions. Reductions in child poverty occurred in periods in which the economy was strong. Between 1993 and 1999, a period of rapid economic growth, the percentage of children in poverty decreased dramatically from 23% to 16%. Since then, during an economic slowdown, the percentage of children in poverty has remained constant.[1]

U.S. Census Bureau statistics for 2001 indicate many differences between those who were in poverty and those who were not. There were substantial differences in the risk of child poverty for different racial and ethnic groups. Thirty percent of Black children and 27% of Hispanic children lived in poor families. In contrast, only 10% of White Non-Hispanic children and 11% of Asian children were poor. However, the reductions in poverty in the mid- to late-1990s were largest for those groups of children with the highest levels of poverty—Black and Hispanic children.[1]

Poverty is not spread equally across the country, but concentrated in central cities and parts of the United States that are outside of metropolitan areas. In 2001, 24% of children in central cities lived in families with income below the poverty threshold, and 20% of children living outside metropolitan areas were in poverty. In contrast, only 11% of children living in suburbs were poor. The distribution also varied by region of the country with the highest concentration occurring in the south central states of Alabama, Arkansas,

> **Poverty, especially extended poverty, is associated with many adverse health outcomes for children.**

Source: Census 2000

Percentage
- 0% - 13%
- 14% - 20%
- 21% - 29%
- 30% - 54%

Alaska

Hawaii

Map 21.1: Percentage of Children Under 18 in Poverty, 2000

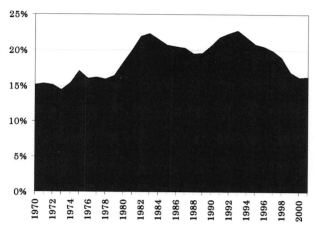

Figure 21.1: Percentage of Children Under 18 Living in Poverty
Source: Historic Poverty Tables 2003

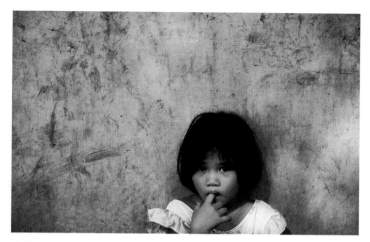

Kentucky, Louisiana, Mississippi, Oklahoma, Tennessee, and Texas. Eighteen percent of families with children in this region were in poverty. One-half as many families (9%) in the New England states of Connecticut, Maine, Massachusetts, New Hampshire, Rhode Island, and Vermont were in poverty. The poverty rate for families in the west north central states of Iowa, Kansas, Minnesota, Nebraska, North Dakota, and South Dakota was also relatively low (10%).[1]

Persons born outside the United States do not always escape poverty by coming to this country. Over one-fifth (21%) of the foreign born who had not become U.S. citizens and who were living in families with children were in poverty. However, the poverty rate for those who had become naturalized citizens was less than half that of the noncitizens. Naturalized citizens also were a little less likely to be in poverty than native-born citizens. (The rate for naturalized citizens was 10%, and the rate for native-born citizens was 12%.)[1]

Not surprisingly, lack of educational attainment was closely linked to poverty. Almost one-third (31%) of families with children were poor when the head of the household had less than 12 years of education. This contrasts sharply with only 3% of families with children when the head of the household had a bachelor's degree or more.[1]

Children in families headed by a single mother comprised one of the largest identifiable groups of children who were living in poverty in 2001. Thirty-nine percent of these

children were poor, compared with only 8% of children living in married-couple families.[1]

The likelihood that children will be in poverty is inversely related to the number of hours their parents work; children's risk of being in poverty goes up as the number of hours their parents work goes down.[2] In fact, one of the greatest disparities between children who were in poverty and those who were not involved the amount of time their parents spent at work. Only 8% of children whose single parent worked at least 20 hours per week or whose two parents worked at least 35 hours per week were in poverty. Fifty-four percent of children whose parents worked fewer hours were in poverty. This huge difference should help delineate one of the most important areas of focus for attempts to reduce child poverty.[3]

However, substantial work activity on the part of parents is not a guarantee of escaping poverty. About 5% of children in married-couple families and 18% of children in single-mother families lived in poverty even though their parents worked the number of hours described above.[3]

For the children who live in poverty, the impacts can be profound and far-reaching. Poverty, especially extended poverty, is associated with many adverse health outcomes for children. For example, children who have experienced persistent poverty were more likely to be shorter for their age than children living in families with higher incomes.[2] Persistent poverty also was associated with lower scores on an index that measured children's physical and motor skills and social development.[2]

Poverty also had a negative association with young children's IQs, verbal ability, and achievement test scores.[4] These negative associations were detected as early as age

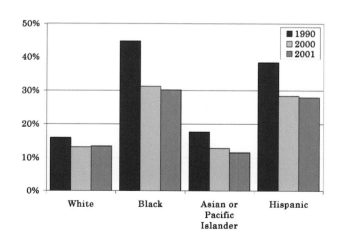

Figure 21.2: Percentage of Children Under 18 Living in Poverty by Race

Source: Poverty in the United States 2003

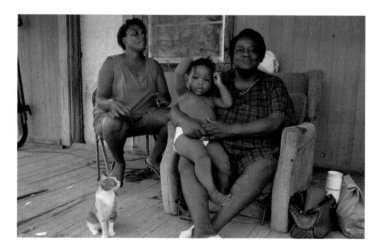

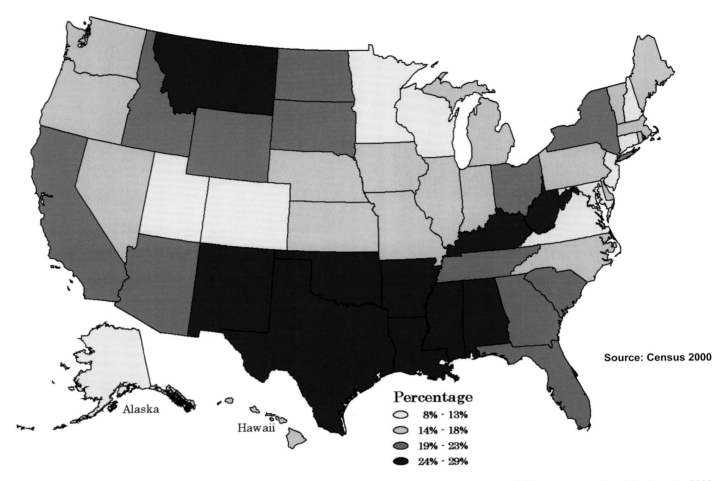

Source: Census 2000

Percentage
⬭ 8% - 13%
⬭ 14% - 18%
⬤ 19% - 23%
⬤ 24% - 29%

Map 21.2: Percentage of Children Under Age 6 in Poverty, 2000

2. Just 1 year of poverty is negatively associated with cognitive skills, and extended periods of poverty and extreme poverty (income less than half of the official poverty threshold) have even stronger negative associations.[4]

A child's chances of graduating from high school were substantially reduced as the number of years spent in poverty increased.[5] Living in poverty as an adolescent was also associated with lower wages as an adult, although much of this association may be due to the characteristics of the parents, family, school, and community rather than poverty per se.

The 1996 federal welfare reform legislation included the explicit goal of increasing the work activity of adults on welfare, and it included work requirement provisions to

achieve this goal. During the strong economic activity of the late 1990s, there was substantial progress on that front, and the Bush Administration has proposed further increases in work requirements for welfare recipients. Simulations by the Heritage Foundation[6] and the Brookings Institution[7] have shown that increasing the

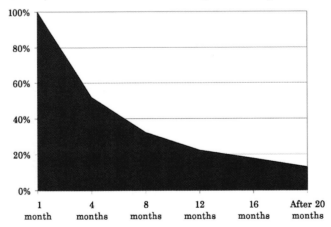

Figure 21.3: Children (Under 18) Entering Poverty in 1996: Percentage That Remained in Poverty by Length of Time

Source: Poverty Dynamics 2003

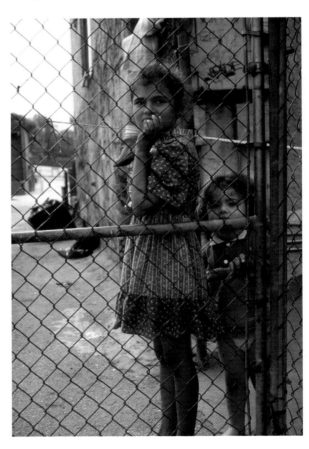

94

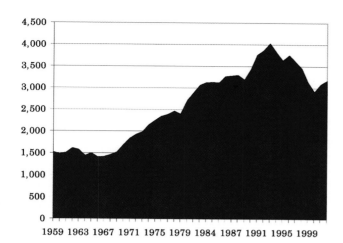

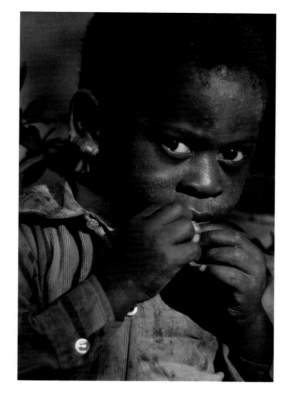

Figure 21.4: Growth in the Number of Female-headed Families Living in Poverty (in Thousands)

Source: U.S. Census Bureau 2003

work effort of poor families would substantially decrease the poverty rate of families and, thus, the poverty rate of children.

Policy approaches that might lead to increases in hours worked by parents in poor families include increasing direct wage subsidies (such as the Earned Income Tax Credit) and indirect wage subsidies (such as child care subsidies for the working poor). These subsidies provide incentives for parents to enter and stay in the work force. Another approach, which is under evaluation by the Department of Health and Human Services, focuses on alternative programs for helping low-income parents work more consistently and for helping them embark on a career path that leads to higher wages and benefits. There is little evidence so far on which type of program is likely to be successful. Each of these supply-side approaches is likely to work best if the economy is strong. Thus, a higher rate of U.S. economic growth and lower unemployment are crucial for reducing poverty.

A possible approach to increase the potential for higher income is to encourage marriage for single parents and preservation of marriage for currently married parents. Two parents working full-time can generally succeed in raising their children out of poverty, even if the parents are

Almost one-third (31%) of families with children were poor when the head of the household had less than 12 years of education.

employed in low-wage jobs. However, there is little rigorous research on how to preserve or promote healthy marriages.

Possible approaches include programs for adults that provide emotional and social support, communication and conflict-resolution training, employment and education services, family planning services, and mental and physical health services. Others include parenting and child development education and services that address domestic violence.

Poverty limits the potential of millions of children in the United States by affecting their physical, emotional, and cognitive development in numerous adverse ways. In addition to the toll poverty takes on those who experience it firsthand, society as a whole suffers when many of our children are prohibited from reaching their full potential and making the contribution they might have made otherwise. Child poverty will remain a major issue until the United States finds a way to greatly reduce it permanently.

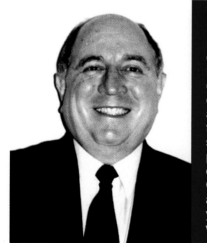

Richard Wertheimer

Richard Wertheimer, PhD, area director for Welfare and Poverty at Child Trends, earned his PhD in economics from the University of Maryland. Dr. Wertheimer directs research projects at Child Trends in four areas: the determinants of teenage childbearing; the economic and social conditions of poor, working families with children; the number and characteristics of vulnerable youth transitioning to adulthood; and the well-being of adolescents whose parents participated in welfare-to-work programs. His recent work includes updates of an assessment of the role of state government policies and programs and socioeconomic factors on teen pregnancy and fertility rates; a descriptive analysis of poor, working families with children using data from the Survey of Income and Program Participation and the Current Population Survey; and state- and city-level data on the conditions of children and their mothers at childbirth. He also recently estimated the number of vulnerable youth who were transitioning to adulthood and the number of kindergarteners who were lagging behind their peers.

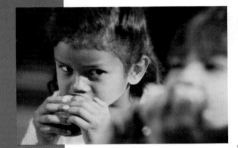

Chapter 22

Patrick H. Casey

Food Insecurity

National experts define *food insecurity* as "limited or uncertain availability of nutritionally adequate and safe foods or limited or uncertain ability to acquire acceptable foods in socially acceptable ways.[1] Conversely, food security is considered a marker of the adequacy and stability of a household's food supply over the preceding 12 months for active, healthy living of all household members.[1,2] The U.S. Household Food Security Scale, an 18-question survey instrument, has been used since 1995 in national surveys (e.g., Current Population Survey) to assess the annual prevalence of food insecurity and hunger in the United States.[3] In the scale, *hunger*, a physiologically uneasy or painful sensation caused by the lack of food, is regarded as the most extreme form of household food insecurity.

In addition to the term food insecurity, researchers have used *food insufficiency* for decades.[4] Food insufficiency is an inadequacy in the amount of food intake due to lack of money or resources. In addition, there have been a number of brief instruments designed to identify hunger.[2] However, the concepts of food insecurity and food security and the U.S. Household Food Security Scale have gained wide acceptance in recent years.[1]

In 2002, the most recent year for which data are available, 11.1% of all households (12.1 million) were food insecure sometime during that year. In 3.5% of U.S. households (3.8 million), one or more household members were hungry sometime during that year because they could not afford enough food.[3] The prevalence of food insecurity was higher in African American (22%) and Hispanic (21.7%) households than in households of other racial and ethnic groups. The rate was even higher in households with family income below the federal poverty line (38.1%). Over 16% of households with children were food insecure at least sometime during the preceding year. Female-headed households with family income less than 130% of the poverty line had the highest prevalence of food insecurity; 47.1% reported food insecurity, and 13.4% reported hunger in at least one household member. Over 12% of children in low-income households were hungry. Approximately 68% of food-insecure households reported

> **Household food insecurity is now a relatively common condition among African American and Hispanic American children, particularly those who live in female-headed households with income below the federal poverty line.**

the condition as recurring, and nearly 20% experienced these conditions frequently or chronically.[5]

There was no consistent trend in the prevalence of food insecurity for 1995 to 1998, but the percentage of all households that were food insecure increased annually from 1999 to 2002. The increase from 10.1% in 1999 to 11.1% in 2002 translates to more than 1.5 million additional food-insecure households. The prevalence of food insecurity with hunger increased from 3% of U.S. households in 1999 to 3.5% in 2002, an increase of more than a half million households. The increase in prevalence existed in all regions of the United States and in all types of households. Households with children had a much greater prevalence of food insecurity than households overall. The prevalence of food insecurity among households with children increased from 14.8% in 1999 to 16.5% in 2002.

Although major events, such as the loss of a job, may jeopardize the budget of any household and result in food insecurity, families who live in poverty are at greater risk. Families of limited income, who typically have no savings to fall back on, have little or no flexible financial resources

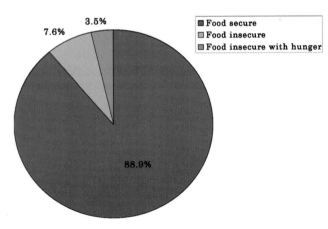

Figure 22.1: United States Households by Food Security Status, 2002

Source: Economic Research Service 2002

3.5%
7.6%
88.9%
- Food secure
- Food insecure
- Food insecure with hunger

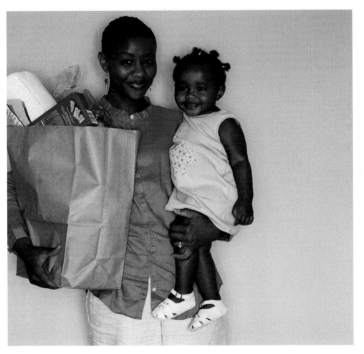

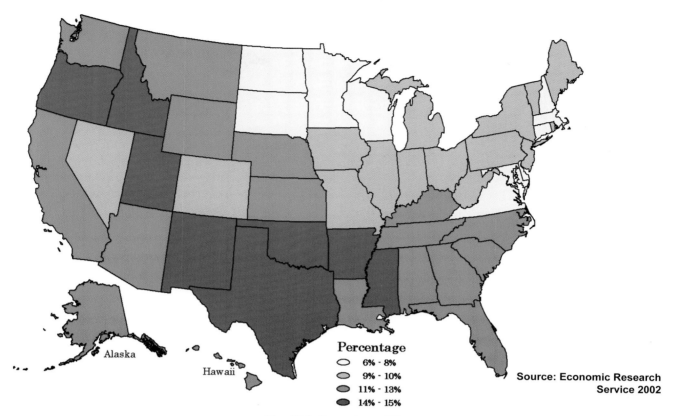

Percentage
○ 6% - 8%
○ 9% - 10%
⬤ 11% - 13%
⬤ 14% - 15%

Source: Economic Research
Service 2002

Map 22.1: Percentage of Households Experiencing Food Insecurity, 2000-2002

to deal with unexpected changes in monthly expenses. Increased expenses associated with price fluctuations in gasoline, home heating or cooling, housing or medical costs, or the loss of food stamps or children's school breakfast and lunch programs during the summer may exceed such families' monthly budgets. Cutting back on the quality or volume of food purchased may be the path of least resistance to get through the month. In addition, healthy, prudent diets that include fruits and vegetables, seafood, and lean meats cost considerably more than energy-dense (high-calorie), less nutritious diets that

contain more fat or added sugar. It is easy to imagine that families with restricted income may ration food, regulate frequency of meals, and/or utilize low-cost, energy-dense foods at times of financial constraints, particularly at the end of the month.

Thus, depending on its severity and duration, food insecurity is an important characteristic that may have significant negative impacts on the nutrition and health status of household members.[6] However, since poverty is known to be associated with lower nutrition and adverse

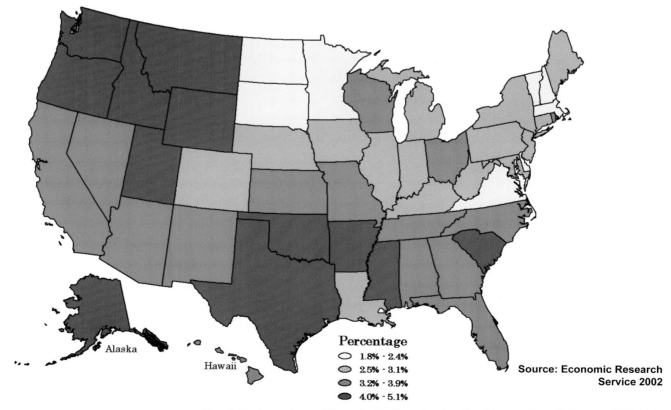

Percentage
○ 1.8% - 2.4%
⬤ 2.5% - 3.1%
⬤ 3.2% - 3.9%
⬤ 4.0% - 5.1%

Source: Economic Research
Service 2002

Map 22.2: Percentage of Households Experiencing Food Insecurity with Hunger, 2000-2002

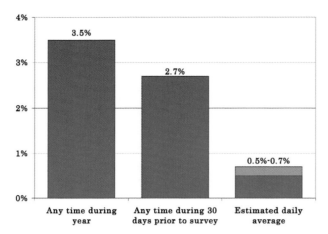

Figure 22.2: Prevalence of Households having Food Insecurity with
Hunger, Dec. 2002

Source: Economic Research Service 2002

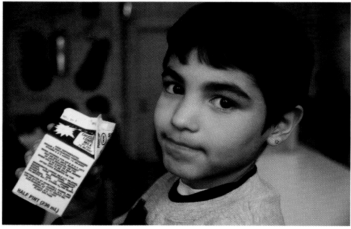

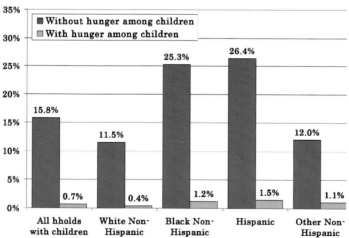

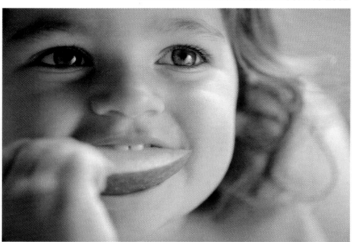

Figure 22.3: Prevalence of Food Insecurity in Households with
Children by Race, 2002

Source: Economic Research Service 2002

health outcomes, it is important to account for the associated effects of poverty while evaluating the independent effects of food insecurity on nutrition and health status.

Understanding of the independent effect of food insecurity and insufficiency on nutrient intake and health status is rapidly advancing. Weekly per-person expenditures on food were much lower in food-insecure households than in food-secure homes ($27.50 vs. $38.57).[3] Fifty-two percent of households that were food insecure reported they occasionally could not afford balanced meals for their children, and 81% reported restricted meals of low-cost food for their children due to financial constraint. However, empirical research has not documented significant negative impacts on reported intake of macronutrients (those needed in relatively large quantities) and micronutrients (those needed in smaller quantities such as trace elements) of children in food-insecure households. In a national survey, there were no significant differences between children in low-income, food-insufficient and low-income, food-sufficient households in total energy, protein, carbohydrate, fat, or cholesterol intake.[7] However, one report found Hispanic children from food-insecure households had significant decreases in meat and energy intake as payday approached.[8] On the other hand, adults in food-insecure households have lower macronutrient and micronutrient intakes, independent of household demographic characteristics like family income.[9,10] The assumption is that adults defer to their children and preferentially feed them during times of food shortage.

In addition, food insecurity has been found to be independently associated with poor adult general physical health, poor mental health, and chronic health conditions.[11] For example, in a national survey of more than 1 million adults in Canada, individuals in food-insufficient households were more likely to report poor or fair health, poor functional health, restricted activities, major depression and distress, and more chronic conditions of heart disease, diabetes, and high blood pressure than those from food-sufficient households. These differences were present even after adjusting for age, sex, education, and income adequacy.[12] Obesity has been associated with food insecurity and insufficiency in women but not in men.[13]

Independent of demographic characteristics, children in food-insecure or food-insufficient households have lower general health status, more negative general health symptoms, and more iron deficiency than other children. For example, in the National Health and Nutrition Examination Survey (1988-1994), a study of more than 11,000 children, those in food-insufficient households were more likely to have poor or fair general health status and were more likely to report stomachaches, headaches, and colds when poverty, past health status, and environmental factors were controlled.[14] In addition, food insufficiency was significantly associated with mental health problems and academic difficulties in children.[15] In another study that used the National Health and Nutrition Examination Survey data, school-age children in food-insufficient households had significantly lower

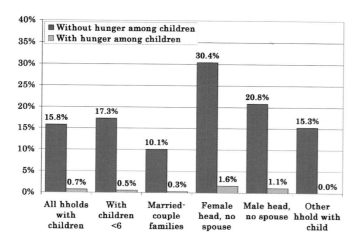

Figure 22.4: Family Composition of Households with Food Insecurity, 2002

Source: Economic Research Service 2002

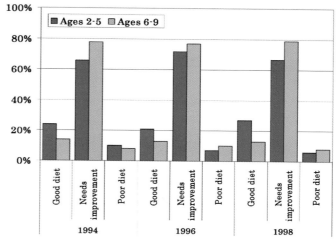

Figure 22.5: Diet Quality Based on Healthy Eating Index

Source: Federal Interagency Forum on Child and Family Stats 2002

arithmetic scores and were more likely to have repeated a grade, have seen a psychologist, and have difficulty getting along with other children.[16] Teens in food-insufficient households were more likely to have seen a psychologist, have been suspended from school, and have difficulty getting along with other children. Although often the topic of discussion and of considerable theoretic concern, an association between food insecurity and childhood obesity has not been confirmed.[8,17,18]

Household food insecurity is now a relatively common condition among African American and Hispanic American children, particularly those who live in female-headed households with income below the federal poverty line. Given the increase in prevalence from 1999 to 2002, there is concern among child advocates and child health clinicians that this trend will worsen as a result of the downturn in the U.S. economy and as a consequence of welfare reform activities.[19] A recent report indicated that children in families whose welfare was terminated, reduced by sanctions, or decreased administratively due to increased family income had a greater likelihood of being food insecure.[20] Loss of food stamps in this context is of particular concern since food stamps have been shown to increase the nutrient intake of children in impoverished families.[21] A recent study showed that school-age girls in food-insecure households who

Households with children had a much greater prevalence of food insecurity than households overall.

participated in federal food assistance programs, like food stamps, had a lower risk of being overweight than girls from households that did not participate in these programs.[22]

While research has not shown that food insecurity is an independent cause of negative child and adult physical and mental health status, one can conclude that food insecurity is independently associated with negative physical and mental health status. Researchers, clinicians, and policymakers should consider food insecurity as one of the important cumulative risk factors for children, particularly those who live in families in poverty.

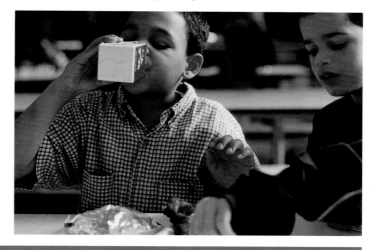

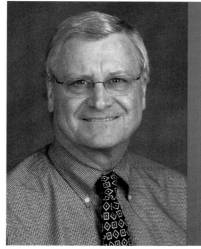

Patrick H. Casey

Patrick Casey, MD, is the Harvey and Bernice Jones Professor of Developmental Pediatrics, director for the Center for Applied Research and Evaluation, and chief of the Division of Developmental/Behavioral Pediatrics at Arkansas Children's Hospital. He is an active clinician and directs the Growth and Development Program, a multidisciplinary referral clinic for children with failure-to-thrive and developmental problems. He is the medical director of the KIDS FIRST program, a statewide system of center-based, early intervention programs for medically vulnerable children. His research interests include normal growth and development of infants; failure to thrive and malnutrition in infancy; the effect of infants' home environment on long-term growth, development, and behavior; and effects of various clinical and nutritional interventions on growth and development. He is the principal investigator for one site of the Lower Mississippi Delta Nutrition Intervention Research Initiative, a project on the health and nutritional status of residents of the delta region of Arkansas, Louisiana, and Mississippi. Dr. Casey is also an investigator in the U.S. Department of Agriculture-supported study of the psychological and psychophysiological consequences of failure to thrive and early malnutrition.

Part Three: About Their Health

Maintaining optimal health of children and youth requires recognition of the multiple factors that determine health. There have been impressive improvements in the health status of children in our country and in many others over the past century. However, challenges to optimal health remain, reflecting the increased occurrence of specific diseases, the impact of violence, and the emergence of issues affecting behavior and emotions. The following section looks at some health problems of increasing significance and identifies some of the challenges that children will be facing in the decades ahead.

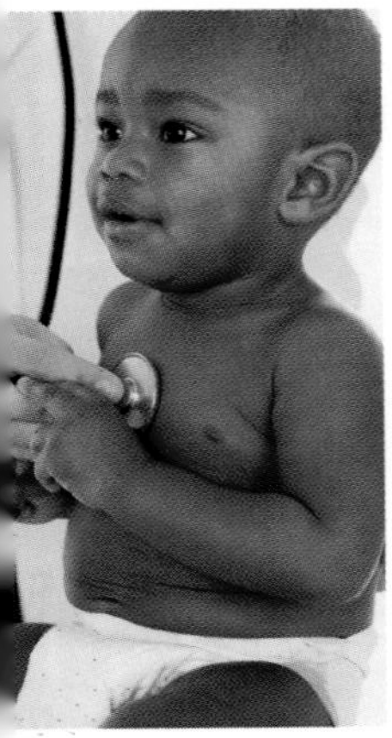

Chapter 23

Child Health:
An Evaluation of the Last Century

*Bernard Guyer
and Alyssa Wigton*

The improvements in the health status of American children (and adults) over the course of the 20th century were nothing short of spectacular. During this period, the life expectancy of Americans increased by 56%, from 49.2 years in 1900 to 76.5 years in 1998. The overall age-adjusted death rate declined by 74%, and the greatest single contribution to the increased longevity of Americans occurred with the decline in infant and child death rates. Unfortunately, such impressive improvements in the overall measures of child health can obscure not only confounding disparities associated with race, class, and geography, but also continuing and emerging health problems of American children.

The purpose of this chapter is to describe the trends in child health over the 20th century and to take stock of the health problems facing American children at the beginning of the 21st century. This will be accomplished by using information from the National Center for Health Statistics, which compiles data from birth and death certificates registered in all states and the District of Columbia, and by using national survey data.

The infant mortality rate (IMR), defined as deaths in the first year of life per 1,000 live births, declined exponentially during the 20th century. In 1915, approximately 100 infants per 1,000 live births died in the first year of life, while in 1998, the IMR was 7.2 deaths per 1,000 live births. The forces driving this 95% decline included, in the early part of the century, improvements in environmental conditions, the provision of a safe milk supply, parenting information, and improved housing. Medical advances, including antibiotics, fluid and electrolyte replacement therapy, blood banks, modern family planning methods, and neonatal intensive care, accelerated the decline in IMR in the latter part of the century. More recently, IMR declines reflect the introduction of surfactant—a complex substance that coats the inside of premature infants' immature lungs to prevent or reduce the severity of respiratory distress syndrome—and the adoption of "back to sleep" practices

In 1900, more than 30 in 1,000 children died between their 1st and 20th birthdays; today, less than 2 in 1,000 die.

that have reduced mortality related to sudden infant death syndrome. It should be noted, however, that little of the decline in IMR resulted from a reduction in the birth rate for low birth weight, high-risk infants. Despite impressive advances in obstetric and prenatal care, the birth weight distribution of American infants has changed little over the century.

For children older than 1 year of age, the overall decline in mortality experienced during the 20th century was spectacular. In 1900, more than 30 in 1,000 children died between their 1st and 20th birthdays; today, less than 2 in 1,000 die. Again, much of this decline took place during the first half of the century when few antibiotics or modern vaccines and medications were available, and it reflects the influences of improved sanitation and living standards on deaths from diarrheal disease, tuberculosis, and other infections.

It should be noted, however, that the decline in child mortality is not uniform across all age groups. For the youngest age groups, 1- to 4-year-olds, 5- to 9-year-olds, and 10- to 14-year-olds, mortality declined by 98%, 96%, and 93%, respectively. The adolescent age group, 15- to 19-year-olds, declined more slowly (85% overall) and has shown a tendency to plateau since 1960. In 2000, the death rate was 32.9 per 100,000 among children 1 to 4

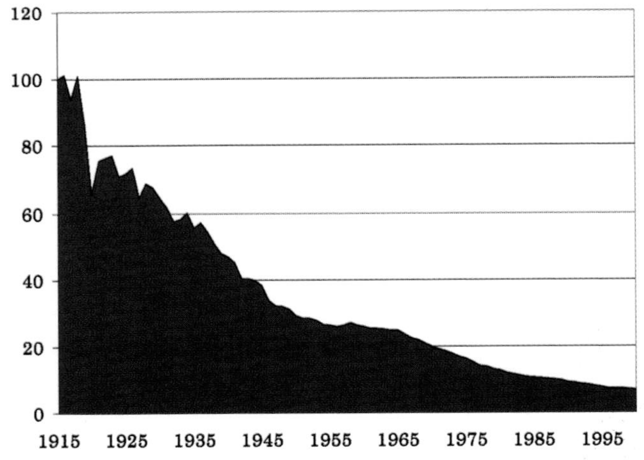

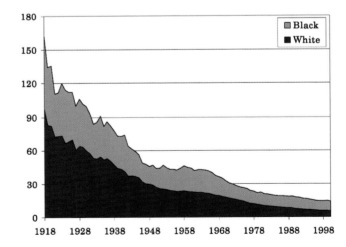

Figure 23.1: Overall Infant Mortality Rate per 1,000 Live Births

Source: National Center for Health Statistics 1996, Murphy 2000, Centers for Disease Control and Prevention 2002

Figure 23.2: Infant Mortality Rate by Race per 1,000 Live Births

Source: National Center for Health Statistics 1996, Murphy 2000, Centers for Disease Control and Prevention 2002

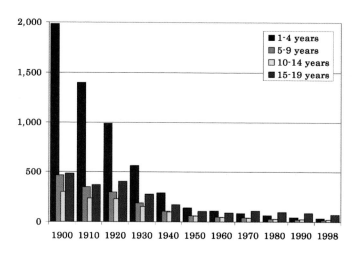

Figure 23.3: Childhood Mortality Rates by Age at Death per 100,000

Source: National Center for Health Statistics 1900-1998

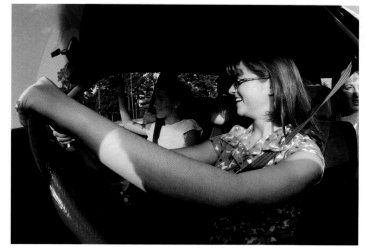

years old, 16.4 among children 5 to 9 years old, 20.9 among children 10 to 14 years old, and 68.2 among youth 15 to 19 years old. As these rates indicate, adolescents continue to be at substantially higher risk for death, primarily due to preventable causes such as accidents and injuries.

By the end of the 20th century, child mortality from infectious diseases declined 99.7%, despite the emergence of HIV/AIDS, which accounted, in 1998, for less than 0.3% of child deaths. Accidents and injuries have emerged as the leading causes of child death, accounting for 43.9% of all child deaths in 1998. The widespread adoption of powerful new vaccines and anti-infectious agents in the latter decades of the century explains these trends.

In contrast to the infectious diseases, accidents accounted for only 6% of child deaths in 1900, but 44% in 1998. Overall, the rate of injury-related child death changed relatively little over the century, but the patterns of causes shifted. At the beginning of the century, child injury deaths occurred principally on the farm, in factories, and from burns. Motor vehicle-related deaths were unheard of in 1900, but now account for more than

half of all child injury deaths, with the child as either a passenger or pedestrian. Motor vehicle-related death is the leading cause of death in adolescence (5,198 deaths in 1999). In addition, increasing numbers of child deaths from violence, including both homicide and suicide, emerged by the end of the 20th century. These intentionally inflicted injuries accounted for nearly 10% of child deaths in 1999 (4,760 deaths). Firearms, as the agent of both accidental and intentional injury deaths, accounted for about 7% of all injury deaths among children ages 1 to 19 in 1999 (3,274 deaths).

While most American children are healthy, disparities by race, ethnicity, socioeconomic status, and geography persist. For example, although infant mortality rates have declined overall, the gap in infant death rates between White and African American infants continues and, in fact, has even widened since the early part of the 20th century.

Recent research indicates that this persisting disparity reflects racial and socioeconomic inequalities in American society. African American families are more likely to be poor and living in communities where chronic economic disadvantage, unemployment, racial discrimination, drugs, and political powerlessness influence the fabric of life. In addition, African American women are more likely to have high-risk pregnancies characterized by infection,

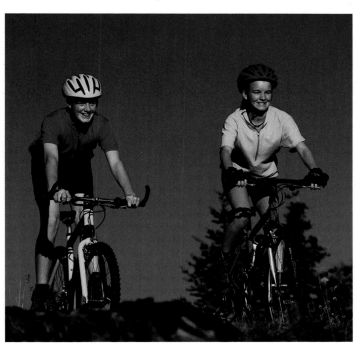

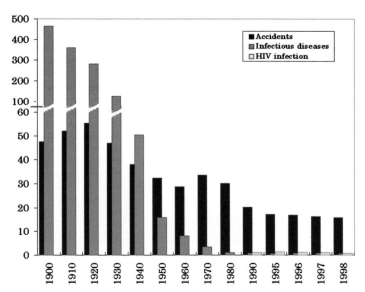

Figure 23.4: Death Rates for Children Ages 1 to 19 by Cause of Death per 100,000

Source: Vital Statistics of the United States 1900-1998

103

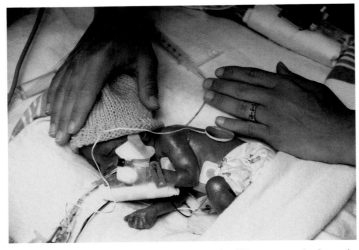

poor nutrition, pre-existing chronic illness, and chronic stress. All of these factors contribute to a higher incidence of preterm birth and low birth weight among African American newborns.

A national survey of American children in 1994 (National Health Interview Survey 1994 Disability Supplement) found that between 15% and 18% of children younger than 18 years old had at least one chronic condition. Among these 20 million children with a chronic condition, 65% were considered mild, 29% moderate, and 6% severe. Rates of asthma and obesity, in particular, are increasing at an alarming rate among American children.

Asthma is among the most severe childhood health conditions, affecting approximately 5 million U.S. children (13%). The impact of asthma on children's health seems to be growing. In just the past two decades, asthma prevalence increased more than 160% among children under age 5. Further, on average, 14 million school days are missed each year, and asthma is now the third leading cause of hospitalizations among children under 15 years of age.

African Americans continue to have higher rates of emergency department visits, hospitalizations, and deaths due to asthma than do White Americans. When compared to Hispanic children, African American children are nearly twice as likely to have had an asthma attack in the past 12 months. Children from low-income families, single-parent families, and minority families also experience disproportionately higher morbidity and mortality due to asthma. Although the exact cause of asthma is unknown, the most important triggers of an asthma attack are environmental tobacco smoke, dust mites, outdoor air pollution such as that caused by industrial emissions and automobile exhaust, cockroaches, pets, and mold.

In addition to asthma, childhood obesity currently affects many American children. The number of overweight American children (defined as those with an age-appropriate body mass index at the 95th percentile or higher) ages 6 to 11 has more than doubled since 1980, while the number of overweight adolescents has tripled during that time. In 2000, about 15% of American children ages 6 to 19, approximately 9 million, were overweight. In addition, more than 10% of preschool children ages 2 to 5 were overweight, up from 7% in 1994. An additional 15% of children ages 6 to 19 were deemed to be at risk of overweight, with their body mass index scores falling between the 85th and 95th percentiles.

Children who are overweight have a 70% chance of becoming overweight adults; that risk rises to 80% if at least one parent is overweight. Being overweight increases the risk for several chronic diseases including heart disease, type 2 diabetes, high blood pressure, some cancers, stroke, and depression. Type 2 diabetes, previously considered a chronic disease primarily affecting adults, is now on the rise among children.

Another chronic condition increasingly recognized in recent years among U.S. children is attention deficit hyperactivity disorder (ADHD). Although a single, consistent, and standard case definition has not yet been implemented, ADHD is estimated to affect 3% to 5% of American children and is the most common neurodevelopmental disorder of childhood. ADHD is considered a serious public health problem not just because of its high prevalence, but also because it can have a substantial impact on school performance and socialization. In addition, children and youth with ADHD are more likely to engage in risky behaviors such as substance abuse. Although there is no definitive cause for ADHD, research has identified prenatal alcohol use, prenatal smoking, low

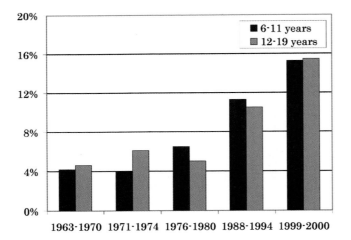

Figure 23.5: Percentage of Children and Adolescents That Were Overweight

Source: Pastor, Makue, Reuben, Xia 2002

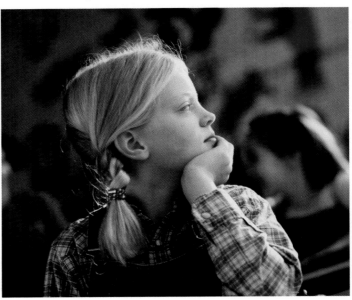

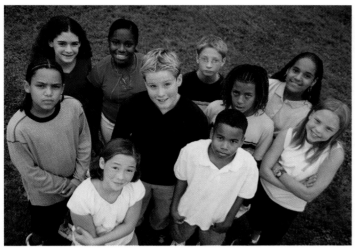

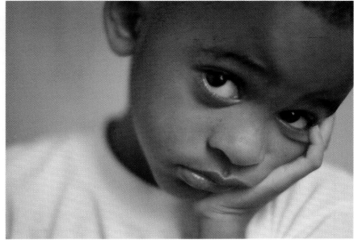

birth weight, and a family history of ADHD as possible contributing factors.

Finally, one cannot adequately discuss the health of American children over the 20th century without considering the impact of the HIV/AIDS epidemic. By the early 1990s, over 1,000 infants were born with HIV infection each year in the United States, and by 2001, perinatal exposure represented 91% of all AIDS cases among children under the age of 13 years. Following the availability of perinatal preventive treatments such as zidovudine (AZT), perinatally acquired AIDS cases declined significantly, showing a reduction of 75% between 1992 and 1998 alone.

The rate of AIDS cases among children under 13 years of age varies significantly by race and ethnicity. While White Americans made up 61% of the population of U.S. children in 2001, they represented only 19% of AIDS cases in children. In contrast, African Americans accounted for only 14% of U.S. children, but represented 65% of AIDS cases in children. Hispanic Americans made up 19% of U.S. children, but represented 15% of AIDS cases in children. Racial and ethnic disparities in HIV infection exist among older children

While most American children are healthy, disparities by race, ethnicity, socioeconomic status, and geography persist.

and youth as well. Of all HIV infections ever reported in the United States for the 13- to 24-year-old age group, African Americans account for 56%. Gender differences also exist; females represent 61% of HIV infections among young people ages 13 to 19 years old, while males represent 39%.

In many ways, children are better off now than they ever have been. There are, however, new and emerging child health problems that warrant special attention, such as asthma, obesity, ADHD, and HIV/AIDS. Further, while overall rates of childhood mortality and morbidity have declined, important disparities by race and income continue to exist and, in some cases, have actually increased since the early 1900s. To a large extent, these health disparities are the consequence not only of differences in access to health services, but of the broader socioeconomic context in which minority and low-income children live. As we embark on a new century certain to provide further advancements in child health, consideration must be given to ensuring that these disparities become a part of the past. In the 21st century, all American children should be able to achieve their optimal health and well-being.

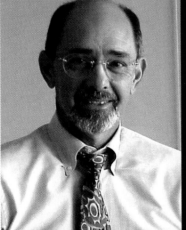

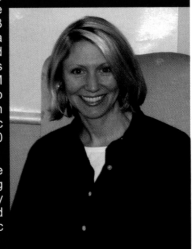

Bernard Guyer and Alyssa Wigton

Bernard Guyer, MD, MPH, is a Zanvyl Krieger Professor of Children's Health in the Department of Population and Family Health Sciences at the Johns Hopkins Bloomberg School of Public Health. From 1989 to 2003, he served as department chair. Dr. Guyer was the recipient of the *"Golden Apple" Teaching Award* in 2003 as well as the *2003 Martha May Eliot Award*. He is a member of the Institute of Medicine (IOM) and chaired the IOM Committee on National Immunization Policies and Practices. Dr. Guyer currently chairs the IOM Committee on the Poison Control System. From 1979 to 1986, Dr. Guyer directed the Maternal and Child Health Agency in the Massachusetts Department of Public Health. In addition, he is the author of more than 200 published papers.

Alyssa Wigton, MS, MHS, has a master of health science degree from the Johns Hopkins University Bloomberg School of Public Health and a master of science in medicine degree from the University of Cape Town. She is currently pursuing her PhD in the Department of Population and Family Health Sciences at the Johns Hopkins University Bloomberg School of Public Health.

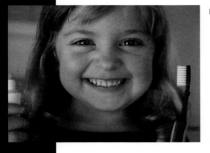

Chapter 24

Burton L. Edelstein

Tooth Decay:
The Best of Times, the Worst of Times

One of the great public health and societal successes for American children is the rapid and remarkable decline in children's experience with tooth decay and its consequences. For baby boomers and their parents, tooth decay was an almost universal experience—so common that it was thought to be a normal part of growing up. Ordinary tooth decay is the primary reason that a quarter of U.S. seniors are missing all of their teeth (*Healthy People 2010*). Unlike these seniors, millions of children today grow up completely free of such dental problems. They are the beneficiaries of better understanding of the decay process, healthier diets, fluoride in all forms, dental sealants, and preventive dental care. For them, this has become the best of times.

For millions of other children, however, dental caries is a daily nightmare of pain, eating difficulties, unsightly smiles, and distraction from play and learning. In fact, tooth decay remains the single most common chronic disease of childhood—5 times more common than asthma according to the U.S. Surgeon General's report, *Oral Health in America*. Tooth decay among America's children may be on the rebound as groups of children with highest rates of dental disease, particularly Latino children, are now growing in population faster than other groups of children. The federal government's *Healthy People 2010* project reports that nearly one in five children between the ages of 2 and 4 years has visible cavities (18%). More than half of all children between the ages of 6 and 8 have visible cavities (52%). An estimated 5 million children have dental disease extensive enough to be consequential to their daily lives. These are children who suffer toothaches and symptoms of infection in their gums, lips, and faces. For them, this continues to be the worst of times.

While early childhood is a time of tremendous promise, it is also a time when disturbances in health or social welfare can take a toll that is expressed throughout life. It is a period when missed opportunities to prevent disease, through positive health behaviors and quality health care, can spell chronic dysfunction and disability. Tooth decay is just such a condition. It is a disease that is typically established during the first 2 years of life. Its early prevention holds promise to limit disease throughout life. The time has now come to put an end to this completely preventable disease—a disease that the

Surgeon General has called a "silent epidemic" and that too many young children experience as personal suffering.

The most common form of early dental disease—early childhood caries (ECC)—begins destroying a child's teeth as early as the first birthday and typically progresses to pain and infection within a year or two. Previously known as "baby bottle tooth decay" or "nursing bottle mouth," this aggressive and rapidly destructive form of tooth decay occurs in children from families of all incomes and social conditions. Its cause, a combination of decay-causing bacteria in plaque combined with dietary sugars, is not different biologically from the more common, slowly progressing tooth decay experienced by many other children. But it is dramatically accelerated by the frequent ingestion of sweetened liquids, most commonly by inappropriate and frequent use of the baby bottle or "sippy" cup as a pacifier.

Children most susceptible are those who, early in life, acquire the bacteria needed to transform sugars into acids that destroy the teeth. These bacteria, called cariogenic bacteria, are typically acquired by an infant or toddler from its mother by direct salivary transmission. Common modes of transmission are sharing a feeding spoon, cleaning a dropped pacifier in the mother's mouth, or allowing a child to put its hand in the mother's mouth and then

> **The most common form of early dental disease—early childhood caries—begins destroying a child's teeth as early as the first birthday and typically progresses to pain and infection within a year or two.**

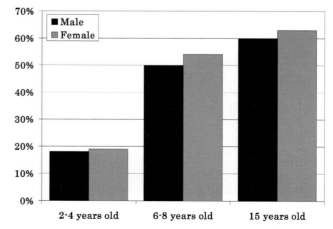

Figure 24.1: Dental Caries Experience of Children by Age and Gender, 1988-1994

Source: Healthy People 2010, 2000

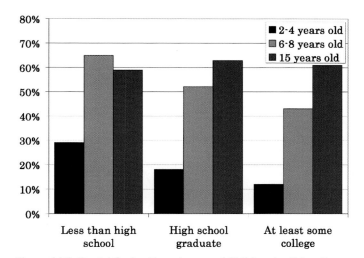

Figure 24.2: Dental Caries Experiences of Children by Education Level of Head of Household and Age, 1988-1994

Source: Healthy People 2010, 2000

into its own mouth. The risk of developing ECC is higher for those children whose mothers have higher amounts of cariogenic bacteria in their mouths and those children who experience a larger number of transmissions of bacteria. The risk also goes up as the amount of sugar in the diet increases to better support the implantation of bacteria on the teeth. The level of these bacteria in a child's mouth can be measured with a simple culture technique.

The first indication that ECC is developing is the presence of dental plaque along the gum line on the front surface of a young child's front teeth. That sign is soon followed by the appearance of opaque white spots in the same area (see photo below) as well as between the front teeth, if they are touching, and on the back side of the front teeth. At these stages, the disease is still reversible by stopping the source of the frequent sugar and applying fluoride to the affected areas using prescription medications and small amounts of toothpaste. But soon these weakened areas start to collapse and cavities become evident, leaving the teeth pitted, rough, discolored, and susceptible to further destruction.

Because baby teeth are small and thin, progression of decay can quickly reach the internal nerves of the teeth, causing pain and infection that spread to adjacent tissues. Unless ECC is noticed and treated early enough and aggressively enough, affected preschoolers may require extensive and costly dental repair, often while under general anesthesia in the hospital operating room.

As with many other childhood problems, "an ounce of prevention is worth a pound of cure," especially because affected children remain at higher risk for cavities throughout their childhood and into their adulthood. Exposure to optimally fluoridated water is the single most effective public health method for reducing caries occurrence, yet EEC occurs even in fluoridated areas if destructive bacterial and feeding conditions are present. That is why the American Academy of Pediatrics, the American Academy of Pediatric Dentistry, the American Public Health Association, and other leading national health groups all support establishing dental care for children at the time of their first birthday. That is also why efforts are underway across the country to enable pediatricians; family practitioners; Special Supplemental Nutrition Program for Women, Infants, and Children (WIC) nutrition workers; home health visitors; and others who come in contact with young children to identify at-risk children and help ensure early care. The importance of early care also underscores a growing effort to prepare today's dental students and practicing general dentists to assess and manage dental conditions of young children. With pediatric dentists comprising

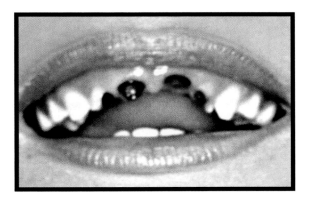

If it pains you to look at this picture, imagine how the child feels.

An estimated 2,500 Rhode Island children between the ages of six months to four years old suffer from Early Childhood Tooth Decay.* But not a single one of them has to. That's because Early Childhood Tooth Decay is preventable. It occurs when children's teeth are harmed by frequently drinking from bottles or sippy cups that contain sweetened milk, juice and soda or other sugary liquids. So if your baby needs comforting, try a bottle of water, a pacifier, a favorite blanket or toy. Be the best parent you can be and help prevent Early Childhood Tooth Decay. It'll make you and your baby feel a lot better.

*Source: Rhode Island Department of Health, Oral health Program; January, 2001.

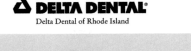
Delta Dental of Rhode Island

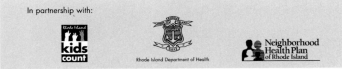

Figure 24.3: Example of Early Childhood Caries Public Service Announcement

Source: Reprinted courtesy of Delta of Rhode Island copyright 2003

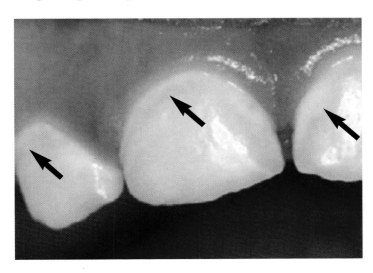

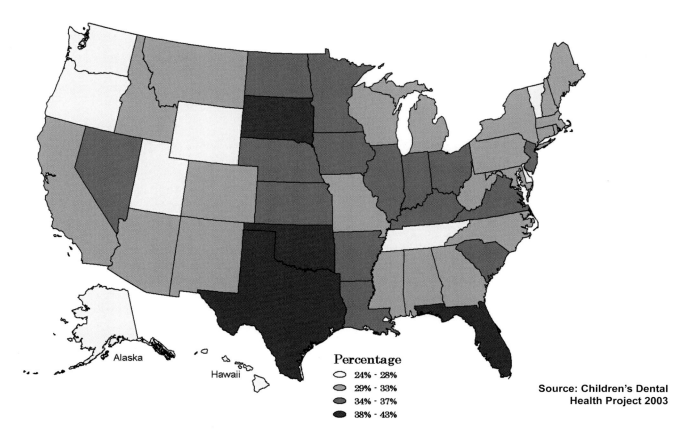

Percentage
○ 24% - 28%
● 29% - 33%
● 34% - 37%
● 38% - 43%

Source: Children's Dental
Health Project 2003

Map 24.1: Estimated Percentage of Children Under 19 without Dental Insurance, 2000-2001

only 3% of all dentists and only about 1 pediatric dentist for every 12 pediatricians in the United States, too many young children cannot access a pediatric dentist, even when needs for specialty care are pressing.

The future holds strong potential for tremendous progress in identifying which children are at high risk for early dental problems, even before those problems are evident. As this risk assessment becomes better refined, protocols can be developed for tailoring care to the individual needs of each child. These risk-based protocols hold strong promise to reduce disease burden among America's children by linking individual levels of risk to individualized preventive interventions including family education about dietary content and patterns, home use of fluorides and antibacterial preparations, and frequency of professional care. Economic modeling based on this science suggests that screening all young children for caries risk followed by intensive, early preventive care for high-risk children can result in overall cost savings.

Ensuring that children, particularly young children at high risk for tooth decay, can obtain meaningful dental care remains a tremendous challenge because of the shortage of available dentists and because of systemic problems with dental care financing. Ideally, every child will have an identified dentist of his or her own who provides regular, ongoing, comprehensive oral health care throughout the child's growing years. This "dental home" parallels the "medical home" concept advanced by the American Academy of Pediatrics wherein every child enjoys uninterrupted access to a single source of care from which all needed services are ensured and coordinated. Such a medical or dental home is important to families as they negotiate the complexities of the health care delivery system.

Ironically, children with the greatest needs for dental care also have the least access to care. Preschoolers in families of poverty are more than twice as likely to experience tooth decay. They experience, on average, more than twice the number of cavities. Parents of these children are twice as likely to report that their child had a toothache or other dental problem. Yet

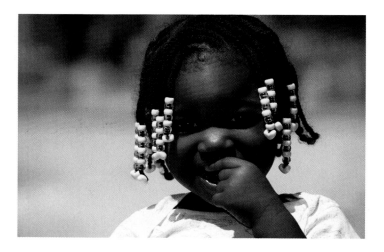

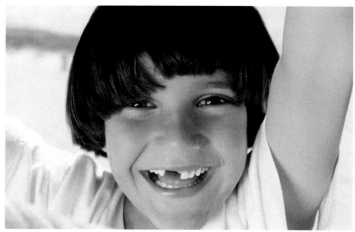

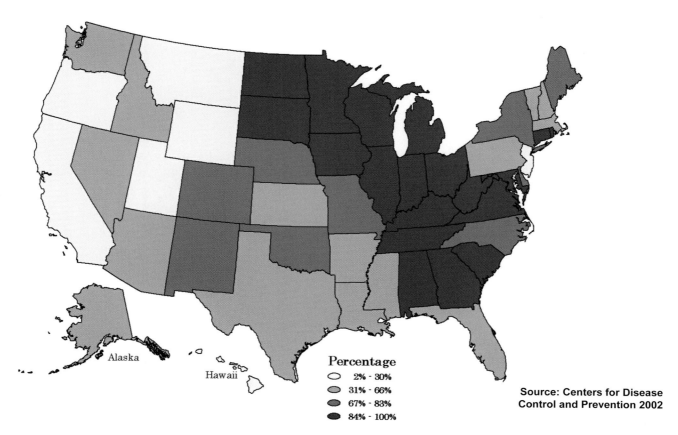

Percentage
○ 2% - 30%
◔ 31% - 66%
◑ 67% - 83%
● 84% - 100%

Source: Centers for Disease
Control and Prevention 2002

Map 24.2: Percentage of Population Receiving Optimally Fluoridated Water, 2000

these young, disadvantaged children are only half as likely to visit the dentist. This is largely because Medicaid—the health insurance program for low-income kids covering nearly one in four children in the United States—too often fails to deliver on its legal requirement to ensure available dental care to low-income children. Children covered by Medicaid are only about one-quarter as likely to obtain a dental visit in a year as they are to obtain a medical visit. Access is compromised by too few dentists participating in Medicaid, overburdened health center dental programs, and, notably, inadequate funding for this form of dental insurance. In addition, an estimated 25 million children lack dental insurance—2½ times more than lack medical coverage, and coverage trends in many states are negative. The odds of any child having dental coverage varies considerably across the United States, reflecting significant variation in state policymakers' commitment to dental

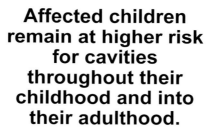

Affected children remain at higher risk for cavities throughout their childhood and into their adulthood.

coverage and differences in levels of employment-based dental insurance.

Nonetheless, there are some remarkably successful efforts to address the problems of dental disease and dental care. Among the success stories at the state level are the *Smile Alabama* program, Michigan's *Healthy Kids* program, and Washington State's *Access to Baby and Child Dentistry* project. Hundreds of local programs involving foundations, physicians, faith-based groups, dental societies, health centers, day care centers, outreach workers, WIC, and more are helping to make a difference for the children fortunate enough to be involved.

Giving America's children something to smile about, and something to smile with, can be accomplished now so that the dramatic decline in dental disease that has occurred for some can soon occur for all.

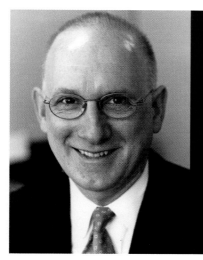

Burton L. Edelstein

Burton L. Edelstein, DDS, MPH, is a board-certified pediatric dentist and professor in the School of Dental and Oral Surgery and the Mailman School of Public Health at Columbia University in New York City. At the dental school, he is chairman of the Section on Social and Behavioral Sciences. He is the founding director of the Children's Dental Health Project, a nonprofit policy organization in Washington, DC, that advances children's oral health and access to dental care. Dr. Edelstein practiced pediatric dentistry in Connecticut and taught at Harvard for 21 years before committing to full-time health policy practice. He has served as a Robert Wood Johnson Health Policy Fellow in the U.S. Senate, worked with the U.S. Department of Health and Human Services on its oral health initiatives, chaired the U.S. Surgeon General's Workshop on Children and Oral Health, and authored the child section of the U.S. Surgeon General's Report on Oral Health in America. Dr. Edelstein is a graduate of SUNY Buffalo School of Dentistry, Harvard School of Public Health, and the Boston Children's Hospital pediatric dentistry residency program.

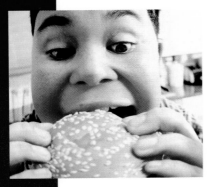

Chapter 25

William H. Dietz

Overweight:
An Epidemic

Few other pediatric health problems have increased as rapidly or pose such grave concerns as the epidemic of overweight among children and adolescents. Although many cultural and societal forces impact this epidemic, families can employ a number of strategies to help their children grow normally.

In the National Health and Nutrition Examination Survey that was completed in 2000, 15% of children 6 years of age or older were overweight.[1] Furthermore, between 1980 and 2000, the prevalence of overweight children

doubled, and the prevalence of overweight adolescents tripled. Boys and girls seem to have been equally affected, but African Americans and Mexican Americans of both genders were at greater risk than Caucasians.[1]

To assess overweight in children, clinicians use a measure called body mass index (BMI). Unlike BMI for adults, BMI for children is gender and age specific due to differences in body composition between the sexes and at different ages. BMIs for children are plotted on charts by gender and age. The location of a child's BMI on the appropriate chart is the indication of whether the child is at a healthy weight since BMI in children and adolescents increases with age. Overweight in children and adolescents is defined as a body mass index at or greater than the 95th percentile for youth of the same age and gender.

Two periods of the life cycle seem associated with an increased risk of overweight that is likely to persist into adulthood. Infants whose birth weight is 4,000 grams (8.8 pounds) or greater are more likely to become overweight children or adults than infants whose birth weight is low or within the normal range.[2] The risk that overweight in a child will persist into adulthood rises

> **Between 1980 and 2000, the prevalence of overweight children doubled, and the prevalence of overweight adolescents tripled.**

steadily throughout childhood and adolescence and seems greatest among adolescents.[3] Furthermore, overweight in adolescence has been associated with an increased risk of death among adult males and a variety of diseases such as diabetes and cardiovascular disease in both male and female adults.[4] These consequences of overweight in adolescence appear independent of the effect of adolescent weight on adult obesity.[4] Although only 25% of adult obesity begins in childhood, childhood onset of overweight that persists into adulthood seems to increase the severity of obesity in adults.[5] For example, the mean adult BMI of people who were overweight prior to 8 years of age and who became obese adults was greater than 40, or approximately 100 pounds or more overweight. Class III obesity (BMI ≥40) in adults is increasing more rapidly than lesser degrees of obesity and may reflect the impact of childhood obesity on the severity of adult obesity.[6]

Although overweight in childhood is often considered a cosmetic problem, it has substantial health consequences. In one study, over 60% of overweight 5- to 10-year-olds had at least one additional cardiovascular risk factor such as elevated blood pressure, elevated cholesterol or triglycerides, or elevated insulin levels;

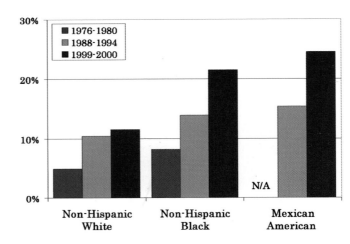

Figure 25.1: Percentage of Children, 6 to 18 Years Old Who Are Overweight

Source: Forum on Children and Family Statistics 2003

Figure 25.2: Percentage of Children, 6 to 18 Years Old Who Are Overweight by Race and Ethnicity

Source: Forum on Children and Family Statistics 2003

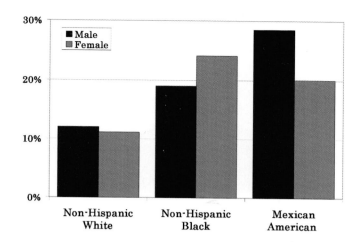

Figure 25.3: Percentage of Children, 6 to 8 Years Old Who Are Overweight by Gender and Race and Ethnicity, 1999-2000

Source: Forum on Children and Family Statistics 2003

25% had two or more cardiovascular risk factors.[7] In adults, the cluster of obesity, hypertension, hyperlipidemia (high cholesterol), and abnormal glucose tolerance has become known as the metabolic syndrome.[8] Approximately 4% of adolescents have findings consistent with this syndrome. The recent emergence of type 2 diabetes among children and adolescents represents a consequence of obesity that previously was thought to occur only in adults. Newly diagnosed type 2 diabetes in adolescents accounts for up to 45% of all new cases of diabetes in some settings.[9] The cumulative incidence of nephropathy (a kidney disorder) after onset of type 2 diabetes in adolescence approximates 40% after 15 years.[10] Therefore, the adverse consequences of type 2 diabetes will occur among adults at much younger ages than in the past. A recent review of pediatric hospitalizations for obesity-related diagnoses indicated that between 1979 and 1999, the number of patients with diabetes nearly doubled, the number with gall bladder disease and obesity tripled, and the number with sleep apnea increased five-fold.[11] The annual costs of obesity-associated diagnoses increased from $35 million (0.43% of hospital costs) in 1979 to 1981 to $127 million in constant dollars (1.7% of hospital costs) in 1997 to 1999.

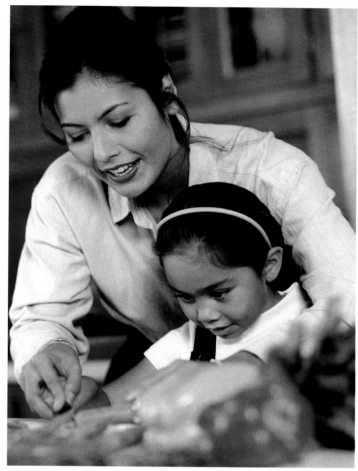

Sufficient evidence exists to justify increased physical activity, control of television time, and breastfeeding as prevention strategies for childhood obesity. In addition, a division of responsibility between parents and children regarding food choices offers a reasonable approach to reduce conflicts about eating and influence food choices by children. An advantage is that these strategies seem to have no major adverse consequences.

Substantial reductions in opportunities for children to be physically active have occurred over the last 20 years. The number of schools that offered daily physical education programs declined from 42% of schools in 1991 to 29% in 1999.[12] Nonetheless, an evidence-based review of strategies to increase physical activity recommended physical education in schools.[13] Lifestyles

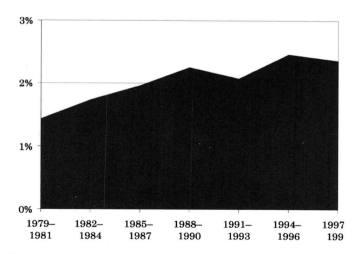

Figure 25.4: Trends in Diabetes-associated Hospital Discharges Among Children 6 to 17 Years Old

Source: Wang and Dietz 2002

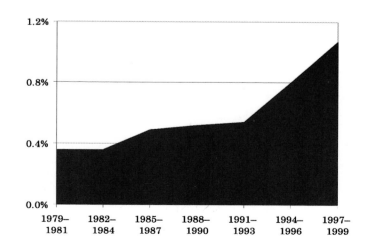

Figure 25.5: Trends in Obesity-associated Hospital Discharges Among Children 6 to 17 Years Old

Source: Wang and Dietz 2002

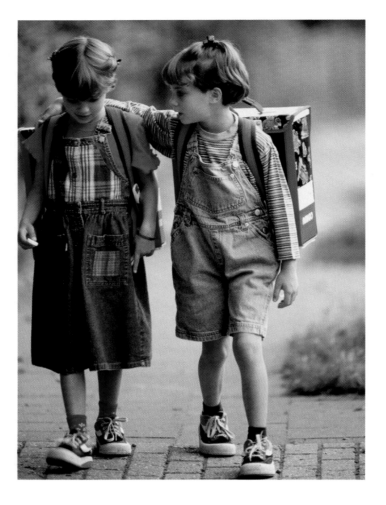

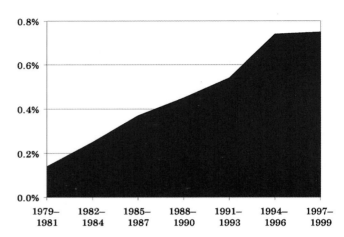

Figure 25.6: Trends in Sleep Apnea-associated Hospital Discharges Among Children 6 to 17 Years Old

Source: Wang and Dietz 2002

have also changed. For example, 20 years ago, most children walked to school. Today, fewer than 30% of children who live within a mile walk to school.[12] Some of the decline in the frequency with which children walk to school may be attributable to changes in community design that have placed schools on the edge of communities or failed to provide neighborhood sidewalks. Construction of new schools in locations accessible to multiple safe modes of transportation besides cars may offer one way to begin to restore daily physical activity to children's lives.[14]

Several studies have demonstrated an association between television viewing and overweight in children.[15-17] Furthermore, epidemiologic, clinical, and intervention studies indicate that reductions in television time seem to be an effective way to reduce the likelihood of excess weight gain[18] or to decrease weight among children or adolescents who are already overweight.[19,20] Whether television leads to excess weight through advertising's influence on food intake or by the displacement of more vigorous physical activity remains uncertain. Nonetheless, efforts to implement the American Academy of Pediatrics' recommendation to limit television time to 1 to 2 hours per day seem highly appropriate.[21]

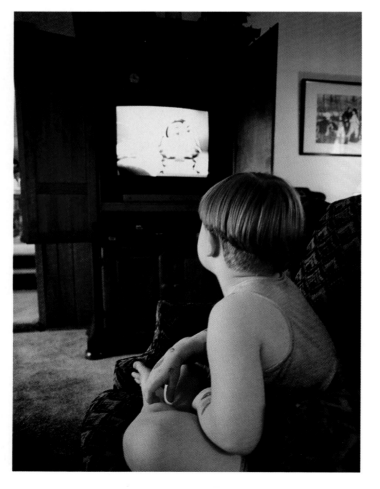

Breastfed babies seem to have a lower risk of overweight in early childhood.[22] The mechanism that explains this association remains uncertain but could involve the increased insulin-like growth factors observed in formula-fed infants, overfeeding that may result when parents urge infants to finish their bottles, or improved recognition of their infant's satiety by nursing mothers.

Other strategies that seem promising to prevent or treat overweight children include reductions in soft drink consumption, reductions in portion size, and increased fruit and vegetable consumption. At this point, there is less evidence that these strategies are effective, but there seems to be no major adverse consequences of putting these strategies in place.

The final potential strategy for the prevention of overweight is the division of responsibility for feeding.

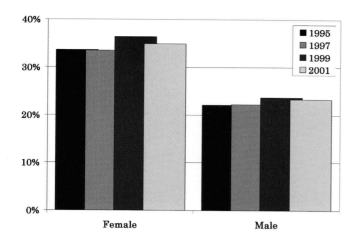

Figure 25.7: Percentage of 9th- to 12th-Grade Students Who Described Themselves as Slightly or Very Overweight by Gender

Source: Youth Risk Behavior Surveillance Survey 1995-2001

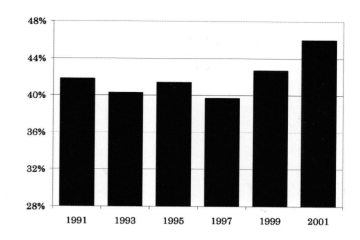

Figure 25.8: Percentage of 9th- to 12th-Grade Students Who Were Trying to Lose Weight

Source: Youth Risk Behavior Surveillance Survey 1991-2001

Parents should be in charge of what children are offered, and children should be allowed to choose what to eat among the foods offered by parents and how much to eat.[23,24] Although no data yet demonstrate that this approach prevents obesity, it may substantially reduce conflicts around feeding. Several important qualifications apply to the division of responsibility. For example, after a parent has offered foods to a child, it is not up to the parent to ensure that the child eats the food that has been offered or to make sure that the child eats enough of the food. Parents are often concerned that if the child chooses not to eat the food, he or she will be hungry. That is exactly the point. Many children have not learned that hunger is the logical consequence of their refusal to eat what is served. In early childhood, parents often are not persistent enough in their efforts to offer children new foods. Multiple attempts may be necessary before children accept a new food in their diet. Other strategies designed to regulate children's food intake may paradoxically increase the desirability of certain foods. For example, "forbidden foods" are a common strategy that parents employ to avoid giving their child high-calorie foods. However, when foods are forbidden, especially when they are available in the

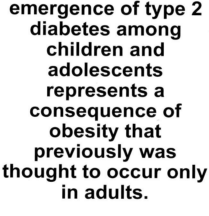

The recent emergence of type 2 diabetes among children and adolescents represents a consequence of obesity that previously was thought to occur only in adults.

house but denied to the child, those foods often become more attractive to children and more likely to be overconsumed when the child has access to them.[25] It is the child's responsibility to decide whether to eat what is offered and how much. Some research suggests that parents who try to control the quantity of their child's food intake may have children who are less capable of controlling their food intake themselves.[26] Another common strategy that parents employ to increase the intake of healthful foods such as vegetables is to make dessert contingent on how much the child consumes. This strategy may also be counterproductive because it promotes overconsumption by the child and may suggest to the child that the food he or she is being encouraged to eat is not a good food.

The emphasis here has largely been on family-related strategies to prevent obesity. It is not clear that these strategies alone will be successful in an environment that promotes inactivity and increased food consumption. Additional preventive and therapeutic strategies will likely require alterations in school and community environments that reinforce the strategies that families employ to prevent overweight and its progression.

William H. Dietz

William H. Dietz, MD, PhD, is the director of the Division of Nutrition and Physical Activity in the Center for Chronic Disease Prevention and Health Promotion at the Centers for Disease Control and Prevention (CDC). Prior to his appointment to the CDC, he was a professor of pediatrics at the Tuft's University School of Medicine, director of Clinical Nutrition at the Floating Hospital of New England Medical Center Hospitals, a principal research scientist at the Massachusetts Institute of Technology (MIT)/Harvard Division of Health Science and Technology, associate director of the Clinical Research Center at MIT, and director of the Boston Obesity/Nutrition Research Center. Dr. Dietz received his MD from the University of Pennsylvania. Following an internship at Children's Hospital of Philadelphia, he spent 3 years in the Middle America Research Unit of the National Institute of Allergy and Infectious Disease in Panama. After the completion of his residency at Upstate Medical Center, he received a PhD from MIT. He has received numerous awards and is the author of over 150 publications in the scientific literature. He is the editor of two books, including *A Guide to Your Child's Nutrition.*

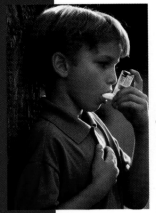

Chapter 26

H. William Kelly

Asthma

Asthma, the most common chronic disease among children in the United States today, affects approximately 5 million children. Over the past two decades, the prevalence of asthma in all children increased by 75%, while the rate in children under age 5 increased by 160%.[1] In the United States, as in other Western industrialized countries, the prevalence of asthma has reached epidemic proportions. Based on the increase in rates from 1980 to 1995, the Pew Environmental Health Commission projects that the number of people in the United States affected with asthma will exceed 20 million by 2010.[2]

One of the few encouraging signs regarding childhood asthma comes from a National Center for Health Statistics analysis that suggests that the prevalence of asthma exacerbations, commonly called asthma attacks, remained relatively stable from 1997 to 2000.[3] This possibly is due to improved therapies that help prevent exacerbations for many children. However, asthma is the third leading cause of preventable hospitalization in the United States, and hospitalizations for asthma among children 0 to 17 years old increased 1.4% per year between 1980 and 1999. Total hospitalizations for all causes for this age group actually decreased during the same time period.[4]

Asthma is a chronic inflammatory disorder of the airways that results in variable degrees of obstruction—creating coughing, wheezing, labored breathing, and shortness of breath.[5] Although the type of cells in the airways that are affected by asthma are the same in the majority of cases (and are consistent with those cells affected by allergies), asthma is expressed in sufficiently heterogeneous ways to lead some experts to call it a syndrome (a group of diseases with similar clinical symptoms). The symptoms can have a variable course from patient to patient and change significantly over time within a patient. Asthma symptoms can be intermittent, producing minimal inconvenience, or they can be persistent, creating

The prevalence of disabling asthma in children increased 232% over the past 20 years.

significant, ongoing disability. Some children experience severe disabling symptoms infrequently and have a lack of symptoms for long periods. Approximately 1.4% of all U.S. children experienced some degree of disability (inability to participate in usual activities such as school or play) from asthma in 1994 to 1995. Indeed, the prevalence of disabling asthma in children increased 232% over the past 20 years while the prevalence of disability due to all other chronic conditions in childhood increased by 113%.[6]

For children with asthma, exacerbations are the leading cause of illness, health care utilization, and direct medical costs. Indirect costs, such as loss of parental work time, also occur when a child experiences asthma exacerbations. In 1994, the total cost of asthma in children under 17 years old was estimated to be $2.25 billion.[7] However, the direct health costs of asthma are only part of the picture as non-asthma-related health costs are higher for children with asthma than for children without asthma.

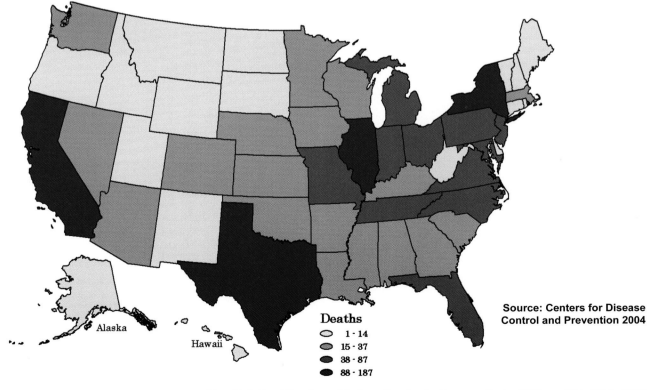

Source: Centers for Disease Control and Prevention 2004

Deaths
- 1 - 14
- 15 - 37
- 38 - 87
- 88 - 187

Map 26.1: Total Number of Asthma Deaths for Persons Under 20 Years Old, 1994 - 2000

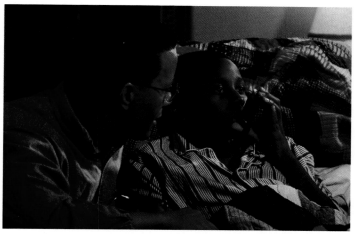

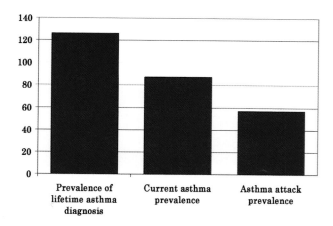

Figure 26.1: Asthma Prevalence per 1,000 for Children Under 18, 2001

Source: Centers for Disease Control and Prevention 2001

Although asthma can occur at any time, it is principally a pediatric disease with most patients being diagnosed by the age of 5 years. Up to 50% of children have symptoms as early as the age of 2 years. Up to 80% of children with asthma have allergies. In fact, the strongest predictors of the development of asthma in infants who wheeze are testing positive to respiratory allergens or having a family history of allergy or asthma.[8]

Although heredity plays a role in the risk for developing asthma, the disorder seems to develop from a combination of inherited risk and environmental factors. Exposure to secondhand tobacco smoke in infancy is one of many environmental factors that are associated with asthma.

The exact causative environmental components still elude researchers, but increasing evidence suggests that urbanization and decreased exposure to common childhood infectious agents (the so-called "hygiene hypothesis") predispose the genetically susceptible individual to have allergies and asthma when the allergic immunologic system develops instead of the immunologic system used to fight infections.[9] The first 2 years of life seem to be the most likely time for the environment to alter the immune

response system. Support for the hygiene hypothesis for asthma comes from studies that indicate that children who live on farms, and are presumably exposed to relatively high levels of bacteria, have a lower risk of developing asthma than children who live in non-farm settings. Additionally, the risk is lower for children with a large number of siblings, those enrolled into child care at an early age, and those exposed to cats and dogs early in life. The amount of antibiotics that children take also plays a role; those who take fewer have a lower risk of developing asthma.[9]

Black children have a higher prevalence of asthma than White children. In fact, between 1997 and 2000 when the prevalence rates of asthma remained relatively constant for children overall, the rates for Black children increased. However, in a study that looked at poverty, race, and urban residence as risk factors associated with pediatric asthma, being Black by itself was not independently associated with increased risk of asthma, neither was being economically disadvantaged. Rather, both Black and White children in urban settings, regardless of

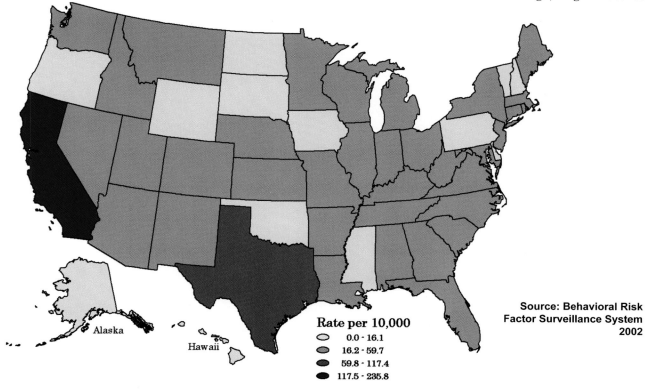

Rate per 10,000
- ○ 0.0 - 16.1
- ◐ 16.2 - 59.7
- ◑ 59.8 - 117.4
- ● 117.5 - 235.8

Source: Behavioral Risk Factor Surveillance System 2002

Map 26.2: Asthma Prevalence in Children Ages 17 and Under, 2002

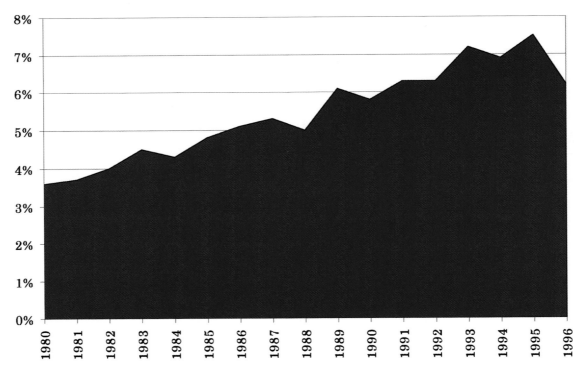

Figure 26.2: Rates for Children Under 18 with a 12-Month Prevalence of Asthma

Source: National Health Interview Survey 1999

income, were at increased risk when compared to children in nonurban settings.[10] In general, Hispanics have a lower prevalence of asthma than Non-Hispanics. However, this may change as urbanization of new immigrants occurs. For example, inner-city Puerto Rican children have a very high prevalence of asthma.[11] Very little information is available for American Indians, although a recent study indicated higher rates of hospitalization for asthma in American Indian and Alaskan Native infants younger than 1 year than for White infants.[12]

The impact of asthma is frequently greater for Black children than for others. Black children are 4 to 5 times more likely to die from asthma than White or Hispanic

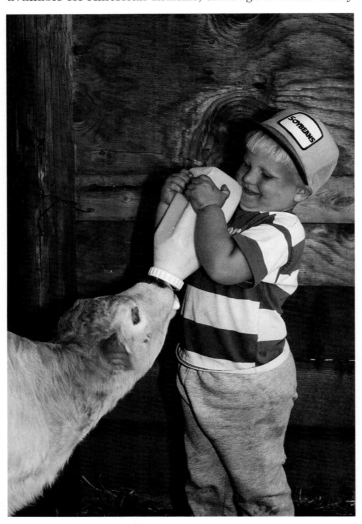

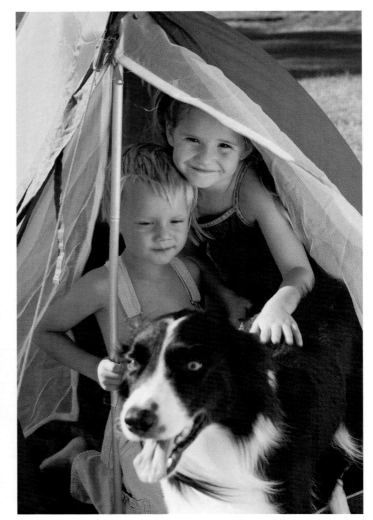

116

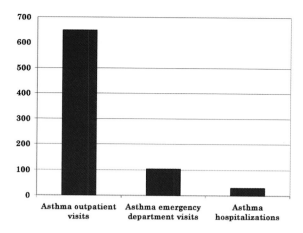

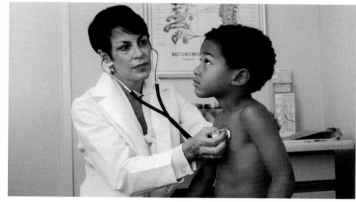

Figure 26.3: Health Care Utilization Rate by Children Under 18, Rate per 10,000 persons, 2000
Source: National Health Interview Survey 2003

children.[4] Prevalence of emergency department visits and hospitalizations reflect a similar disparity, with Black children having 3 to 4 times the rates of White children. During a 10-year period in St. Louis, 59% of all admissions for asthma in children were readmissions, demonstrating the chronic nature of asthma. Twenty-four percent of those admissions were for children with three or more admissions.[13] Black children disproportionately made up the admissions, and multiple admissions were strongly associated with being Black.

The therapy of asthma has evolved over the last 15 years to emphasize the use of preventive, anti-inflammatory medication instead of bronchodilators that treat the symptoms.[5] Prescribing anti-inflammatory therapy, principally the inhaled corticosteroids, has clearly reduced severe exacerbations of asthma that result in emergency department visits, hospitalizations, and death. Yet, studies have consistently found under-use of appropriate controller medication in Blacks and Hispanics compared to Whites of similar socioeconomic status, and poor inner-city children often do not use home management plans for acute asthma exacerbation.[14] This is due to under-prescribing by physicians as well as to issues that may be present in some economically disadvantaged families. These families may have a distrust or fear of the health

The Pew Environmental Health Commission projects that the number of people in the United States with asthma will exceed 20 million by 2010.

care system for various reasons, they may have language difficulties, and they may not see a primary physician, but wait to receive care in an emergency department when the situation is worse. Clearly, the lack of quality primary care for those with asthma is a leading contributor to the poor outcomes seen in some populations.

Recognizing the disparity in outcomes among those with asthma and the lack of successful treatment on the part of some caregivers, the National Institutes of Health and the World Health Organization have developed guidelines for the appropriate management of asthma.[5,15] These reports present the latest information on assessment and monitoring of asthma, control of factors contributing to asthma severity, pharmacological therapy, and education of patients. They stress that successful asthma control and outcomes depend on partnerships between caregivers and patients.

Additionally, a committee of national experts on asthma and health policy developed a blueprint for improving asthma outcomes in children in the United States[16] The committee identified 11 policy recommendations that encompass health care financing, patient and health care practitioner education, and strengthening of the public health infrastructure. These experts recognize that it will take a broad-based approach with coordination of activities at the national, state, and local levels to reduce the risk and burden of asthma in children as well as reduce the inequalities of asthma outcomes in underserved children.

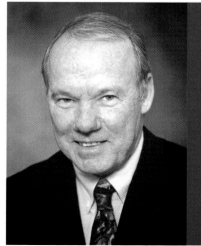

H. William Kelly

H. William Kelly, PharmD, BCPS, FCCP, is a professor emeritus of pediatrics and pharmacy at the Department of Pediatrics, School of Medicine, University of New Mexico Health Sciences Center. His bachelor's degree in pharmacy is from Washington State University, and he finished his doctorate in pharmacy and his clinical pharmacy residency at the University of Minnesota. He is director of the Albuquerque site of the Childhood Asthma Management Program, a large National Institutes of Health multicenter, longitudinal trial of treatments for asthma in children. Dr. Kelly has published over 80 research articles, reviews, and book chapters on the pharmacotherapy of asthma. He was co-editor of *Pediatric Asthma*, part of the Lung Biology in Health and Disease Series. He is a member of the National Institutes of Health's National Asthma Education and Prevention Program Science Base Committee and Expert Panel that authored the *Guidelines for the Diagnosis and Management of Asthma Update on Selected Topics 2002*. He also was a consultant for the National Heart, Lung, and Blood Institute and World Health Organization's Global Initiative for Asthma that published *Pocket Guide for Asthma Management and Prevention in Children*.

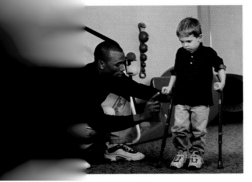

Chapter 27

Polly Arango

Special Health Care Needs

Fifty years ago, many children born with severe disabilities or serious health conditions either died in infancy or, if they survived, were often placed in institutions. Children with less severe disabilities tended to be limited in their activities and isolated at home. Fortunately, times have changed. Today in the United States, millions of children with special health care needs live with their families, go to school, overcome various challenges, and contribute to the richness of our communities.

For decades, health professionals, researchers, and policymakers struggled with ways to define and count children who have chronic health conditions and/or disabilities. In the 1980s, pediatricians and researchers created the actual phrase, "children with special health care needs." Then in the late 1990s, the federal Maternal and Child Health Bureau developed a definition: "...those who have or are at increased risk for a chronic physical, developmental, behavioral, or emotional condition and who also require health and related services of a type or amount beyond that required by children generally." A more limiting definition comes from the 1996 Supplemental Security Income Program (SSI). To determine eligibility in the program, SSI uses the following criteria: "An individual under the age of 18 shall be considered disabled for the purposes of this title if that individual has a medically determinable physical or mental impairment, which results in marked and severe functional limitations, and which can be expected to last for a continuous period of not less than 12 months."

The most common childhood disabilities are respiratory diseases (usually asthma), followed by speech and mental impairments and mental and nervous system disorders. Specific chronic conditions or disabilities can include cerebral palsy, cystic fibrosis, hearing or sight impairments,

Today in the United States, millions of children with special health care needs live with their families, go to school, overcome various challenges, and contribute to the richness of our communities.

sickle cell anemia, autism, muscular dystrophy, behavioral disorders, and hundreds of other common or rare diagnoses. In addition, many children are medically fragile and depend on devices to eat and breathe. Children with physical impairments often require wheelchairs or computerized communication equipment to carry out their daily activities.

How many children in the United States have special health care needs? Using its broad definition, the Maternal and Child Health Bureau originally estimated that 18% of all Americans under the age of 18 (12.6 million children) fell into this category. In 2000, the National Center for Health Statistics conducted the first national telephone household survey about children with special health care needs. Results showed that more than 9 million children, or 13% of all children living in the United States, had special health care needs. The federal government now uses this figure for policies and programs involving children with special health care needs.

Who are these children? The 2000 National Health Survey indicated that almost 17% of Native American children, 14% of Non-Hispanic White children, 13% of Non-Hispanic Black children, and almost 9% of Hispanic children had special health care needs. However, studies about ethnicity and disability are not

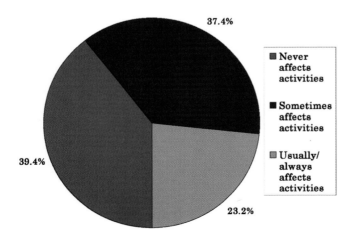

Figure 27.1: Impact of Child's Special Health Care Needs on Functional Ability, 2000

Source: Health Resources and Services Administration 2003

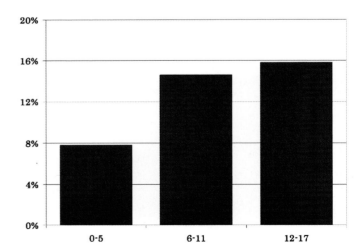

Figure 27.2: Percentage of Children with Special Health Care Needs by Age, 2000

Source: Health Resources and Services Administration 2003

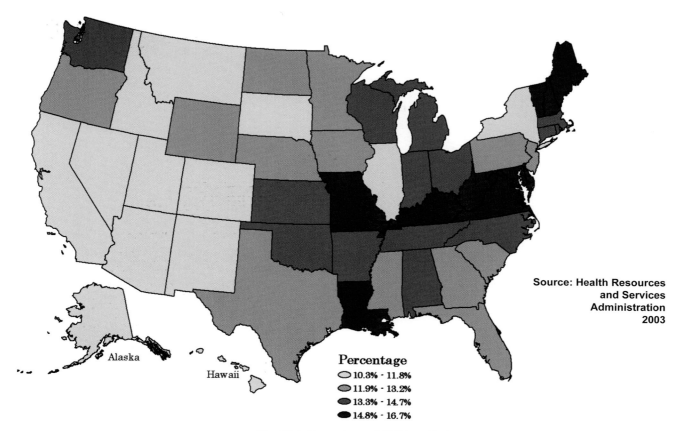

Percentage
- ⬭ 10.3% - 11.8%
- ◗ 11.9% - 13.2%
- ⬤ 13.3% - 14.7%
- ⬤ 14.8% - 16.7%

Source: Health Resources
and Services
Administration
2003

Map 27.1: Percentage of Children Under 18 with Special Health Care Needs, 2000

conclusive and are often contradictory. In addition, screening tools to find children with special health care needs often do not identify Hispanic and Black children as effectively as they do other children.

Children from low-income families are nearly twice as likely to have a serious mental or physical disability as those children whose parents have higher incomes. In addition, children with special health care needs who live in poverty have an 80% greater likelihood of being limited in their activities because of their condition than children with a similar diagnosis who are not poor. Children living in single-parent families are more likely to have special health care needs than those who live in two-parent families.

When a child has special health care needs, almost every aspect of family life is impacted: the parents' marriage, sibling relationships, finances, employment, health insurance, leisure time, and child care. Almost 21% of U.S. families who have children with special health care needs report financial problems, and close to 17% of parents have had to cut back on their work hours. Thirteen percent have stopped working altogether in order to attend to their child.

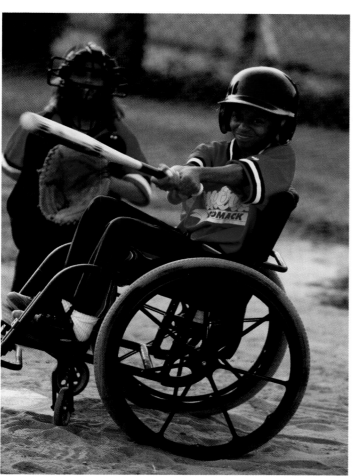

Because of the complexities of their conditions, children with special health care needs usually use more than one health care clinician and often more than one health care system. For example, an adolescent boy with cerebral palsy might retain the services of his hometown primary care physician, receive speech and physical therapy at school, and travel frequently to a large city to see his neurologist and orthopedist. In addition, children with chronic conditions are often sick. They make 26 million more visits per year to the doctor than typical children and spend 5 million more days in the hospital annually, with many restricting their daily activities for slightly more than 2 weeks per year. The public and private systems serving these children can be complicated, so one parent often becomes the case manager for the child, negotiating with the insurance plan, scheduling therapies, and meeting with special educators. More than 20% of families reported spending at least 6 hours per week providing or coordinating health care for their children. Over half the families said they provide specific health care, including

119

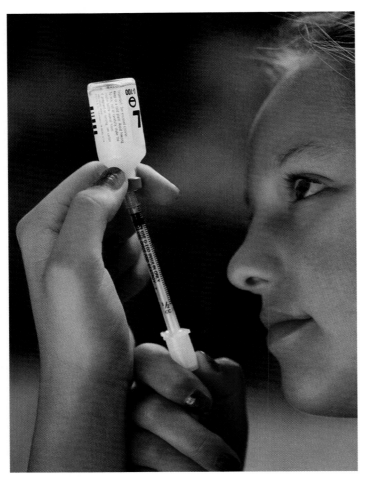

therapy, equipment repairs, and dressing changes, sometimes up to 20 hours per week.

Family-centered care, based on the premise that the family is a child's primary caregiver, has become recognized as the optimum approach by professionals who serve children with special health care needs. The principles of family-centered care include strong family-professional partnerships, information sharing, cultural competence, and consistent quality health services within a medical home for every child.

In order to receive medical care, children with special health care needs must have health insurance, either through their parents' employer-based insurance or a government program. However, almost 12% of these children did not

have health insurance at one time during a 12-month period in the year 2000. And almost 34% of families whose children had disabilities or chronic conditions indicated that the child's health insurance was inadequate; this is most likely to occur when the child is covered only by private insurance.

The following government programs are designed to assist children with special health care needs:

State Children with Special Health Care Needs Programs/Title V is the federal-state program responsible for this group of children. Depending on the state, Title V provides direct services, such as screening, diagnosis, or orthopedic services, or it works with other agencies to ensure that public and private programs are available and coordinated.

Medicaid is the federal-state health insurance program for people with disabilities or people living in poverty and offers excellent benefits to children with special health care needs. In most states, the Katie Beckett waiver can provide medical coverage and support services to children with special health care needs. Some children with complex conditions who have private health insurance can also qualify for Medicaid.

The State Children's Health Insurance Program (SCHIP) was a first step for providing health insurance to every child in America. However, there are still about 10 million children in the United States without insurance. Every state has a different name for SCHIP as well as different income requirements. Some states enroll SCHIP children in Medicaid, while others use private insurance plans.

Supplemental Security Income Program (SSI) is a federal program designed to assist families by providing monthly cash benefits to help cover the extra costs that a child with a severe physical, mental, or emotional disability adds to a family's expenses. In most states, SSI recipients also qualify for Medicaid.

Because parents find it hard to understand and negotiate this health care maze, a national grassroots organization, Family Voices, provides information at www.familyvoices.org. The Federation of Families for Children's Mental Health also provides information at www.ffcmh.org.

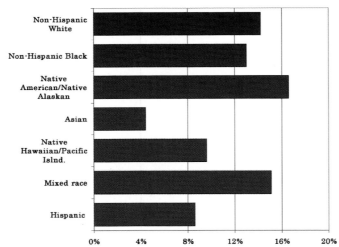

Figure 27.3: Percentage of Children with Special Health Care Needs by Race and Ethnicity, 2000

Source: Health Resources and Services Administration 2003

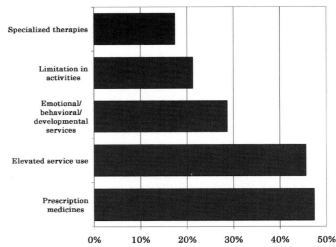

Figure 27.4: Percentage of Children with Special Health Care Needs by Type of Need or Condition, 2000

Source: Health Resources and Services Administration 2003

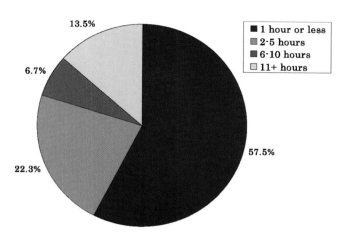

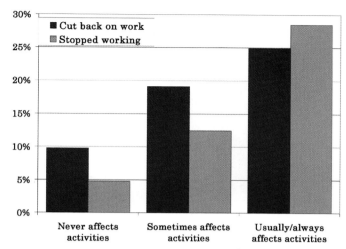

Figure 27.5: Time Spent Providing, Arranging, or Coordinating Care for a Special Health Care Needs Child per Week, 2000

Source: Health Resources and Services Administration 2003

Figure 27.6: Percentage of Parents Cutting Back or Stopping Work by Functional Ability of Special Health Care Needs Child, 2000

Source: Health Resources and Services Administration 2003

Developmental and educational programs for children with special health care needs, regulated by a federal law, the Individuals with Disabilities Education Act (IDEA), also vary across the country. An infant identified as at risk for a disability in one state might be enrolled immediately in an early intervention program for child development and family support. In another state, infants with similar conditions might be served only if they have a specific diagnosis. Toddlers with disabilities can be enrolled in developmental preschool programs.

IDEA requires that public schools provide a free and appropriate educa-tion in the least restrictive environment for all students, regardless of their disability or health condition. The purpose behind IDEA is that all supports necessary, including therapies, buses with lifts, and specially trained teachers, must be available so that every child in every school has the opportunity to learn. Because IDEA is a federal law, students and their families can pursue its implementation through legal channels if necessary. It is important to consider that an analysis of the effects of disability on children showed that these children

Almost 21% of U.S. families who have children with special health care needs report financial problems, and close to 17% of parents have had to cut back on their work hours.

missed more than 20 million days of school in 1 year in the late 1990s.

Employment practices, school district policies, state insurance regulations, and even urban planning can have positive or negative impacts on children with special health care needs and their families. Can a father take time off to attend medical appointments or school meetings for his daughter? Can youth with disabilities find summer jobs? Do neighborhood schools welcome all children, or are some students bussed away to special schools? Will a mother's health insurance cover her son's special health needs? Do neighborhood playgrounds have equip-ment that children with physical disabilities can safely use? Does a town have respite programs that give parents who have children with special needs a break from caregiving?

America's children with special health care needs are first and foremost children, living with their families, attending school and places of worship, and making friends. They are resilient and determined to grow up to be productive adults. Like all children, they are gifts to their communities and promises for our future.

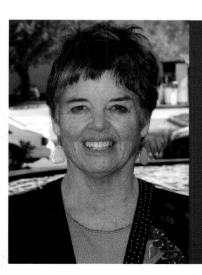

Polly Arango

For more than 20 years, Polly Arango, BA, has been a writer, speaker, and advocate for children and families in New Mexico and across the country with a special focus on making family-centered systems of care a reality for youngsters who, like her son Nick, have special health care needs. In 1992, she cofounded Family Voices, a national grassroots network with 45,000 families and friends working together to improve care for children and youth with special health needs. Arango served as its first executive director. Arango represents families and family-centered care issues in her own county and state, as well as on many national boards and commissions and in international forums. She is the coauthor of *New Mexico, a New Guide to the Colorful State; Touring New Mexico; Family/Professional Collaboration;* and *Partners at Work,* as well as many articles on health care, New Mexico, and family.

Chapter 28

Frederick P. Rivara

Impact of Injuries

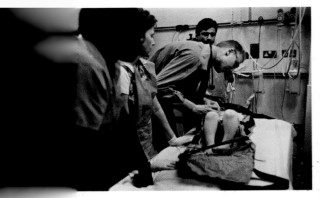

With the remarkable success of immunizations and advances in the understanding of tumor biology, the traditional causes of death from infectious diseases and cancer have been replaced by problems that may seem as insurmountable as polio 50 years ago. Injuries are now the most common cause of death and disability to children and adolescents in the United States, as well as in all industrialized countries of the world. Nearly 150,000 people of all ages die from trauma each year in the United States. For infants under 1 year, the number of traumatic deaths ranks higher than the next 10 leading causes combined. Over the last two decades, substantial progress has been made to decrease the death toll from injuries. In fact, between 1981 and 2000, the rate

of unintentional injuries among children and adolescents 19 and younger dropped by 39%. There also has been a dramatic decline in deaths due to violence. For the same age group (0-19), the violent death rate has dropped 36% from its peak 10 years ago, although this trend now seems to be plateauing.

Nevertheless, there are many indicators that we can do far better. The rate of fatal injuries among children in many countries is much lower than in the United States. For example, among children under 15 years, the rate in the United States in 1998 was more than twice that in England, Wales, and the Netherlands. Only New Zealand had a higher rate than the United States among the 11 industrialized nations studied. The overall mortality rates do not reflect the serious disparities in injury mortality rates between minority and White children in the United States. The overall rates of fatal injuries

> **Injuries are now the most common cause of death and disability to children and adolescents in the United States.**

among the 0- to 19-year-old White population are nearly twice those among their Asian counterparts. However, rates for African American children are nearly three-fold higher than those for Asian children. American Indians and Alaskan Natives have rates profoundly higher than that of Whites. These differences are even more striking for homicide; African American children and adolescents die from homicide nearly 8 times more frequently than do Asians. The fatality rate of African American children due to injury is comparable to that for children living in low- and middle-income countries, while the rates for White and Asian children are nearly as low as that of any country in the world.

The rate of injuries among males are two- to three-fold higher than among females for all racial groups, reflecting risk-taking behavior by males and our society's acceptance of it. This risk-taking behavior seems to begin

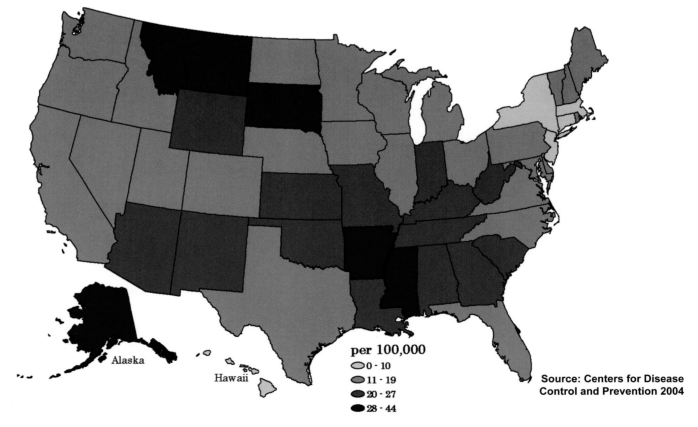

per 100,000
- ⬭ 0 - 10
- ⬤ 11 - 19
- ⬤ 20 - 27
- ⬤ 28 - 44

Alaska

Hawaii

Source: Centers for Disease Control and Prevention 2004

Map 28.1: Rate of Fatal Injuries for Children 0 to 17 Years Old, 2000

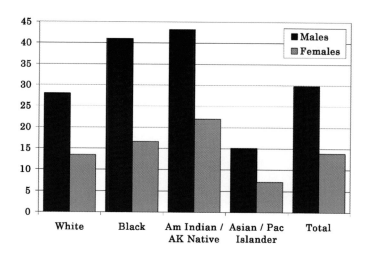

Figure 28.1: Fatality Rate From Injuries for Children Ages 0 to 19, (per 100,000), 2000

Source: Centers for Disease Control and Prevention 2004

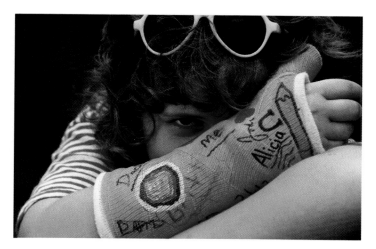

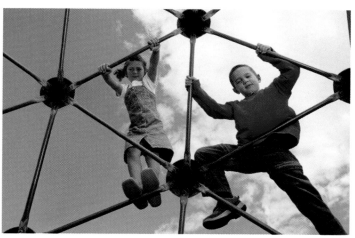

very early in the first decade of life and continues well into adulthood. It manifests itself in many different ways—drinking while driving, speeding, carrying a weapon, or using illicit drugs—all of which can lead to an increased risk of injury.

The science of injury control that has built up in the last 35 years has rightfully moved away from unfruitful searches for "accident proneness" and emphasis on parental supervision to an emphasis on the role of the environment as a modifiable risk—or protective factor—for injury. Perhaps the most important of the environmental risk factors for injury is poverty. Children living in poverty have a greater risk of nearly every type of injury than non-poor children. This includes pedestrian-motor vehicle collisions, fires and burns, drowning incidents, falls from heights, and violence. Poverty and parental educational differences account for nearly all of the increased risk of fatal injury among African American and Latino children. Poverty often means that children live in firetraps and dilapidated housing, in tenements with no

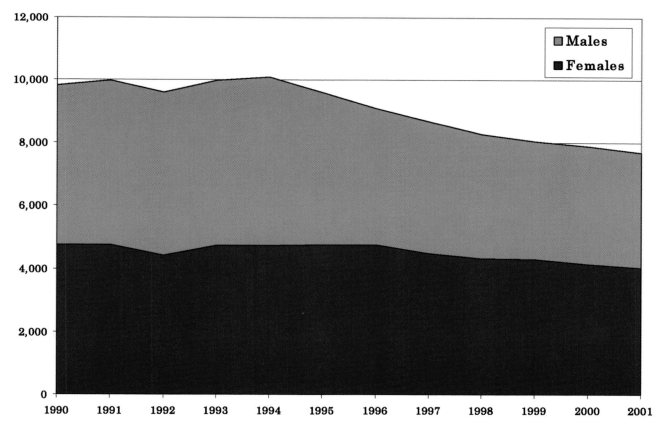

Figure 28.2: Total Fatalities From Injury for Children 17 and Under by Gender

Source: Centers for Disease Control and Prevention 2004

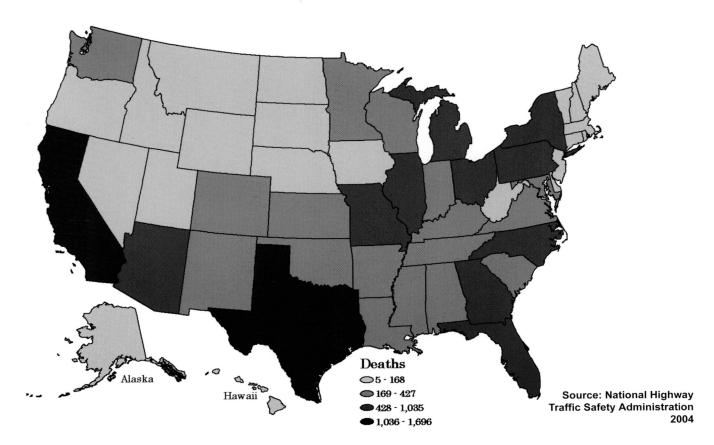

Deaths
- ○ 5 - 168
- ◔ 169 - 427
- ◑ 428 - 1,035
- ● 1,036 - 1,696

Source: National Highway
Traffic Safety Administration
2004

Alaska

Hawaii

Map 28.2: Total Automobile Accident Fatalities for Children 0 to 17 Years Old, 2002

air-conditioners, and in neighborhoods built for motor vehicles, rather than for pedestrians or bicyclists. Poverty also can mean that children live in neighborhoods with high crime rates and easy access to guns and with low levels of neighborhood cohesion and sense of self-efficacy. Lower levels of parental education mean that these children are less likely to use protective gear such as bike helmets, car seats, and personal flotation devices.

The geographic variations in injury reflect the racial and socioeconomic composition of the population. For example, the high rate of homicides in the southern United Stated is primarily due to the low socioeconomic status of African Americans in these states. Once rates are adjusted for poverty, these racial and geographic differences nearly disappear. The higher rate of fire and burn injuries in the southern United States reflects the lower income of the population and the type of housing in which children live. Geographic variations in seatbelt and car seat use are due to racial and socioeconomic differences in the population.

The response to the problem of injuries has been a relatively muted one. Just 10 years ago the Centers for Disease Control and Prevention created the National Center for Injury Prevention and Control. Today its budget is not commensurate with the magnitude of the injury problem. For example, the medical cost for hospital-admitted injuries of individuals under age 21 in the state of California alone is estimated at $822 million dollars annually. In contrast, the National Center for Injury Prevention and Control's 2003 budget was approximately $150 million and is facing cuts in 2004. There is no National Institute for Injury Control at the National Institutes of Health; injury research is scattered across different institutes and agencies within the federal government. Private foundations have largely ignored the

problem of injuries, with rare exceptions such as the Brain Trauma Foundation created by families of victims to improve injury prevention and care of people with brain injuries.

This lack of proportionate attention to the problem of injuries is surprising given the success of injury control efforts, especially those for injuries to children. Wearing bicycle helmets can reduce the risk of head injuries by 85%, and bicycle helmet promotion programs have sprung up across the country over the last decade. The promotion of motor vehicle occupant protection for children has resulted in nearly universal use of car seats for infants and a 52% reduction in fatal motor vehicle injuries in this age group, although there is almost a universal lack of use of booster seats for 4- to 8-year-olds. The 1967 Flammable Fabrics Act made children's sleepwear flame retardant and has resulted in a virtual disappearance of these types of

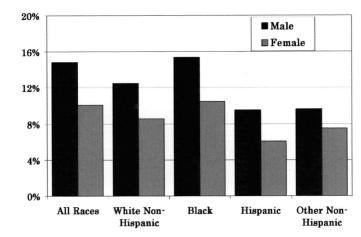

Figure 28.3: Percentage of 0 to 17 Year Old Children Experiencing Injuries, 2000

Source: Centers for Disease Control and Prevention 2004

burns. The Poison Packaging Prevention Act and the advent of poison centers have nearly eliminated fatal poisoning to children under the age of 5. Agreement by appliance manufacturers to preset water heater temperatures to safe levels has almost eliminated tap water burns to children.

Changes in behavior and attitude require time and perseverance, as evidenced by the slow but steady decline in drunk driving deaths in the United States. Over the last 10 years, for example, intoxication rates for drivers of all ages involved in fatal crashes decreased on the order of 20%. The National Highway Traffic Safety Administration estimates that minimum drinking age laws have saved more than 20,000 lives since 1975.

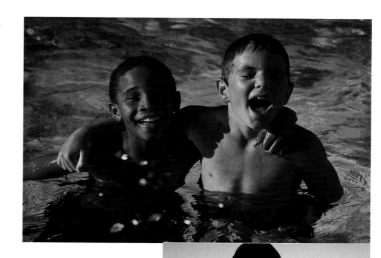

One of the most important tasks in reducing injury rates is to fully implement the strategies that have been shown to reduce injuries to children and adolescents. As many as one-third of injury fatalities in this age group could be prevented through the full implementation of available prevention strategies: motor vehicle occupant protection, traffic calming to prevent pedestrian injuries, use of bicycle helmets, safe storage of guns, adequate pool fencing and use of personal flotation devices, use of smoke detectors, and adoption of self-extinguishing cigarettes. Some of these intervention strategies require behavior change on the part of the individual, while others require behavior change at the level of com-

As many as one-third of injury fatalities. . . [to children and adolescents] could be prevented through the full implementation of available prevention strategies.

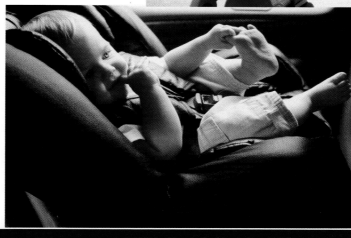

munities and legislatures. With injuries, as with many other parts of medicine, a critical need is for the fruits of the last few decades of research to be translated into actual improved health of the population. Other nations have much more fully implemented these strategies throughout their society. It is time for the United States to take the necessary steps to achieve the low injury rates seen in many other countries. Perhaps the most important change is in attitudes. All injuries to children must be viewed as preventable if we are to reduce disparities and the toll of trauma.

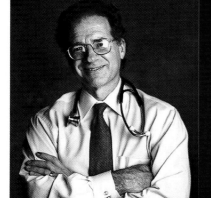

Frederick P. Rivara

Frederick P. Rivara, MD, MPH, former director of the Harborview Injury Prevention and Research Center in Seattle for 13 years, is a world-renowned expert in the field of injury prevention. The founding president of the International Society for Child and Adolescent Injury Prevention, his contributions to the field have spanned more than 25 years. Dr. Rivara received his medical degree from the University of Pennsylvania and a masters of public health degree from the University of Washington. He was a resident at the Children's Hospital Medical Center in Boston and the University of Washington. Dr. Rivara's current appointments include the George Adkins Professor of Pediatrics at the University of Washington School of Medicine, adjunct professor of epidemiology, vice-chair of the Department of Pediatrics, and Head of the Division of General Pediatrics at the University of Washington School of Medicine. He is also editor of the *Archives of Pediatrics and Adolescent Medicine*, the oldest pediatrics journal in the United States.

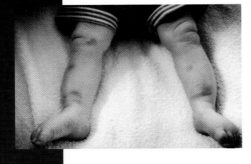

Chapter 29

Robert W. Block
and Robert M. Reece

Maltreatment

The National Child Abuse and Neglect Data Systems of the Administration for Children and Families in the U.S. Department of Health and Human Services indicated there were 903,000 known cases of child maltreatment in 2001. This translates to a rate of 12.4 victims out of every 1,000 children in the United States. As alarming as these figures are, they do not completely reflect the extent of child maltreatment and the terrible toll it takes on our children since many cases go unreported or unsubstantiated. There were 1,300 confirmed deaths due to child maltreatment in 2001, but professionals in the field believe the number was higher. Despite the prevalence of child maltreatment, funding for research, prevention, intervention, and treatment is grossly inadequate.

Child maltreatment is behavior that causes physical or emotional harm and can result from acts of commission or omission. Categories of child maltreatment include physical abuse, sexual abuse, neglect (including some forms of failure to thrive), and emotional abuse.

Physical abuse consists of inflicted, non-accidental injuries ranging from minimal to fatal. Bruising is the most commonly encountered form of physical maltreatment. Acts that cause minor physical harm frequently escalate to more damaging acts that result in severe injuries. During infancy and through early childhood, abusive head trauma is the greatest cause of mortality and long-term morbidity from physical abuse. Fractures are frequently the result of abuse, especially in the preambulatory age group. Some fracture types are particularly indicative of maltreatment. Intentional burns constitute one-fifth of all serious burns in infants and young children. Less commonly reported injuries include abdominal and chest trauma,

> **The highest rates of abuse and neglect [in 2001] were in the very youngest children—from birth to 3 years old.**

intentional poisoning, microwave burns, and insertions of foreign objects into the body.

Sexual abuse is the involvement of a child in an experience designed to bring sexual gratification or power and control to an adult or someone who is more than 4 years older than the victim. In 2001, 9.6% of victims of maltreatment had been sexually abused. There are three considerations in the diagnosis of sexual abuse. The first and most important is the child's statement (the "disclosure"). The second is the child's behavior since some sexualized behaviors are highly suggestive of sexual abuse. The third consideration is the medical examination. Although some forms of sexual maltreatment are obvious and particularly brutal, most are subtle and cause no significant anatomic changes that can be seen upon physical examination, particularly since most disclosures occur days to weeks after the abuse.

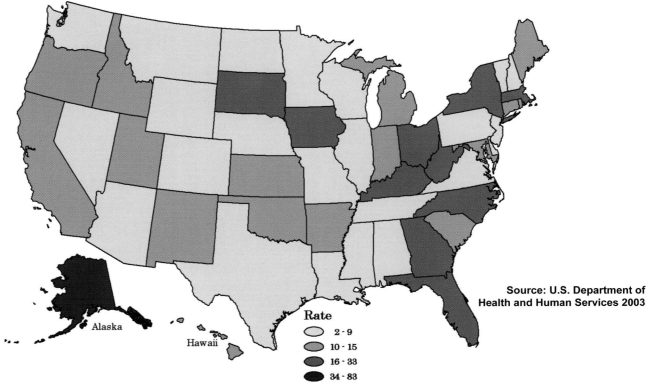

Source: U.S. Department of Health and Human Services 2003

Rate
- 2 - 9
- 10 - 15
- 16 - 33
- 34 - 83

Map 29.1: Rate of Substantiated Abuse per 1,000 Children Under 18, 2001

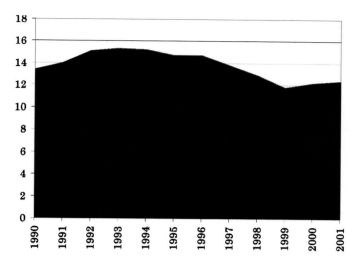

Figure 29.1: Child Victimization Rates per 1,000 Children Under 18

Source: U.S. Department of Health and Human Services 2003

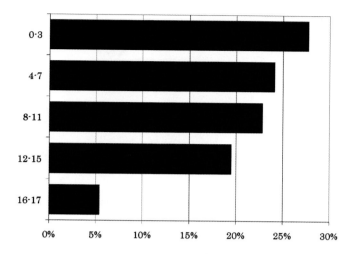

Figure 29.2: Percentage of Child Abuse Victims by Age, 2001

Source: U.S. Department of Health and Human Services 2003

Neglect refers to the failure to meet a child's basic needs or other acts of omission by adults responsible for the care of a child. Over 59% of the victims of maltreatment in 2001 experienced neglect. Approximately one-third of child fatalities that resulted from maltreatment were due to neglect. Essentially, neglect is the failure to provide food, clothing, shelter, health care, education, supervision, safekeeping, protection, and nurturing. Children who are failing to thrive may be victims of nutritional neglect, especially if poverty, psychological disorders in a parent or caregiver, or other risk factors for maltreatment are involved. Dental health neglect and exposure to vaccine-preventable diseases without immunizations may also be forms of child maltreatment. A chaotic home, domestic violence, drug use and manufacture, and other environmental factors may contribute to neglect.

Emotional abuse is a repeated pattern of damaging interactions between parent or caregiver and child that becomes typical of the relationship. In some situations, the pattern is chronic and pervasive, while in others the pattern occurs only when triggered by alcohol or other potentiating factors. Occasionally, a very painful incident, such as an unusually contentious divorce, can initiate psychological maltreatment. Psychological maltreatment of children occurs when a person conveys to a child that he or she is worthless, flawed, unloved, unwanted, endangered, or only of value in meeting another's needs. If severe or repetitious, the following behaviors may constitute psychological maltreatment: spurning (belittling, degrading), terrorizing, exploiting or encouraging inappropriate behaviors, denying emotional responsiveness, rejecting, and isolating. Victims of emotional abuse comprised almost 7% of all victims of child maltreatment in 2001.

The National Child Abuse and Neglect Data Systems indicated there were 2,672,000 reports of possible child abuse or neglect in 2001. Sixty-seven percent of these reports (approximately 1,802,000) merited investigation, and authorities substantiated 903,000 (32%) of these cases. The highest rates of abuse and neglect were in the very youngest children—from birth to 3 years old. Boys and girls were almost equally at risk for maltreatment; 48% of the victims were males, and 51.1% were females.

Children who had been victims of maltreatment in earlier years were twice as likely to experience maltreatment again.

Just over half (50.2%) of the victims in 2001 were White, 25% were African American, and 14.5% were Hispanic. Two percent of the victims were American Indians and Alaska natives, and 1.3% were Asian-Pacific Islanders. The perpetrator of all types of maltreatment was most often a woman (59.3% of all perpetrators), except in cases of sexual abuse. Mothers accounted for 40.7% of all those who committed child maltreatment, and a mother or father acting alone accounted for 80.9%.

There is no single cause of child maltreatment, but there are repeated themes in medical and sociological reviews that emphasize risk factors of parents and other caregivers. Among these are the following:

- **isolation**—a parent or caregiver living apart from or without a spouse, extended family, empathetic neighbors, or other support individuals and groups;

- **poverty**—a parent or caregiver living in a socioeconomic situation that creates barriers to access of health care, adequate day care, education, and other necessities;

- **psychological disorders**—a parent or caregiver whose abilities to nurture are compromised by depression or other mental health issues

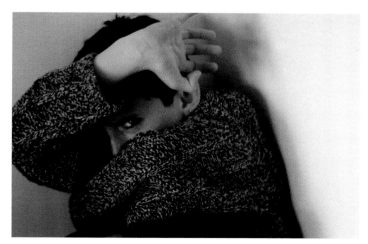

Neglect

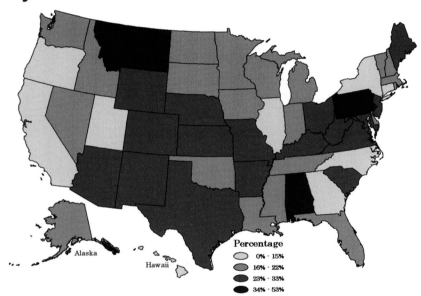

Percentage
- 0% - 28%
- 29% - 47%
- 48% - 69%
- 70% - 90%

Physical Abuse

Percentage
- 0% - 15%
- 16% - 22%
- 23% - 33%
- 34% - 53%

Sexual Abuse

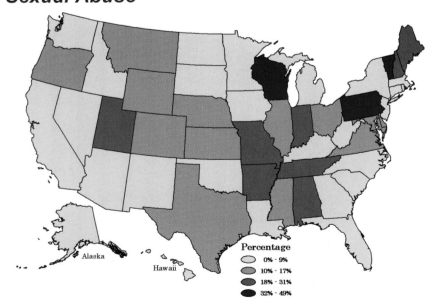

Percentage
- 0% - 9%
- 10% - 17%
- 18% - 31%
- 32% - 49%

Map 29.2: Percentage of Total Maltreatment Victims by Type of Abuse, 2001

Source: U.S. Department of Health and Human Services 2003

creating barriers to appropriate parenting;

- **alcohol and drugs**—a parent or caregiver with lifestyle habits or addictions that preclude appropriate priorities in daily living;

- **domestic violence**—a parent or caregiver living in fear, needing to make impossible choices between protecting children or self;

- **history of child maltreatment**—a parent or caregiver who was a victim of maltreatment during childhood; and

- **young age**—a parent or caregiver who is young, unprepared, and at higher risk for parenting stress and abusive reactions to infants and children.

Recognition and reporting are the first steps in dealing with child maltreatment, and appropriate personnel must then intervene in an attempt to prevent further harm to the child. Comprehensive, interdisciplinary intervention teams may include some or all of the following: a child protection services professional to receive and investigate reports of maltreatment by parents or other immediate family members; a law enforcement officer to receive and investigate cases where injury is noted and to investigate other cases that are outside the mandate of child protection services; a health care professional to perform an examination and provide treatment, if necessary; a mental health professional to facilitate accurate recall by children or to deal with the child and family, or both; and a district attorney (or similar official) to accept filings of abuse and to determine prosecutorial action. Unfortunately, many locales do not have sufficient intervention teams, and lack of funding is often the reason.

Despite warnings from expert panels that the condition is epidemic, the federal government and state governments have not recognized child maltreatment as an important priority. Well over a decade ago, the U.S. Advisory Board on Child Abuse and Neglect attempted to raise awareness with the publication of *Child Abuse and Neglect: Critical First Steps in Response to a National Emergency*. In a subsequent report, the advisory board described the system for child protection as "overwhelmed and on the verge of collapse—a collapse so grave that children will be even more seriously at risk than they are now." These reports were ignored.

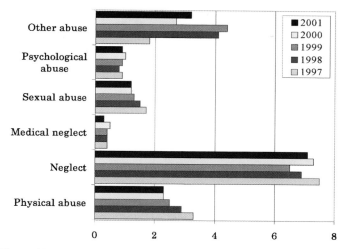

Figure 29.3: Child Victimization Rates by Abuse Type, per 1,000 Children Under 18

Source: U.S. Department of Health and Human Services 2003

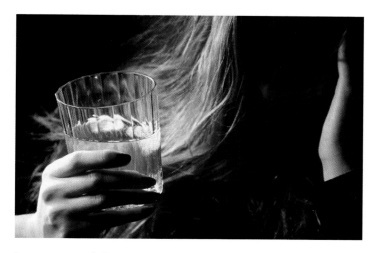

Media coverage, which could be a source of information about the incidence of child maltreatment and the facts of particular cases, is lacking. Because child maltreatment is unpleasant, sometimes journalists are reluctant to report these stories, and many times, they create a media circus that loses the true tragedy in the midst of diversions by lawyers or others. Some reporters and news journals distort fact in favor of market share. Further obscuring the public's knowledge about the extent of child maltreatment are the Web sites and postings on the Internet that argue vehemently about false allegations, witch hunts, child abuse intervention "cults," and other issues.

Mothers accounted for 40.7% of all those who committed child maltreatment [in 2001], and a mother or father acting alone accounted for 80.9%.

A 2002 query to a National Library of Medicine database using the term *child abuse* yielded 44,087 titles of medical journal articles, while *childhood cancer* yielded only 16,868. Almost half of the cancer citations indicated studies supported by the U.S. government's Public Health Service, but few child maltreatment studies receive government support. Large, multi-site, long-term, follow-up studies are common in cancer research, but not one exists for the more prevalent health harm of child maltreatment. Prioritized funding of research on child maltreatment prevention, intervention, and treatment would optimize child health and safety.

A growing number of health care providers, scientists, and others recognize that there is an urgent need for attention to child maltreatment in the United States. They understand that there must be publicly funded, carefully designed studies in areas including, but not limited to, the biomechanics of injury to infants and children; the incidence of inflicted, non-accidental injuries of various types at different ages; new diagnostic techniques, imaging, and laboratory testing; risk factors; intervention plans that are most effective; and cost-effective prevention efforts. While a few studies are underway, total funding for these badly needed projects is not enough to help turn the tide of child maltreatment. Legislators and other policymakers must recognize and understand the toll that child maltreatment is taking on our smallest and most vulnerable citizens.

Robert W. Block and Robert M. Reece

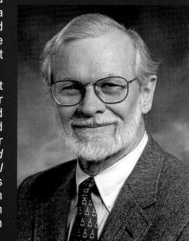

Robert W. Block, MD, is the chair of the American Academy of Pediatrics Committee on Child Abuse and Neglect. He is professor and Daniel C. Plunket Chair, Department of Pediatrics, University of Oklahoma, Tulsa Campus. He is the chief child abuse examiner for the state of Oklahoma, serving on the Board of Child Abuse Examination and the state's Child Death Review Board. Dr. Block helped develop the Tulsa Children's Justice Center, a multidisciplinary child abuse evaluation center affiliated with the University of Oklahoma and the Child Abuse Network, Inc., a not-for-profit community agency that coordinates the center team.

Robert M. Reece, MD, is clinical professor of pediatrics at Tufts University School of Medicine and visiting professor of pediatrics at Dartmouth Medical School. He has worked as a clinician, teacher, and researcher in child maltreatment since the early 1970s. Dr. Reece is the editor of the books *Child Abuse: Medical Diagnosis and Management* and *Child Abuse Treatment: Common Ground for Mental Health, Medical and Legal Professionals*. He edits *The Quarterly Child Abuse Medical Update*, has published 39 medical journal articles, and contributed 20 book chapters. The American Academy of Pediatrics recognized him for outstanding service to maltreated children in 2000, and the Helfer Society presented him the award for distinguished contributions in the field of child maltreatment in 2003.

Chapter 30

Paul M. Darden

Immunization Delivery

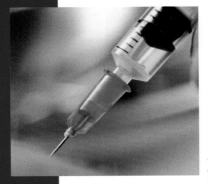

The impact of immunization on the health of children is perhaps best indicated with this quotation: "The two public health interventions that have had the greatest impact on the world's health [are] clean water and vaccines."[1] In the past 50 years, vaccine-preventable childhood diseases have gone from common and unremarkable (though sometimes deadly) to uncommon and remarkable.[2,3] Perhaps the most notable achievements in immunization delivery have been the eradication of smallpox and the planned eradication of polio from the world.[4-6]

There have been many changes, some failures, and numerous successes in the delivery of immunizations to U.S. children in the last 20 years.[7,8] We have substantially increased the types of vaccines and the immunization rates of

preschool children.[7-9] Even with our successes, we remain short of our goals.[10,11] Yet as we reach our goals, we cannot be complacent. Vaccine-preventable diseases will return if our commitment to immunization wanes.[12,13]

The childhood immunization schedule in the United States has changed substantially over the last 20 years. In 1985, three separate vaccines protected against seven diseases. A child received only one injection during an immunization visit and only five injections over the first 2 years of life.[14] Today, the immunization schedule is much more complex. There are now seven recommended vaccines that protect against eleven diseases. With the introduction of the combination

> **Perhaps the most notable achievements in immunization delivery have been the eradication of smallpox and the planned eradication of polio from the world.**

vaccine for diphtheria, tetanus, pertussis, hepatitis B, and polio,[15] the number of injections recommended at a visit has declined for the first time in many years. Now, instead of five injections at some visits in the first year of life, as was the case just a few years ago, there is a maximum of three injections per visit.[14,16-19] A common complaint of both immunization providers and parents is too many injections at one visit.[20,21] Combination vaccines can and should be used to reduce the number of injections.[22,23]

Private health providers immunize most children in the United States.[24] In 2002, 60% of 2-year-old children received all immunizations from the private sector, with an additional 25% receiving

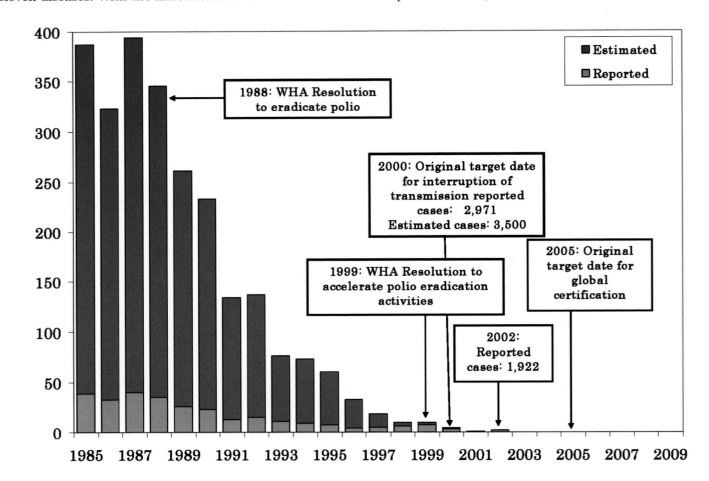

Figure 30.1: Worldwide Progress in Polio Eradication, Number of Estimated and Reported Polio Cases (in Thousands)

Source: World Health Organization 2003

About Children

Disease	Baseline 20th century annual morbidity*	2000 morbidity	Percent decrease
Smallpox	48,164	0	100.00
Diphtheria	175,885	1	99.99
Pertussis	147,271	7,867	94.70
Tetanus	1,314	35	97.30
Polio (paralytic)	16,316	0	100.00
Measles	503,282	86	99.98
Mumps	152,209	338	99.78
Rubella (CRS)	823	9	98.91
Haemophilus influenza	20,000	1,398	93.01

*Baseline time periods vary by disease depending on the date the appropriate vaccine became available and the availability of data.

Figure 30.2: Annual Morbidity for Nine Vaccine-preventable Diseases

Source: Centers for Disease Control and Prevention 1999, 2000

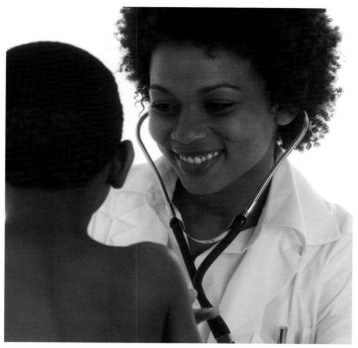

immunizations from a mix of public providers (such as state health departments) and private providers or in other settings.[25]

The U.S. Department of Health and Human Service's Healthy People 2010 goals include goals for immunization of children. The objective for a series of vaccines is to increase to 80% the proportion of young children and adolescents who receive all vaccines that have been recommended for at least 5 years for universal administration.[11] For young children ages 19 to 35 months, this means that they should have received four injections of the combination vaccine for diphtheria, tetanus, and acellular pertussis (previously known as DTP and now called DTaP), three of polio vaccine, one of measles vaccine, three of *Haemophilus influenzae* type b (Hib) vaccine, three of hepatitis B vaccine (Heb B), and one of varicella vaccine. In 2002, only 66% of children were up-to-date on this series of vaccines. However, the varicella vaccine has only recently been recommended for routine use,[26,27] and the proportion of children who receive this vaccine is increasing rapidly.

The Healthy People 2010 goal for selected individual vaccines (DTaP, Hib, HepB, measles-mumps-rubella [MMR] vaccine, polio vaccine, and varicella vaccine) is that 90% of 2-year-olds receive all recommended doses.[11] The United States is already achieving the goal of 90% for the Hib vaccine, MMR vaccine, and polio vaccine and is at 89.9% for a fourth, the HepB vaccine. We have not met the goal for the combination vaccine for diphtheria, tetanus, and pertussis (DTaP) and the varicella vaccine. However, coverage of the recently introduced varicella vaccine increased by over 14 percentage points to 80.6% between

2001 and 2002 and should achieve 90% coverage well before 2010.[7,28] Achieving the recommended four doses of the DTaP vaccine has been an elusive goal. Four doses of the previous DTP vaccine and now the DTaP vaccine have been recommended in the first 2 years of life for more than 20 years.[14] The maximum coverage for four DTaP doses occurred in 1998 when the United States reached an 83.9% immunization rate.[27] In 2002, only 81.6% of 2-year-olds had received at least four doses of DTaP.[28]

Measles and the measles vaccine illustrate the benefits and potential pitfalls of immunization. Prior to the

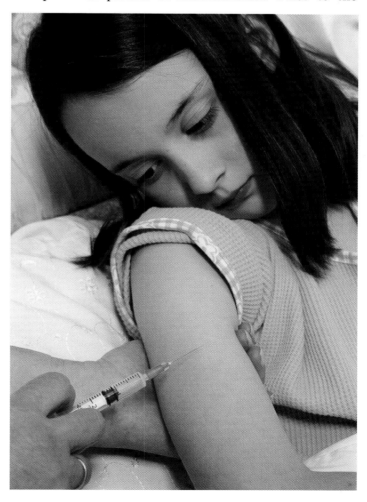

Factor	Year				
	1985	1995	2003*	2004**	2004***
Diseases	7	9	11	11	12
Vaccines	3	5	7	7	8
Maximum injections at one visit	1	2 or 3	5	3	3 or 4
Injections over the first 2 years	5	8-12	20	14	16-17

* Without the combination vaccine (Combvax) for influenza and hepatitis B
** With the combination vaccine (Pediarix) for diphtheria, tetanus, acellular pertusis (Dtap), polio (IPV), and hepatitis B (HepB)
*** Routine influenza vaccine to be introduced in the second half of 2004

Figure 30.3: Number of Diseases, Vaccines, and Injections by Year

Source: Centers for Disease Control and Prevention 1983, 1986, 1995, 2004

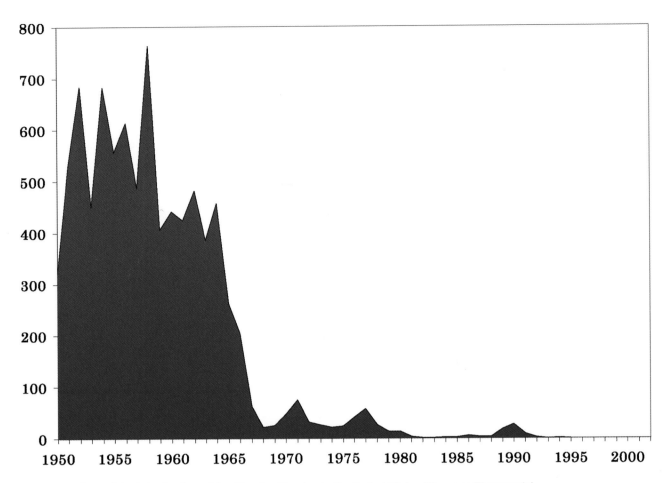

Figure 30.4: The Effect of the Introduction of the Measles Vaccine in the United States (Cases in Thousands)

Source: Centers for Disease Control and Prevention 1999, 2004

introduction of measles vaccine, there were an estimated 3 to 4 million cases of measles annually with 500,000 cases and 500 deaths reported to the Centers for Disease Control and Prevention (CDC).[29] After the licensure of the first measles vaccine in 1963, the incidence of measles fell precipitously, and, in 1983, only 1,497 cases of measles were reported. There was a resurgence of measles cases in 1989 to 1991; over those years, there were 55,622 cases and 123 deaths reported. The major reason for this epidemic of measles was unvaccinated children.[8,30-32] With the subsequent redoubling of immunization efforts spurred by this epidemic, measles incidence substantially decreased.[33] In fact, today the transmission of measles within this country has ended; in 2002, there were only 44 cases of measles reported in the United States. Most of the 44 cases were imported or directly linked to an imported case of measles.[30]

Polio should be the next disease eradicated from the world.[5,6] With the introduction of poliovirus vaccine in the United States in 1955, cases of polio dramatically decreased. The last case in the United States caused by wild virus occurred in 1979, and the last cases in all of the Americas were in 1991.[34,35] The current target for the interruption of transmission of poliovirus worldwide is 2004 to 2005.[5,6]

Children who live in poverty are much less likely to receive all routine immunizations when compared to children above the poverty level.[36-38] Minority children in the United States, especially Black children, are less well-immunized than White children.[39-41] Recently, data from the CDC's 1999 National Immunization Survey documented a

continuing racial disparity in immunization rates with 81% of White children being fully immunized as opposed to 74% of Black children.[42]

Parents can refuse to have their children vaccinated on religious or philosophical grounds in most states.[43,44] The exemptors, as the unvaccinated children are called, are not randomly distributed and occur in clusters. Exemptors are more likely to get disease, and schools with a greater proportion of exemptors are more likely to have outbreaks of disease. Less intuitive is that vaccinated children are also at risk from exemptors. In a study of a measles outbreak, at least 11% of the children who had the disease

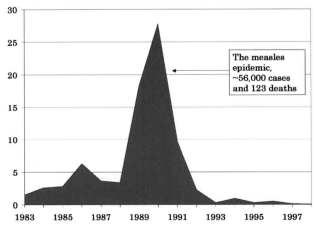

Figure 30.5: The Measles Epidemic in the United States (Cases in Thousands)

Source: Centers for Disease Control and Prevention 1999, 2004

had been vaccinated but still acquired infection from an exemptor.[43]

There are proven methods to increase immunization rates, and interventions that affect immunization rates can act at different levels of the system. The CDC's Task Force on Community Preventive Services has published assessments of interventions and recommendations for interventions to improve immunization rates.[45,46] It is clear that education alone is not effective in increasing rates. Reminding parents and children that they are due or overdue for immunizations, requiring immunization by law to attend school or daycare, and implementing programs that educate the community and include other interventions have all been found to be effective.[46] There also is strong evidence that reducing immunization costs to the family and expanding access to immunization services increase immunization rates.[46]

The U.S. Public Health Service's National Vaccine Advisory Committee has published standards for pediatric immunization practices based on evidence and expert opinion.[47] The standards target health care professionals, including the many people in clinical settings other than providers who share responsibility for vaccinating children. These standards address the availability of services, assessment of vaccination status, communication of vaccine benefits and risks, handling and administration of vaccines, and the implementation of strategies to improve vaccination coverage.[47]

Providers should implement the CDC's Task Force on Community Preventive Services' recommendations and the Public Health Service's Standards for Pediatric Immunization Practices. Using methods of quality improvement of service delivery in providers' offices is an effective means to implement these interventions.[48-50] Bordley et al., in a trial of office-based quality improvement in eight practices in North Carolina, found a 12 percentage point improvement in complete immunizations in 2-year-old children.[48]

Immunization registries, which are computerized information systems that collect data about all children within a geographic area such as a county or state, have

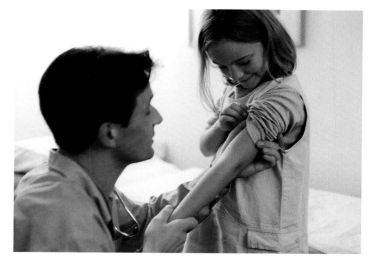

tremendous potential for assessing and improving immunization rates.[51-54] Identifying areas with low immunization coverage would facilitate targeting intervention efforts where they are most needed. One of the Healthy People 2010 objectives is that 95% of children less than 6 years of age become part of an immunization registry.[11] Registries have been in development in the United States for over a decade. While considerable planning and resources have been devoted to their development, information on their current status and use is hard to obtain.[55-57]

The successes and opportunities in immunization delivery are tremendous. The use of immunization registries is the most likely way that the United States will progress from its present plateau in immunization rates. For registries to be effective, doctors in private practice must participate since they are the immunization providers to most children. Ensuring that all immunization providers participate in registries will require that the federal government and professional organizations take a leadership role to make sure that registries are useful, easy to use, and affordable. The success of registries also will depend on the commitment of resources to enable entry of existing information to create a viable tool for immunization providers and others. This country must provide the infrastructure to ensure optimal delivery of the powerful tool of immunization.

> **The use of immunization registries is the most likely way that the United States will progress from its present plateau in immunization rates.**

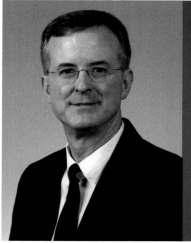

Paul M. Darden

Paul M. Darden, MD, is professor of pediatrics at the Medical University of South Carolina where he also has a joint appointment in the department of biometry and epidemiology. Dr. Darden is a past president of the Ambulatory Pediatric Association, an editorial board member of *Ambulatory Pediatrics*, and a reviewer for numerous professional journals. Among his five ongoing research projects are two funded by the Centers for Disease Control and Prevention to address issues of immunization delivery. Dr. Darden is widely published in the professional literature, most frequently in the areas of pediatric epidemiology, immunization delivery, and health care services.

Dr. Darden received his MD at the University of Texas Southwestern Medical School and completed his residency at the Children's Medical Center in Dallas. He has held fellowships at McGill University in Montreal and at the University of North Carolina.

Chapter 31

Peter G. Szilagyi

Health Insurance

A merica is unique among developing countries in terms of its health insurance system. In most countries, the government provides health insurance. In the United States, however, a patchwork of private and public programs that vary greatly in terms of policies, covered benefits, restrictions, and prices comprise our health insurance system. Some insurance plans have broad coverage that includes hospital, outpatient, and home-based services. Other plans cover only limited health care services and require families to use certain providers. To provide coverage for their children, many parents must learn how to sign up for health insurance, select among plans, maintain their coverage, find health services consistent with their coverage, pay for certain services up front or afterwards, deal with changes in benefits, and generally advocate for their children within their health insurance system. Although the system

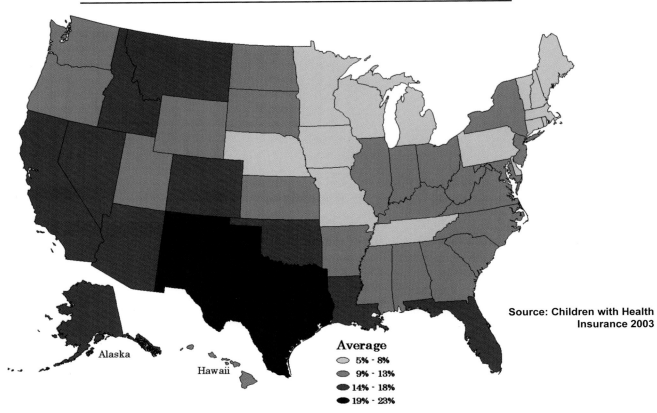

Source: Children with Health Insurance 2003

Average
- 5% - 8%
- 9% - 13%
- 14% - 18%
- 19% - 23%

Map 31.1: Percentage of Uninsured Children in 2001

works well for many American children, millions are left out entirely, or their families struggle to maneuver within the complicated programs.

In 2001, over 68% of the children in the United States less than 19 years old were covered by private insurance. Of those covered by private insurance, 93% were in employer-based health plans in which parents obtained health insurance for their children through their employment. Government-sponsored programs covered more than one-fourth of the children; most (86%) of these children were enrolled in Medicaid or the State Children's Health Insurance Program (SCHIP). Younger children were more likely than older children to have government-sponsored health insurance; therefore, a higher percentage of older children were uninsured. Twelve percent of all children below 19 years of age, or 9.2 million children, had no insurance coverage at all.

> **Although the system works well for many American children, millions are left out entirely, or their families struggle to maneuver within the complicated programs.**

The percentage of children who lacked health insurance varied widely across states. In some states (Minnesota, Missouri, Rhode Island, and Vermont), less than 6% of the children were uninsured, while in other states (New Mexico and Texas), more than 20% had no coverage. Some of this variation reflects demographic differences in children. Certain populations were more likely to be uninsured: adolescents, poor children, racial and ethnic minority children (particularly Hispanic children), foreign-born children, and children residing in central cities. It is important to note that even though Non-Hispanic White children were less likely than other racial and ethnic groups to be uninsured, there were more Non-Hispanic White children than children of other races and ethnicities; therefore, the largest group of uninsured children consisted of Non-Hispanic White children. In addition, 28% of young adults (18- to 24-year-olds) were uninsured.

Between 1987 and 1997, the percentage of children who lacked health insurance remained relatively stable despite some efforts to expand Medicaid coverage for low-income children. The SCHIP program began in 1997, and, in the ensuing 4 years, the percentage of children who were uninsured declined. Recent data from the 2002 Census show that the overall percentage of children who were uninsured dropped slightly from 12.1% in 2001 to 11.6% in 2002, even though the percentage of adults who were uninsured increased during this period (14.6%-15.2%).

Several major forces have shaped the health insurance experience of American children. One is Medicaid, the government health insurance program for low-income children that started in 1965 and expanded substantially in the 1980s. Medicaid now insures more children than any other single insurance provider. It covered more than 24 million children less than 20 years of age in 2000. More than 40% of low-income children and one in five children overall were covered by Medicaid or SCHIP. While eligibility depends on income and varies widely across states, the benefits package of Medicaid is generally very broad. Medicaid covers services often not covered by private insurance such as developmental, school, and specialty services and home health care. With the economic downturn since 2000 and rising Medicaid costs, states are under increasing pressure to reduce benefits or otherwise restrict Medicaid expenditures. One often misunderstood fact is that although children comprise the largest group of Medicaid enrollees (47% in 1999), they consume a small proportion of Medicaid expenditures (16%).

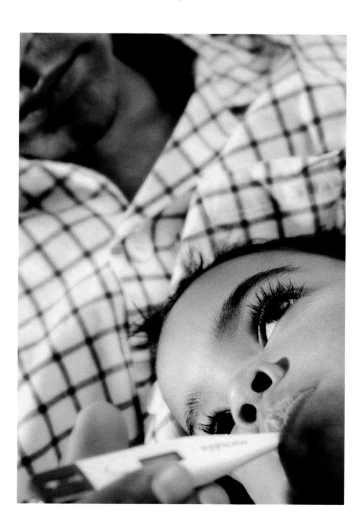

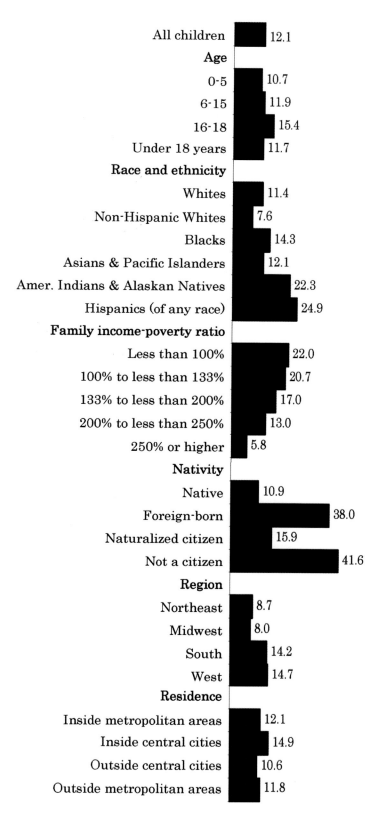

Figure 31.1: Percentage of Children Who Were Uninsured in 2001
Source: Children with Health Insurance 2003

A second major force in health insurance is SCHIP. This program began in 1997 in a national attempt to provide insurance for low-income, uninsured children whose family incomes were high enough to make them ineligible for the usual Medicaid benefits. Benefits through SCHIP can be administered through an expansion of Medicaid that incorporates some children who were previously ineligible or through private insurance that is paid for by the SCHIP program. Like

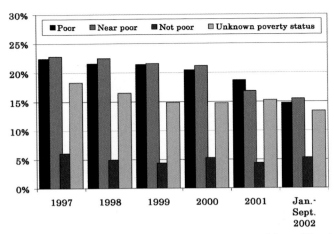

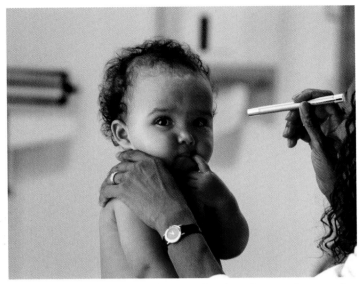

Figure 31.2: Percentage of Persons Under 18 Years of Age without Health Insurance Coverage, by Poverty Status

Source: Trends in Health Care Coverage 2003

Medicaid, SCHIP is a state-run program in which eligibility, type of program, and benefit structure all vary across states. This important source of insurance for mostly low-income, working families reached more than 5 million children in 2002. However, many children who are eligible for either Medicaid or SCHIP are not enrolled. Enhanced outreach and reduction of barriers could increase enrollment in these public programs and reduce the ranks of the uninsured.

A third major force in children's health insurance involves the rise in managed care plans. These diverse plans range from staff model health maintenance organizations (HMOs), in which salaried physicians provide primary care to defined populations, to independent practice association arrangements, in which an open-panel organization of independently practicing physicians contracts for services with an HMO. The major trends regarding HMOs involve (a) a rapid rise in the number of these plans in the 1980s and 1990s, (b) initial cost savings followed by smaller cost savings more recently, (c) increased consumer sovereignty and concerns about restrictions of services due to HMOs, and (d) increasing variety and complexity of the makeup of managed care organizations. Multiple studies have demonstrated that different managed care arrangements can affect the utilization of services for children in both positive and negative ways depending on the level of

benefits, the amount of cost-sharing for patients, the types of physician payments, the level of restrictions regarding referrals, and other factors. Managed care will continue to evolve, but it is here to stay. In 2001, about 28% of U.S. children less than 18 years old were enrolled in HMOs, and 52% of Medicaid enrollees less than 20 years old were enrolled in Medicaid managed care plans.

Health insurance does matter for children and adolescents. Numerous studies that compare insured and uninsured children have indicated that uninsured children have poorer access to health services, fewer visits to health providers, less preventive care, poorer quality of care in many instances, and, often, worse health outcomes. Furthermore, studies of Medicaid programs, Medicaid program expansions, pre-SCHIP state programs, and, very recently, SCHIP programs have shown that providing health insurance to children enhances their receipt of health care services, particularly preventive and ambulatory services. Insurance reduces unmet needs for health services and improves quality in several areas such as immunization delivery, receipt of preventive care, continuity of care with the same provider, asthma treatment, receipt of medications, and parent satisfaction.

Health insurance is particularly important for certain vulnerable populations of children. One such population is children with special health care needs, which includes

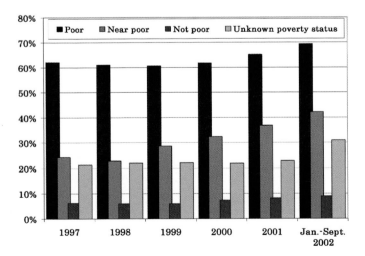

Figure 31.3: Percentage of Persons Under 18 Years of Age With Public Health Plan Coverage, by Poverty Status

Source: Trends in Health Care Coverage 2003

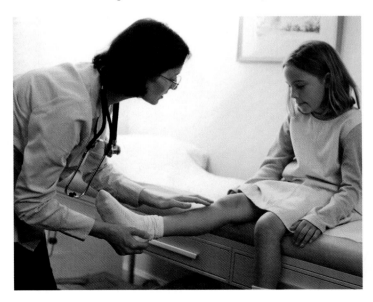

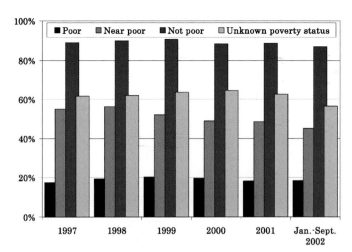

Figure 31.4: Percentage of Persons Under 18 Years of Age with Private Health Insurance Coverage, by Poverty Status

Source: Trends in Health Care Coverage 2003

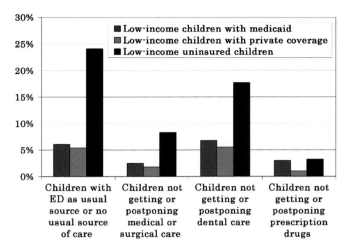

Figure 31.5: Access to Care Among Low-income Children, by Insurance Status, 1997

Source: Health Care Access and Use 2001

children with chronic medical, behavioral, developmental, or mental health problems. This group requires higher use of services, as well as more specialized and ancillary health services such as home nursing and developmental services. They also frequently require durable medical equipment. Although children with special health care needs are a bit more likely to have health insurance than other children, the uninsured special-needs children are at greater risk for poor outcomes than are other uninsured children. Special-needs children who have inadequate benefits from their insurance plans are also at risk for poor outcomes. Adolescents, who are more likely to be uninsured and also more likely to engage in risky behaviors, are another vulnerable population. This group would benefit from preventive care and counseling during health visits. A third vulnerable population involves immigrant children and their families. This group has a high rate of being uninsured as well as language, cultural, and, often, logistical barriers to the receipt of health care.

To help ensure that children receive the health care they need, state-based incremental reforms aimed at strengthening public health insurance programs (Medicaid and SCHIP) could include improving linkages

> **Uninsured children have poorer access to health services, fewer visits to health providers, less preventive care, poorer quality of care in many instances, and, often, worse health outcomes.**

across programs to prevent children from falling through the cracks; streamlining application and administrative procedures to enroll eligible children and prevent children from falling out of the ranks of the insured; providing more outreach to vulnerable populations; monitoring the performance of programs, particularly for vulnerable populations; and improving the funding stream to ensure adequate funding for enrolled and eligible children. Reforms at the private insurance level should involve re-examining the current trend toward greater cost-sharing and more restricted benefits for children's services, providing linkages and coordinated programs to complement other children's services, and monitoring managed care performance. Of course, providers and families should stress cost-effective care and preventive care to minimize unnecessary health care expenses and counter the seemingly inexorable rising costs of health insurance.

A national measure of our commitment to children is how well we provide them with health care. Health insurance opens the door to the needed care. Receipt of adequate health care, in turn, leads to better outcomes, improved development, and reduced health problems down the road.

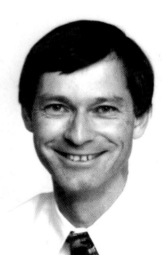

Peter G. Szilagyi

Peter G. Szilagyi, MD, MPH, is professor of pediatrics and chief of the Division of General Pediatrics at the University of Rochester School of Medicine and Dentistry. He is a general pediatrician who provides primary care to his patients within the primary care practice at the medical center. He is also an experienced health services researcher and has done pioneering studies evaluating health care for uninsured children, the impact of managed care, the impact of statewide health insurance programs on the health of children, the impact of the State Children's Health Insurance Program, and the financing of health services for vulnerable children. His research has contributed to state and national health insurance reform. He has served on a variety of advisory boards, including a health systems study section for the Agency for Healthcare Research and Quality. He also has performed numerous advisory roles for the Centers for Disease Control and Prevention regarding vaccine-related issues, and he served on the Subcommittee on Family Impacts of Uninsurance for the Institute of Medicine's Committee on Consequences of Uninsurance. This subcommittee produced the publication *Health Insurance Is a Family Matter*.

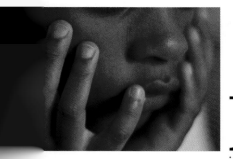

Chapter 32

Kelly Kelleher

Mental Health

Mental health problems are the most common, costly, chronic, and disabling conditions confronting American children today. Dramatic declines were recorded in many of the major infectious and medical problems afflicting children in the last century. However, mental health problems are not declining at all and may be increasing.[1] Most scientists estimate that mental health problems affect one out of five children of school age in the United States[1-4] and an even larger percentage of youth in juvenile justice facilities, child welfare services, special education, and medical facilities.[5-7] In fact, as public mental health institutions and services have diminished over the past 40 years, these other child service sectors have become the de facto mental health systems for children and adolescents.[8-10]

Not only are mental health problems common, they are expensive for families, children, and society. Attention deficit hyperactivity disorder (ADHD) is one of the most common mental health problems diagnosed in school-age children. Costs for ADHD alone are similar to, or exceed, the costs for treatment of asthma, the most common non-mental health, chronic condition in childhood.[11] When the costs for ADHD are combined with other mental health problems, the total societal costs for treatment and management of mental health conditions exceed any other chronic problems of childhood.[12]

The concept of mental health problems as chronic, or long-lasting, among children is a relatively new one. The majority of studies on mental health treatment focus on acute, or short-term, care—as does much of the training for care providers of children and adolescents with mental health problems. However, a growing body of evidence suggests that these are recurrent

> **Most scientists estimate that mental health problems affect one out of five children of school age in the United States and an even larger percentage of youth in juvenile justice facilities, child welfare services, special education, and medical facilities.**

illnesses that may ebb and flow over time for many youth.[13-15] In fact, many children and adolescents with mental health problems will see persistence of the problems into adulthood. Moreover, in many children, secondary mental health problems or substance abuse may become challenging comorbidities, or coexisting problems, that frustrate typical treatments.[16,17]

The extent of disability associated with mental health problems is not as well understood. Several major studies demonstrate that mental health problems, particularly depression, are associated with extremely high levels of disability—more so than any other condition among adults in the United States, except for heart disease.[18-20] Worldwide, mental disorders are the second leading cause of disability for all ages.[10] For children, the data are less clear, but adolescents miss more school as a result of emotional and behavioral symptoms than any other condition.[21] Children and adolescents with

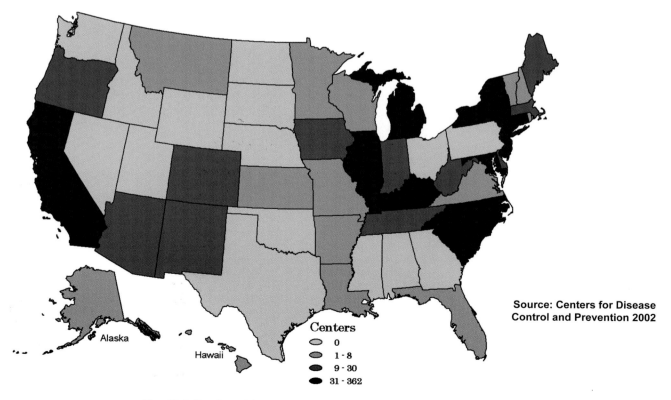

Source: Centers for Disease Control and Prevention 2002

Centers
- 0
- 1 - 8
- 9 - 30
- 31 - 362

Map 32.1: Number of School-based Health Centers Providing Mental Health and Social Services, 2000

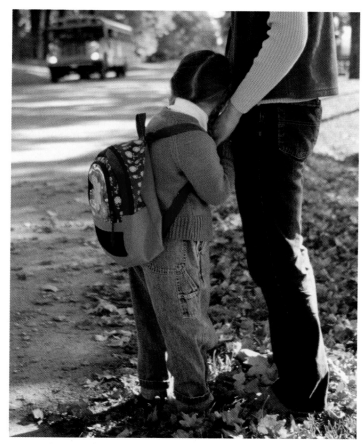

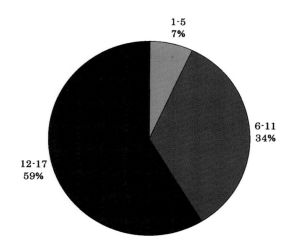

Figure 32.1: Mental Health Costs by Age Groups, 1998

Source: National Advisory Mental Health Council 2001

mental health problems are more likely to drop out of school and fail than any other group of children with disabilities. Similarly, youth in the juvenile justice system with mental health problems experience more recidivism than others.[7] In short, mental health problems produce as much, or more, impairment than almost any other condition. Needless to say, the costs to families and society are enormous. Sturm and colleagues estimate that direct treatment costs of mental disorders alone cost $12 billion in the United States annually.[12] This does not include the lost productivity and school performance, time away from work

for parents and families, and other indirect costs associated with child and adolescent mental health problems. Moreover, families are likely to pay more for mental health care than any other part of their health care expenditures because of inequities in financing for youth mental health care as compared to other kinds of medical care.[22] These inequities in financing include less availability of insurance for mental health care, more restrictions on payments for mental health care and the types of conditions covered, and larger cost sharing by patients and families.

This is unfortunate in light of the explosion in treatment research suggesting that while mental disorders are common, costly, and chronic, they are also increasingly treatable. Innovations and improvements in both psychopharmacology and psychotherapy offer the best hope yet of enhancing the quality of life for children and adolescents with mental disorders. For example, several studies document the efficacy of the new selective serotonin reuptake inhibitors for adolescent depression, while early results suggest that they may be effective for anxiety

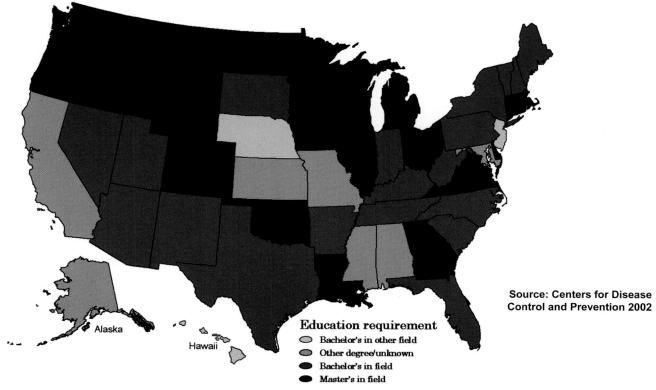

Source: Centers for Disease Control and Prevention 2002

Education requirement
- Bachelor's in other field
- Other degree/unknown
- Bachelor's in field
- Master's in field

Map 32.2: Educational Requirements for Newly Hired Social Workers, 2000

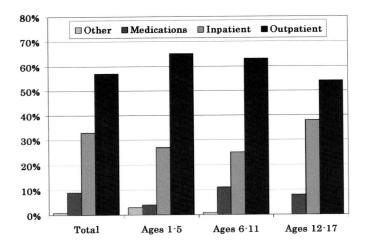

Figure 32.2: Mental Health Costs by Type of Service and Age Groups, 1998

Source: National Advisory Mental Health Council 2001

disorders as well.[23-27] For other conditions like ADHD, the efficacy of stimulants has been known for half a century. However, new improvements like long-acting formulations and stimulant substitutes make finding an acceptable option for children and families easier than ever before.[28]

Improvements in psychotherapy for youth are also appearing in the scientific literature. Cognitive behavior therapy, in particular, seems quite promising for adolescents with, or at risk of, depression. Similarly, those with phobias appear to respond to well-trained therapists following treatment manuals. In all, more than 1,500 studies document the efficacy of child psychotherapy for specific mental health problems.[29]

A related class of treatments, like multisystemic therapy, focuses on classroom, family, and community interventions for disruptive behaviors or aggression. Multisystemic and similar therapies are based upon a belief that children and adolescents operate among and are affected by an entire network of systems. These therapies are efficacious in controlled trials, and multisystemic therapy demonstrates reasonable cost-effectiveness data in some trials.[30]

In addition to the burgeoning literature on successful interventions, there is new information on the increasing number of youth treated for mental health problems. For example, pediatricians and family physicians now recognize more than twice as many youth with psychosocial problems as they did 20 years ago.[1] They are also prescribing more psychotropic or psychiatric medications than ever before. In fact, these medications have increased by an order of magnitude in the past two decades.[31-33] While much has been written about overmedication of children with psychiatric drugs, the majority of the evidence still suggests that most children with mental disorders are undertreated rather than overtreated, although there are exceptions. More children than ever before receive outpatient mental health care from specialists, and schools now provide mental health services for more youth than at any previous time.[8]

However, mental health care in the United States has been called "fragmented" at best and much worse.[34,35] It is clear that routine care in the specialty mental health sector, especially for ongoing medical management, is increasingly available only to those with resources to pay out-of-pocket.

Even with the necessary resources, obtaining care requires skilled families and advocates to seek the best possible services among an eclectic and poorly coordinated specialty system composed of mental health professionals in clinic settings. This leaves the growing number of less well-off youth with mental disorders to seek care in other service sectors like education, child welfare, primary care, and juvenile justice. These settings practice and provide mental health services in an unstandardized and intermittent fashion. Most have been forced to create their own mental health services as adjuncts to community-based mental health specialists. Even for those who are tireless advocates, there are numerous financial and organizational barriers to effective care. Providers infrequently involve families and youth in ongoing care. Little standardized information and treatment based on the best available evidence are provided in routine training programs.[36,37] Most service contracts either preclude or make it difficult to work across multiple service sectors or to share and coordinate information. In short, crisis services may be available for short-term management, but long-term, comprehensive care is rarely an option. Clearly, changes in mental health treatments for children and adolescents are warranted.

Changes in research would make mental health interventions more effective for children and adolescents. Investigators are currently encouraged by funding agencies to conduct small, randomized trials of interventions with volunteer populations that focus on pristine cases without complications or evidence of other problems. These are hardly conditions encountered in routine clinical practice.[38,39] These practices diminish the likelihood that important research areas will be funded—even when those areas are considered priorities by federal agencies.[40] Changing the research incentives and culture to support practice-based research or research on routine treatments

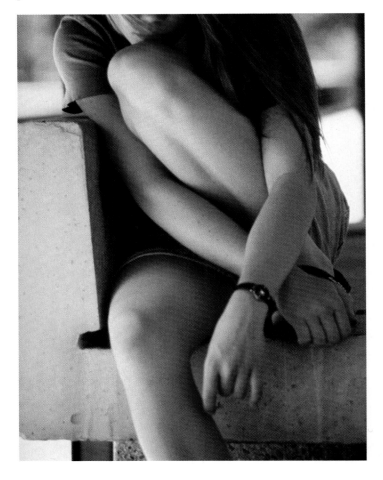

in typical, nonacademic settings is essential to finding real-world solutions. Similarly, studies that focus solely on patient, or possibly patient and provider, behavior will miss key elements of health systems and their organization that play a role in improving child mental health. It is clear from several demonstration projects that changes in treatment practices as well as the larger systems in which they are set are required for sustainable improvements. In short, interventions that are based on meaningful evidence and supported by systems that encourage their use are the only hope of long-term improvement.

Changes in practice would make mental health interventions more effective for children and adolescents. The growing acknowledgment that mental health problems are chronic and recurrent suggests that fundamental changes in care delivery systems are essential to improving care. Current medical care systems are based on a 400-year-old medical model designed to address acute problems. They are provider-centered, visit-based, and patient-initiated. Chronic care systems would be better served by a patient-centered, long-term approach that relies on systems that monitor and track patients across different practices, emergency rooms, and hospitals; clinician- or system-initiated care that does not wait until symptoms are severe before seeking people out; and provider decision support that uses computers to avoid medication dosing errors, drug reactions due to allergies, and poor care standards.[41,42] Although existing technology is available and used in some places, widespread change in practice will require a revolution in training and information services.

Changes in policy would make mental health interventions more effective for children and adolescents. A number of advances that could improve patient care are held hostage to antiquated funding streams developed more than 50 years ago. They include the use of innovative technology such as e-mail or telephone care management to track patient symptoms over time and provide encouragement to comply with treatment recommendations; home visitors to educate patients about their health conditions; and patient and family engagement strategies. Current health and mental health care financing systems

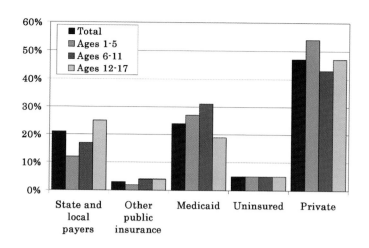

Figure 32.3: Mental Health Costs by Insurance Status and Age Groups, 1998

Source: National Advisory Mental Health Council 2001

pay for volume of care among those seeking services rather than purchasing improved outcomes or better health for populations. Financing practices that take into account delivery systems, accountability, and scientific evidence is only now being considered seriously, in part because of the rapid decline in employer-based insurance coverage and the current public sector funding crises. Long-lasting improvements in mental health care will require radical revision of financing for services and health, including, at a minimum, the equitable treatment of mental health problems as compared to other medical conditions and the elimination of disparities for poor and underserved populations.

In conclusion, mental health conditions among children and adolescents are common and expensive. New treatments offer more hope than ever before that youth with mental disorders and their families can live more fully. Fortunately, more affected children and adolescents are receiving treatment than ever before, even in the face of inadequate financing and delivery systems. However, the next steps toward improving care will require even greater efforts as we seek to change research practices, care delivery, and mental health policy to improve the quality of mental health treatment for youth.

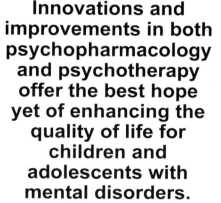

Innovations and improvements in both psychopharmacology and psychotherapy offer the best hope yet of enhancing the quality of life for children and adolescents with mental disorders.

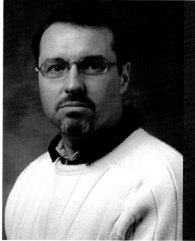

Kelly Kelleher

Kelly Kelleher, MD, MPH, is the director of the Office of Clinical Sciences of Columbus Children's Research Institute and professor of pediatrics at The Ohio State University. He is also adjunct professor of pediatrics, psychiatry, and health services. Formally, Dr. Kelleher was the Staunton Professor of Pediatrics, Psychiatry, and Health Services and director of Child Services Research and Development Program at the University of Pittsburgh School of Medicine and the Children's Hospital of Pittsburgh. He has authored numerous articles appearing in such journals as *Pediatrics*, *JAMA*, and *Journal of Affective Disorders*. Dr. Kelleher is currently studying the effectiveness of treating children's behavioral problems in primary care as well as issues related to child maltreatment. In addition, he is examining the benefits of coordinated research efforts and interaction across a broad range of scientific disciplines and clinical domains.

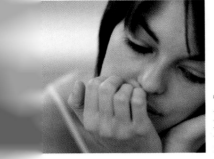

Chapter 33

Ardis L. Olson

Maternal Depression

The well-being of children is strongly influenced by the mental health of their parents. Depression is the most common mental health problem and the most studied parental mental health issue. Existing research has focused primarily on the impact of depression in the mother. While postpartum depression has been recognized as playing an important role in child outcomes,[1] the impact of depression across all of childhood and adolescence has recently become more widely recognized.[2] The effect of maternal depression on the child's mental health and normal development may be subtle[3,4] and go unrecognized by health care providers.[5] A variety of issues or symptoms observed by the practitioner can have maternal depression as a key factor. For example, the clinical problems of

a 1-month-old infant with multiple visits for feeding issues, a 4-year-old boy whose mother is concerned about his out-of-control behavior, and an 11-year-old girl with multiple somatic (physical) complaints may all derive from maternal depression.

Maternal depression is often not recognized as a common problem that may have an impact on many children. Women are nearly twice as likely as men to have an affective (mood) disorder, with a major depressive disorder being most prevalent (9% of women in community samples have a 6-month prevalence).[6] Women during the childbearing ages of 18 to 45 represent the largest group of individuals with major depression. Two-thirds of these women are parents. Women are more prone to depression for multiple reasons, only some of which are fully understood. Hormonal influences and strains from multiple social roles involving children, household, and work all contribute.[7,8] When parenting young children, dissonance between actual work status and expectations also plays a role.[7] While these factors affect most mothers, those who experience additional financial, personal, and social stresses are particularly vulnerable.[9-12]

While a major depressive disorder has the most impact on a mother's offspring, it is important to recognize that depressive symptoms of less severity are a common problem that has considerable impact on children. Though recognition of postpartum depression (associated with parenthood and hormonal changes) is a part of both pediatric and general knowledge, less attention is given to persistent maternal depression. Nearly half of the mothers who screen positive for postpartum depression have had a course of chronic or recurrent depression over the ensuing 2 years. For some mothers, the transition to parenthood and the burden of caring for an infant are specific, destabilizing events leading to depression. For other mothers with a history of past depression, postpartum depression is one episode among several.[13] The birth of the child may be only one more stressor for mothers where high

levels of psychosocial and economic stresses and associated depression already exist. Thus, it is important to recognize that depression, for many mothers, is an issue that persists beyond the first few months of the child's life and is not restricted to the postpartum period.[14]

Individuals with less severe depression still suffer impairments in work, home, and social settings.[15] Mothers with depressive symptoms are more likely to feel less competent as a parent and are less likely to implement preventive health advice.[16,17] They bring their children for more medical visits and have children with more somatic complaints and behavioral problems.[18-20] In the general population, the prevalence of depressive symptoms is 15% to 20%[21]; however, the rates are 2 to 3 times higher in certain populations under additional stress.[20,22]

> **While postpartum depression has been recognized as playing an important role in child outcomes, the impact of depression across all of childhood and adolescence has recently become more widely recognized.**

Circumstance	Increase in risk for depression
Mothers with financial adversity	2-3 times higher
Teenage mothers & single mothers	2 times higher
Mothers with marital or family difficulties present	
Mothers with medical illnesses	2 times higher
Children with chronic illnesses	2-3 times higher
Mothers of young children Postpartum Toddler years	10%-20% 2 times higher

Figure 33.1: Mothers at Greatest Risk for Depression

Source: Olson 2004

The consequences of major maternal depression for the child vary with the child's developmental stage and temperament as well as the social supports available to both mother and child.[18] For infants and young children, both major and subthreshold (low) levels of depression in the mother have been shown to affect emotional and cognitive development. Maternal interactions with their young child are affected. A depressed mother may be either withdrawn and unavailable or hostile and overly intrusive.[23] The infant or child experiences fewer positive parenting experiences (reading, cuddling, singing, etc.), a lack of daily routines, inconsistent discipline and affect (emotional display), and negative discipline.[24] When maternal depression persists, young children are more likely to have ongoing behavioral problems and delays in cognitive development.[25,26]

Children of a depressed parent are at increased risk of developing a psychiatric disorder due to both genetic and environmental factors. Children of a depressed parent are 4 times more likely than other children to develop an affective disorder.[2] Girls are particularly vulnerable when their mother is depressed.[27] In the presence of parental depression, children experience chronic stress in the context of their family environment. They also lack requisite role models to learn appropriate emotional regulation and problem solving.[28] Teenagers, as a result, are more likely to develop a variety of behavioral problems, including depression, somatic complaints, anxiety, and acting-out behaviors.[29]

Maternal depression often goes unrecognized and untreated. Depressed mothers may not regard their moods as a depressive disorder. Pediatric providers, as the health professionals who often have the most contact with mothers, have the opportunity to help mothers recognize their symptoms as depression. However, studies of both adult and pediatric health providers demonstrate that only 50% of women with depression are identified during routine clinical care.[5] Pediatricians react to concerns voiced by mothers, but only 8% routinely ask mothers about depressive

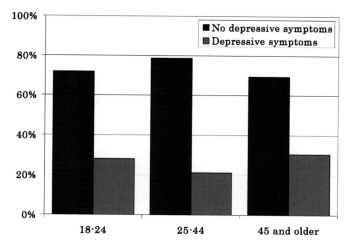

Figure 33.3: Percentage of Women 18 and Older with Child(ren) Under 18 with a Positive Depression Screen by Age, 2002*

Source: McMillen, Southward, Pascoe 2002

symptoms during the postpartum period or at other times.[30] Mothers, on the other hand, have been open to pediatricians' inquiry about their mental health status,[31] particularly in the context of an ongoing, trusting relationship.[32]

While pediatricians perceive themselves as gatekeepers or facilitators of access to mental health services for children, they are less likely to see themselves as having a frontline role in responding to the mental health needs of mothers. Only 57% of nationally surveyed pediatricians felt that it was their responsibility to recognize maternal depression.[30] In

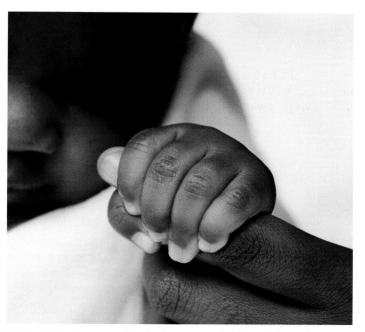

*Note: All the figures in this chapter were derived from information about maternal depression that was obtained using a previously validated three-item screening tool abstracted from the RAND eight-item screening instrument for depressive disorders developed by Burnam et al. Respondents were asked: (1) "On how many days in the past week did you feel depressed?" (2) "In the past year, have you had 2 weeks or more during which you felt sad, blue, depressed or when you lost all interest in things that you usually care about or enjoy?" (3) "Have you had 2 years or more in your life when you felt depressed or sad most days, even if you felt okay sometimes?" If a mother responded "yes" to two or three of the statements, the screen was scored positive; question number 1 was scored a "yes" if the mother felt depressed on 1 or more days in the past week. This screening tool has a sensitivity of 100% and a specificity of 88% when compared to the RAND instrument for detecting the presence of a depressive disorder in the past month in a primary care population.

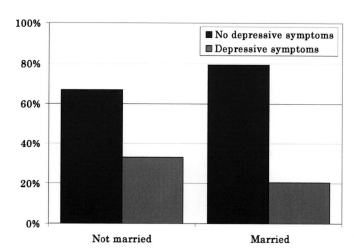

Figure 33.2: Percentage of Women 18 and Older with Child(ren) Under 18 with a Positive Depression Screen by Marital Status, 2002*

Source: McMillen, Southward, Pascoe 2002

143

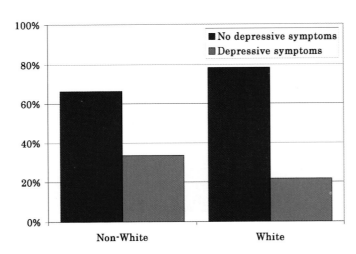

Figure 33.4: Percentage of Women 18 and Older with Child(ren) Under 18 with a Positive Depression Screen by Race, 2002*

Source: McMillen, Southward, Pascoe 2002

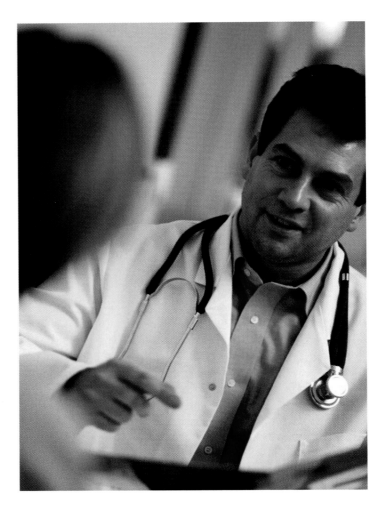

addition, many pediatricians consider their lack of knowledge and skills to be a barrier that limits their involvement.[30] In order to increase the recognition and management of family depression in primary care, pediatric residency training and continuing education need to include more specific training about assessing and intervening when family mental health issues exist. Adult mental health providers caring for parents with depression also seldom assess or provide counseling about the impact of depression on children. Thus, the emerging research regarding methods of promoting resiliency and protection of children from the emotional consequences of parental depression needs to be applied within both the pediatric and mental health professions.

What steps can be taken to help mothers and improve the outcomes for their children? Some key areas could benefit families and, therefore, merit attention by pediatric providers, educators, and policy leaders concerned about children's mental health and development: (a) better education of pediatricians

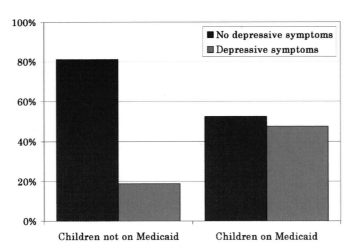

Figure 33.5: Percentage of Women 18 and Older with Child(ren) Under 18 with a Positive Depression Screen by Medicaid Status, 2002*

Source: McMillen, Southward, Pascoe 2002

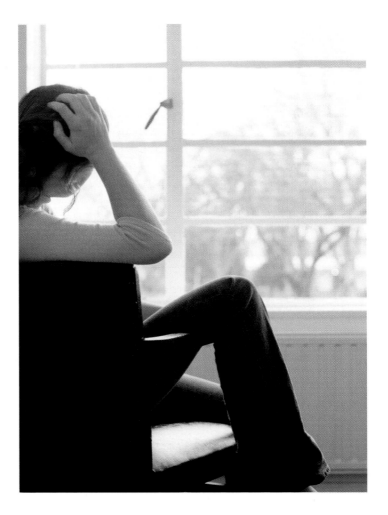

144

about family depression and how it impacts children; (b) increased awareness by adult mental health providers of the impact of depression on parents' offspring; (c) new interventions to enhance the recognition of maternal depression by pediatricians and their staffs; (d) further research into how to prevent adverse outcomes for children in the primary care setting; and (e) development of adequate community services to support parents and families.

Approaches to detection and management of parental mental health problems developed by mental health, child development, and behavioral health providers, in association with pediatricians, must be realistic, yet appropriate. Screening mothers for depression at well-child visits represents one important approach; recent recommendations of the U.S. Preventive Services Task Force supported routine screening of all adults for depression.[33] Screening may be rapidly conducted since inquiry with only two questions has been shown to be as effective as longer screening measures.[34] After detection through screening, mothers need to be linked with community supports and available resources.

New practice models with a proactive approach to supporting mothers with young children represent another way to respond to maternal needs. The national Health Steps Program adds a trained developmental health specialist to the primary care health team. This model has been shown to help depressed mothers discuss their feelings and be more effective parents.[35] Another option is the provision of collaborative care in settings where pediatric care and mental health services are both available, facilitating an effective response to the needs of both the depressed mother and child.

While these recent primary care approaches to enhancing children's health through better family mental health are encouraging, more research is needed to determine how to intervene with mothers and their children in both primary care and mental

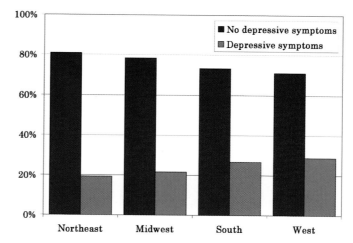

Figure 33.6: Percentage of Women 18 and Older with Child(ren) Under 18 with a Positive Depression Screen by Region, 2002*

Source: McMillen, Southward, Pascoe 2002

health settings. It is particularly important to learn how approaches other than medication can relieve depression and enhance parental functioning. Quality improvement activities by insurers and health care organizations offer an opportunity to implement a systematic practice approach for preventive mental health care services and to decrease the adverse outcomes of family depression. A requisite component of quality improvement is an awareness of the extent and appropriateness of community resources that can support families and an awareness of mental health services necessary for optimal care.

The mental health of parents, especially mothers, is a major factor in the mental health of children. Awareness of the short- and long-term consequences of parental depression on the well-being and development of children mandates a more aggressive and comprehensive approach to prevention, detection, and management. Through the combined efforts of parents, child health professionals, and leaders of health and community organizations, the outcomes for children can be enhanced.

> **The effect of maternal depression on the child's mental health and normal development may be subtle and go unrecognized by health care providers.**

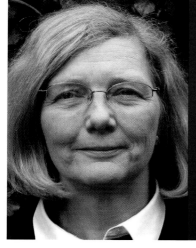

Ardis L. Olson

Ardis L. Olson, MD, is an associate professor of pediatrics and community and family medicine at Dartmouth Medical School. Dr. Olson is the director of the Clinicians Enhancing Child Health network, a practice-based primary care research network of pediatricians and family physicians. She received her undergraduate and medical school training at the University of Minnesota and completed her pediatric residency at the University of Rochester Strong Memorial Hospital in Rochester, NY.

For 30 years Dr. Olson has combined community research, clinical practice, and education. Her focus has been on helping to provide better preventive health care in primary care and community settings. Her research and community-based activities have focused on mothers with depressive symptoms, children and families affected by chronic illnesses, ways to enhance sun protection, and adolescent health risk reduction.

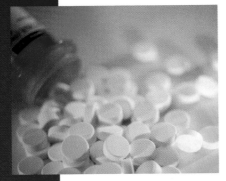

Chapter 34

Ann Doucette

Youth Suicide

Growing up today is an achievement rather than an expectation for many children. We have watched with rapt attention as news correspondents detail facts indicating mental health concerns, problematic interpersonal relationships, and family discord for many of the youth who are associated with suicide and violence. The pain of our youth has come to be the drama that haunts the print media and the nightly news and becomes the substance for made-for-TV miniseries. Far less attention, however, is given to building and to strengthening our ability to identify early risk and warning signs that mediate these unfavorable youth outcomes, as well as to cultivating community foundations that optimize youth development and increase resilience.

Suicide refers to self-chosen behavior to end one's life. Suicidal behavior may reveal itself in terms of thoughts (ideation), suicidal gestures (attempts that are not successful), and suicide (a death that is intentionally accomplished). Youth suicide is a complex issue. There is no simple answer as to why youth commit suicide. While there is some intuitive assumption that youth suicide attempts are motivated by attention-seeking or revenge-seeking behavior—the *"they'll be sorry when I'm no longer here"* scenario—research indicates that attention and revenge are not motives for adolescent suicide attempts. Most adolescent suicides are associated with a desire to escape or stop painful situations.[1]

Most information on youth suicide comes from three sources: (a) psychological autopsies that gather information about the youth from family and friends, (b) school-based surveys, and (c) emergency room reports of treatment for intentional injuries. Much of the existing research on suicide is retrospective, after the suicide or suicide attempt has occurred. It is difficult to get accurate

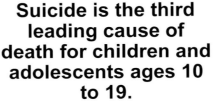

Suicide is the third leading cause of death for children and adolescents ages 10 to 19.

estimates of the incidence of suicides because suicide attempts not requiring medical attention are less likely to be reported. The underreporting of suicide completion is also likely since suicide classification involves conclusions regarding the intent of the deceased. Single vehicular fatalities and many seemingly unintentional injury deaths leave little conclusive evidence of intent. The stigma associated with suicide is also likely to contribute to the underreporting of both attempts and completions.

Research indicates that growing up in socially distressed community and family environments places youth at higher risk for suicidal behavior.[2,3] Changes in family situations like divorce and parental unemployment have been noted as potential risk factors, but little research exists to confirm this assumption. In a 1995 study, C.W. Kienhorst and colleagues found that adolescent suicide attempters perceived less social support and understanding from their parents than did

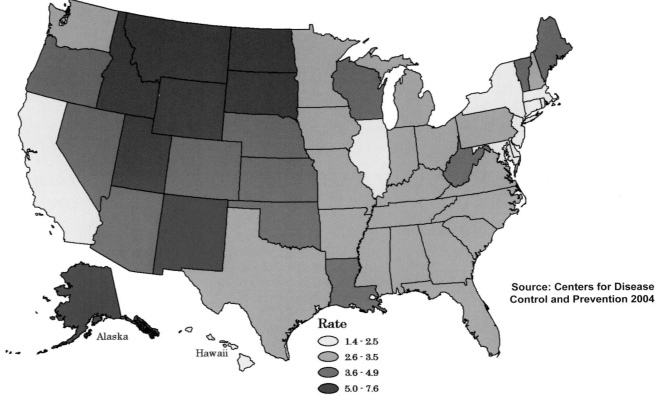

Source: Centers for Disease Control and Prevention 2004

Rate
- 1.4 - 2.5
- 2.6 - 3.5
- 3.6 - 4.9
- 5.0 - 7.6

Map 34.1: Suicide Rate for Children Under 20 Years Old per 100,000, 1990-1993

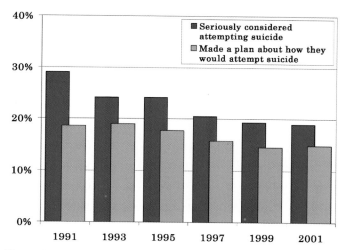

Figure 34.1: Percentage of 9th- to 12th-Grade Students Who Considered Suicide in the Last 12 Months

Source: Youth Risk Behavior Surveillance Survey 1991-2001

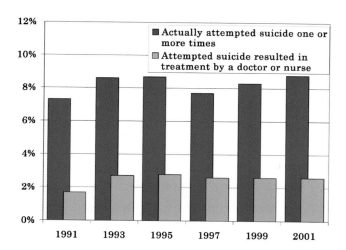

Figure 34.2: Percentage of 9th- to 12th-Grade Students Who Attempted Suicide in the Last 12 Months

Source: Youth Risk Behavior Surveillance Survey 1991-2001

depressed adolescents.[1] Another study revealed that suicidal adolescents rated their family environment as rigid and disconnected.[3] Exposure to family and neighborhood violence also seems to contribute to suicidal risk. Youth may feel helpless in stopping or decreasing the violence and may see suicide as the only way of ending deep psychological pain.

Previous suicide attempts as well as previous ideation are among the most dominant predictors of suicidal behavior. Substance use (alcohol, drugs, etc.) is also a factor. The use of alcohol and other drugs reduces inhibition, alters the cognitive processes that likely influence suicidal behaviors, and impairs the ability of youth to weigh the consequences of those behaviors.[4] Reduced inhibition and cognitive impairment increase the risk for completed suicide.

Adolescence is a time of developmental change that may be stressful.[5] Many studies indicate that adolescents experience feelings of self-deprecation and isolation in response to the developmental tasks set before them[6] and that these tasks may seem overwhelming and upsetting. Suicidal behavior may be mediated by developmental stages, as well as by other psychological factors. Cognitive distortion, misrepresentations of reality, and coping styles have been noted as contributing factors. Orbach, Rosenheim, and Hary note that suicidal youth are less likely to articulate alternative solutions to solving stressful problems.[7] Suicidal youth may be preoccupied with a specific trauma, for example, the rejection of a boy/girlfriend or parental and peer conflict. Often they feel that there is no solution for their problem and that the ultimate resolution is a very restricted one, that of suicide. Research also indicates that suicidal youth are more likely to exhibit more attributional errors,

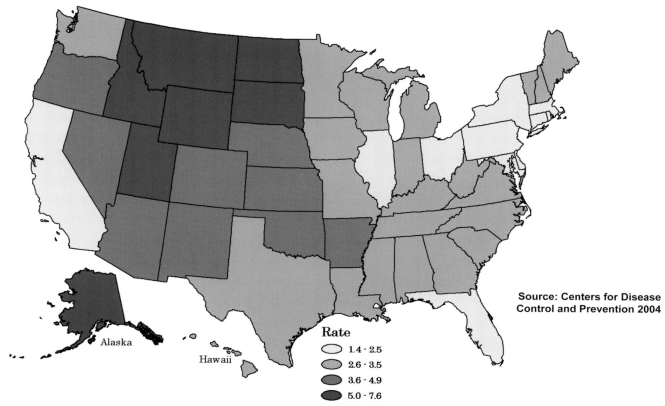

Source: Centers for Disease Control and Prevention 2004

Rate
- 1.4 - 2.5
- 2.6 - 3.5
- 3.6 - 4.9
- 5.0 - 7.6

Map 34.2: Suicide Rate for Children Under 20 Years Old per 100,000, 1995-1998

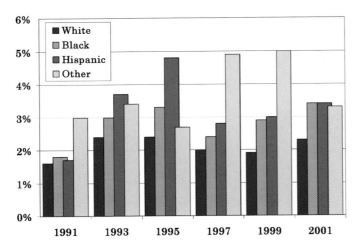

Figure 34.3: Percentage of 9th- to 12th-Grade Students That Required Medical Treatment as a Result of Attempting Suicide in the Last 12 Months by Race

Source: Youth Risk Behavior Surveillance Survey 1991-2001

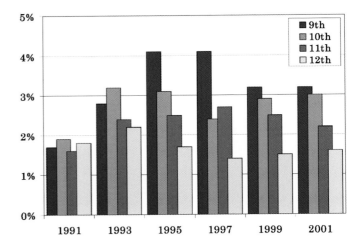

Figure 34.4: Percentage of 9th- to 12th-Grade Students That Required Medical Treatment as a Result of Attempting Suicide in the Last 12 Months by Grade Level

Source: Youth Risk Behavior Surveillance Survey 1991-2001

a belief that things are more unfavorable than they are[8]; to have difficulty in handling emotions and perceiving consequences of behavioral actions[9]; and to be impulsive in terms of resolving problems.[10]

Emotional states are also identified as contributing risk factors. Intuitively there is an assumed relationship between suicide and depression/hopelessness. Suicidal behavior has been linked to bipolar, conduct, and depressive disorders as well as schizophrenia. While depression is one of the strongest correlates of suicidal behavior, the majority of depressed adolescents do not commit or even attempt suicide.[11] In fact, most youth completing suicide were retrospectively identified with a behavioral health problem, but were not actively receiving mental health treatment.

The effect of pubertal changes during adolescence is considered by some professionals to contribute risk for adverse adolescent outcomes. However, the nature of this relationship is unclear. Hamburg notes the phenomenon of *biopsychosocial dysbalance*, the increasingly earlier onset of puberty and the growing lag in psychological and emotional development needed to address the associated developmental tasks.[12] This phenomenon may affect female adolescents more than their male counterparts in terms of suicidal behavior, as pubertal change occurs earlier and more noticeably for girls than for boys. While male adolescent suicide completions outnumber

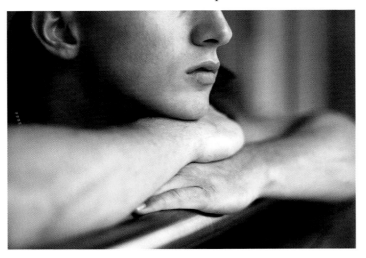

those of adolescent females, suicide attempts are much more likely among adolescent females.

The most basic statistic known about suicide is that suicide risk increases with age. The completed suicide rate for children between 10 and 14 years of age is 1.3 per 100,000. The rate increases to 8 per 100,000 between ages 15 and 19 and to 12 per 100,000 for young adults between 20 and 24 years of age. While these numbers may seem small, suicide is the third leading cause of death for children and adolescents ages 10 to 19.[13] It is preceded by unintentional injuries and malignancies (for 10- to 14-year-olds) and homicide (for 15- to 19-year olds). We also know that suicide attempts far exceed suicide completions. In fact, suicide attempts surpass the number of suicides in adolescents, more than for any other age group.[14] The American Association of Suicidology estimates that in a typical high school classroom, three students (one boy and two girls) are likely to have made a suicide attempt in the past year.[15]

The Centers for Disease Control and Prevention conduct the Youth Risk Behavior Surveillance Survey nationally every 2 years with public middle and high school students. In 2001, this nationally representative survey revealed that 28% of the students reported experiencing a sense of hopelessness for 2 weeks or more that was so severe it prevented them from doing usual activities. Nineteen percent of the students completing this survey indicated that they had seriously considered attempting suicide, and nearly 9% of the students revealed that they had made a serious suicide attempt in 2001. Girls were almost twice as likely to acknowledge having attempted suicide (11.2% of girls, 6.2% of boys); however, boys were almost 5 times more likely to complete suicide.

Available data indicate that there are differential rates of suicidal thoughts and behaviors for racial/ethnic youth groups. Thirteen percent of African American youth completing the 2001 Youth Risk Behavior Surveillance Survey reported seriously contemplating suicide compared to approximately 20% of Caucasian and 19% of Hispanic youth completing this survey. Twelve percent of Hispanic youth revealed they had made a serious suicide

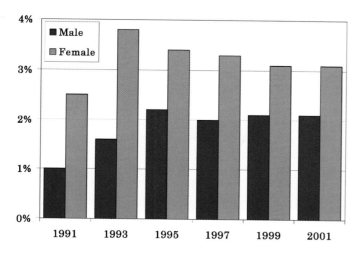

Figure 34.5: Percentage of 9th- to 12th-Grade Students That Required Medical Treatment as a Result of Attempting Suicide in the Last 12 Months by Gender
Source: Youth Risk Behavior Surveillance Survey 1991-2001

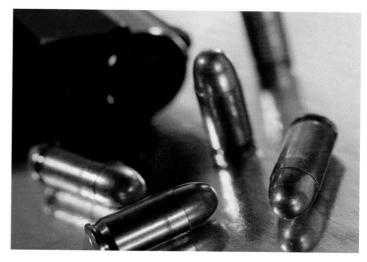

attempt compared to 8% of Caucasian and 9% of African American youth survey respondents.[16]

The lethality of the method used in a suicide attempt affects the likelihood of completion. Youth who use firearms are more likely to complete suicide compared to youth who ingest drugs. The availability of specific suicide methods influences the method of choice and the resulting likelihood of completion.[17] For example, rural, western states have the highest suicide completion rates and also have higher rates of firearm ownership than do more urban states with significantly lower rates of completion. Although most suicide completions are related to firearms, the majority of suicide attempts by youth are the result of self-poisoning such as drug overdose.[1] Adolescent suicide attempters are as likely to use prescription and over-the-counter drugs and inhalants as illegal drugs such as alcohol, marijuana, crack, or cocaine. It is important to consider that access to prescription and over-the-counter drugs and inhalants is easier than access to illegal drugs sold in underground economies.

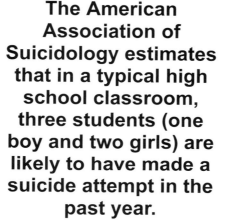

The American Association of Suicidology estimates that in a typical high school classroom, three students (one boy and two girls) are likely to have made a suicide attempt in the past year.

Prevention and intervention efforts have been largely directed at alleviating symptomatology (depression, hopelessness, etc.) or enhancing cognitive skills (coping, problem-solving, impulsivity reduction, etc.) as opposed to targeting a broader conceptual framework. Our efforts to mitigate adolescent suicide are often not called on until tragedy occurs. Furthermore, prevention specialists are not likely to be the individuals whom suicidal youth approach in times of crisis. Youth are more likely to turn to peers or adults they trust—*gatekeepers*. The initial point of contact during a suicidal crisis is critical; it is a time when the recognition of suicidal considerations and/or behavior is crucial and appropriate intervention essential.

Youth suicide is a poignant and traumatic event for the families, friends, and communities (schools, neighborhoods, etc.) left behind. While it remains a relatively rare event, we must remember that the loss of youth to suicide is preventable. Currently, widespread systematic prevention strategies do not exist. To successfully reduce and prevent youth suicide, we must enhance our ability to recognize suicidal youth and refer them to sensitive and appropriate resources, as well as to develop home, school, and community-based strategies to optimize protective factors and reduce risk. Children are 100% of our future; we must not allow suicide to jeopardize that future.

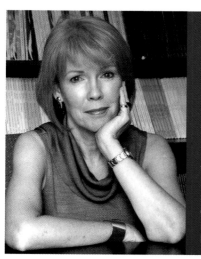

Ann Doucette

Ann Doucette, PhD, is a senior research associate at the Vanderbilt Institute for Public Policy at Vanderbilt University. Dr. Doucette conducts research with children and adolescents at risk of adverse developmental outcomes, particularly youth violence, gang involvement, mental health disorders, and youth suicide. Her work in the area of youth violence prevention focuses on school and community settings and on the role of child/adolescent and family mental health status and family violence in mediating aggressive youth behavior. Dr. Doucette is currently developing a comprehensive, integrated measurement system that assesses both treatment process indicators as well as service intervention outcomes for children and adolescents receiving behavioral health care services. She cochairs the Outcomes Roundtable for Children, supported by the Substance Abuse and Mental Health Services Administration, and chairs the Measurement Specification/Design/Methods Workgroup of the Forum on Performance Measures for Behavioral Healthcare and Related Service Systems. Dr. Doucette received her doctoral training at Columbia University.

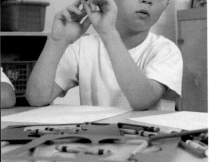

Chapter 35

Mark L. Wolraich

ADHD
Attention Deficit Hyperactivity Disorder

Attention deficit hyperactivity disorder (ADHD) is the most common mental diagnosis in children and is characterized by inattention, hyperactivity, and impulsivity. Although ADHD may appear to be a new condition, particularly because of its recent identification as a disorder that affects adults, it actually has a long history. A mid-19th century German physician, Heinrich Hoffman, incorporated two characters in a children's book that represented the characteristics of ADHD: Fidgety Phil and Harry Who Looks in the Air.[1] Then in 1902, at a meeting of the Royal College of Physicians, George Still described a disease he characterized as resulting from a defect in moral character.[2] He noted that the problem resulted in a child's inability to internalize rules and limits and additionally manifested itself in patterns of restless, inattentive, and over-aroused behaviors. He suggested

that the children likely had experienced brain damage but that the behavior also could have arisen from hereditary and environmental factors.

The connection to brain damage seemed more evident in 1917 to 1918 following a worldwide epidemic of influenza with encephalitis that resulted in symptoms of restlessness, inattention, impulsivity, easy arousability, and hyperactivity in some recovering children.[3,4] Subsequently, when many cases emerged with similar behavioral manifestations but no clear evidence of brain damage, minimal cerebral/brain dysfunction/damage became the name of the disorder for a while.[5]

Because the evidence for definite brain damage was weak in most cases, the more behavior-descriptive names of hyperkinetic impulse disorder and hyperactive child syndrome came into use.[6] In 1980, as a result of the work of Virginia Douglas and colleagues, the focus again shifted to considering inattention rather than hyperactivity as the primary deficit.[7,8] This shift in focus resulted in a change in the diagnostic label to attention deficit disorder[9] and, more recently, to attention deficit hyperactivity disorder.[10,11]

Throughout its history, the core behavioral dimensions of ADHD have remained inattention, impulsivity, and hyperactivity. Attention deficit hyperactivity disorder stems from an interaction between neurologically based central nervous system characteristics and a child's environment. Because the major effective treatments for ADHD, stimulant medications and behavioral interventions, have similar effects on all children regardless of their diagnosis, the determination about whom to treat has been very dependent on the diagnostic process. While there continues to be some debate about defining the criteria for ADHD, particularly in defining cutoff criteria, there is little disagreement among most clinicians about the existence of this condition and the main characteristics of inattention, impulsivity, and hyperactivity.

The fourth edition of the *Diagnostic and Statistical Manual of Mental Disorders*[11] provides the state-of-the-art criteria for the diagnosis of ADHD. It defines two dimensions of core symptoms: inattention and a combination of impulsivity and hyperactivity. Researchers have found these two dimensions consistently, even when studying varied populations of children from different countries. Each dimension consists of nine behaviors:

Inattention

- makes careless mistakes
- has difficulty sustaining attention
- seems not to listen
- fails to finish tasks
- has difficulty organizing
- avoids tasks requiring sustained attention
- loses things
- is easily distracted
- is forgetful

Impulsivity and Hyperactivity

- blurts answers before questions are completed
- has difficulty awaiting turn
- interrupts/intrudes upon others
- fidgets
- is unable to stay seated
- moves excessively (restless)
- has difficulty engaging in leisure activities quietly
- is "on the go"
- talks excessively

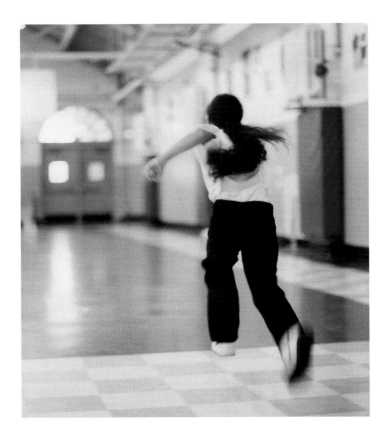

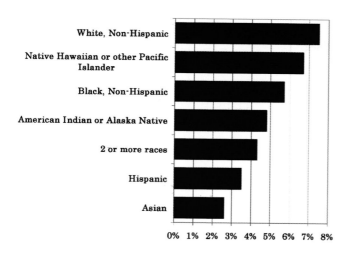

Figure 35.1: Percentage of 3- to 17-Year-Olds Ever Told That They Had ADHD by Race, 2001

Source: National Center for Health Statistics 2003

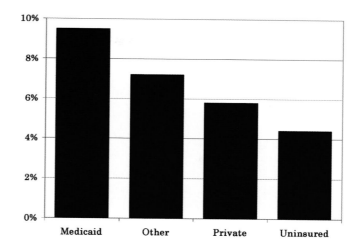

Figure 35.2: Percentage of 3- to 17-Year-Olds Ever Told That They Had ADHD by Insurance Type, 2001

Source: National Center for Health Statistics 2003

Some of the inattention behaviors involve executive functions, which are the functions that help individuals organize activities, sustain attention, and filter out extraneous stimuli to execute their activities appropriately. The impulsivity and hyperactivity dimension consists of three impulsive behaviors (the first three behaviors listed) and six hyperactive behaviors. To have a diagnosis of ADHD, a patient should have at least six behaviors in either dimension that occur inappropriately often for the patient's developmental level. Additionally, the symptoms must have been present for at least 6 months, started before the age of 7 years, caused significant impairment in more than one setting (e.g., school and home), and not been the result of another mental disorder.

ADHD is a heterogeneous disorder in which multiple causes can manifest similar behavioral symptoms. By far the most common cause has been genetic transmission. Studies of twins have demonstrated the genetic transmission of ADHD

Because the major effective treatments for ADHD, stimulant medications and behavioral interventions, have similar effects on all children regardless of their diagnosis, the determination about whom to treat has been very dependent on the diagnostic process.

with a heritability of 0.75.[12] The implication of this finding is that if one twin has ADHD, there is a 75% chance that the other twin also will have it. Family studies have shown that adoptive relatives of children with ADHD are less likely to have the disorder than biologic relatives.[13,14] Biologic siblings have a 2 to 3 times greater risk of having ADHD, and parents of a child with ADHD also have a greater risk than parents who do not have a child with ADHD.[15] Most recently, scientists have identified abnormalities in specific genes, such as a dopamine (a neurotransmitter) transporter gene (DAT1), in a small number of individuals with ADHD, further suggesting genetic transmission.[16-18]

Insults to the brain can result in the behaviors characteristic of ADHD. For instance, children who are born prematurely have a higher incidence of ADHD, probably resulting from a lack of oxygen to the brain before or after birth.[19] Traumatic injuries to the brain, exposures to toxic substances (such as lead), and infections (such as

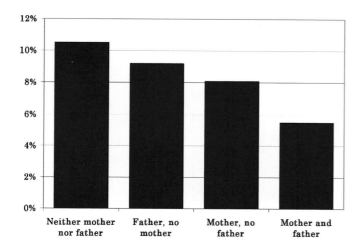

Figure 35.3: Percentage of 3- to 17-Year-Olds Ever Told That They Had ADHD by Family Type, 2001

Source: National Center for Health Statistics 2003

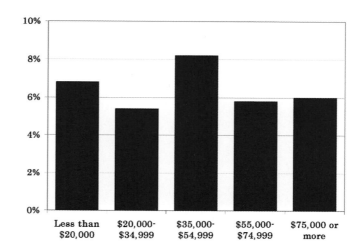

Figure 35.4: Percentage of 3- to 17-Year-Olds Ever Told That They Had ADHD by Family Income, 2001

Source: National Center for Health Statistics 2003

meningitis) can result in similar behavioral symptoms. Exposures in utero (before birth) to alcohol can cause ADHD symptoms that, when most severe, are manifested in fetal alcohol syndrome.

Researchers have identified some of the preliminary central nervous system mechanisms that are associated with ADHD. Studies of brain anatomy have demonstrated that, on average, individuals with ADHD have smaller prefrontal cortexes, basal ganglia, and cerebellar vermix. Brain function studies such as positron emission tomography, single photon emission computed tomography, and functional magnetic resonance imaging have shown decreased brain activity in these areas. Additionally, studies have shown a relationship between the neurochemical dopamine and the brain functions of these areas.[20,21]

While research has progressed significantly in identifying possible underlying mechanisms in individuals with ADHD, it is important to note that the sophisticated assessment techniques now available do not help facilitate the clinical diagnosis. The reason they are not helpful is that there are such wide variations in brain size and brain activity of both individuals with ADHD and those without ADHD (with a good deal of overlap between the two groups) that the assessments cannot adequately determine who has ADHD.

Treatment of ADHD is comparable to treatment of other chronic disorders and has socioenvironmental as well as individual biological components. Two therapies, stimulant medications and behavioral interventions, have demonstrated clear short-term benefits.

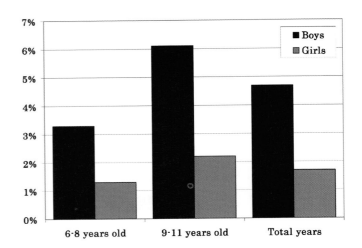

Figure 35.5: Percentage of 6- to 11-Year-Olds with ADHD by Gender and Age, 1997-1998

Source: National Center for Health Statistics 2002

Behavioral interventions must take place both in the school and in the home. They generally consist of encouraging appropriate behaviors and discouraging inappropriate behaviors. A reward system of praise as well as points or tokens encourages appropriate behaviors. Loss of points or tokens or punishment such as "time-out" is the discouragement for inappropriate behaviors. While the approach sounds simple, implementation of successful programs requires specifically trained clinicians in most cases.

Charles Bradley first reported the benefits of stimulant medication in 1937, starting with Benzedrine and focusing on children in inpatient residential care.[22] There was little activity in the field subsequent to Bradley's work until the 1950s when clinicians rediscovered his findings, and the commercial use of methylphenidate (Ritalin) began in 1957. Stimulant medications, primarily dextroam-

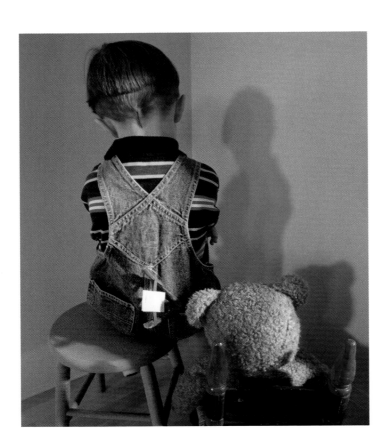

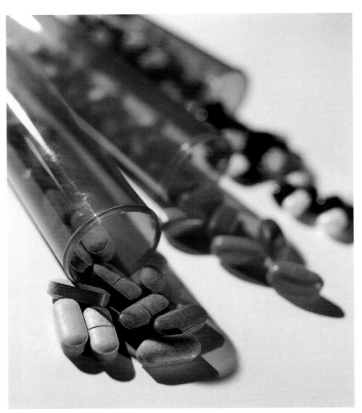

phetamine (Dexedrine) and methylphenidate, have become the mainstays of medication management. A large number of scientific studies have demonstrated the effectiveness and safety of these medications.[23] The stimulants are rapid-acting but only last 4 to 6 hours, requiring the administration of medication at school. However, several delivery systems (Concerta, Metadate CD, and Ritalin LA) have become available recently that extend the time the medication is active. One nonstimulant medication, atomoxetine (Strattera), is now available for treating individuals with ADHD.

All interventions for children with ADHD, both stimulant medication and behavioral interventions, are nonspecific. This means that while the treatments are effective for children with ADHD, children without the diagnosis respond similarly to these treatments. Further, interventions treat the symptoms but do not produce a cure. They are effective mainly as long as they are in use, but research has shown no lasting effects after the medications are terminated.

A major controversy exists among authorities over the appropriate use of stimulant medications to treat children with ADHD. In the past decade, the use of stimulant medications increased rapidly; usage was between 2½ and 5 times greater at the end of the decade than at the beginning.[24] In addition, the number of children treated varies from country to country, region to region, and even from city to city in the United States.[25] The concern is that children are being given stimulant medications inappropriately.[26-28] Some studies have shown that inappropriate treatment also includes not giving these medications to children with the condition who would likely benefit.[29] The American Academy of Pediatrics and the American Academy of Child and Adolescent Psychiatry have developed programs aimed at improving clinicians' abilities to correctly diagnose and treat patients with ADHD.[30,31]

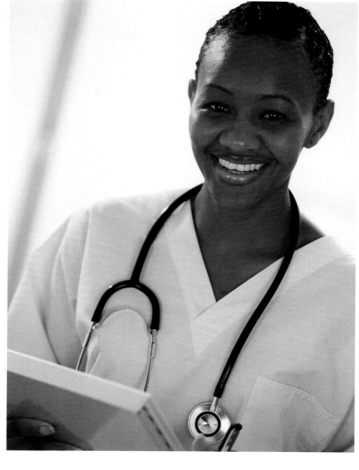

In the past decade, the use of stimulant medications increased rapidly; usage was between 2½ and 5 times greater at the end of the decade than at the beginning.

Researchers and clinicians have made more progress in defining ADHD and treating children with the condition than has been made for any other childhood mental disorder. Studies such as those on genetics and brain function are providing important information about many children with a diagnosis of ADHD. However, much is still unknown, and more research is needed that will lead to a better understanding of the causes of ADHD and to better diagnostic methods and treatments. It is also important for clinicians to become more effective at translating research findings into practice so that individuals with ADHD can receive the most effective care possible.

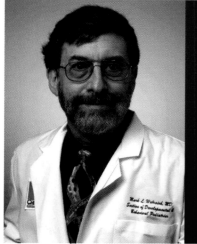

Mark L. Wolraich

Mark L. Wolraich, MD, is the CMRI/Shaun Walters Professor of Pediatrics at the University of Oklahoma Health Sciences Center and the director of the University of Oklahoma Child Study Center. Dr. Wolraich earned his medical degree from the SUNY Upstate Medical Center. He completed his residency in pediatrics at the University of Oklahoma Health Sciences Center and a pediatric fellowship in care of the handicapped child at the Oregon Health & Sciences University Child Development and Rehabilitation Center. He has chaired or participated in a number of national activities including the development of the American Academy of Pediatrics guidelines for the diagnosis and treatment of attention deficit hyperactivity disorder (ADHD) and a national collaborative that trained primary care clinicians in the diagnosis and treatment of ADHD sponsored by the National Initiative for Children's Healthcare Quality. He is a past president of the Society for Developmental and Behavioral Pediatrics. He has received many financial awards to conduct pediatric studies and has authored or coauthored more than 150 journal articles, abstracts, book chapters, and monographs.

Part Four: About Their Roles, Hopes, and Rights

There is a concern about the lives of children—not just about what happens to children when they reach adulthood. If our only marker of success is the extent to which children become productive members of the adult society, we miss the essence of childhood, emergence of individuals, flowering of individual skills, laughter, misgivings, dreams, and hopes. The chapters that follow represent only a small window into the lives of children and youth. Yet they do signify, hopefully, a deep respect for the capabilities, attributes, skills, opinions, and rights of children.

Chapter 36

John P. Bartkowski

Religion Among American Teens: Contours and Consequences

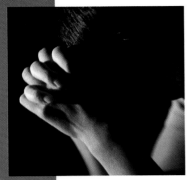

Conventional wisdom suggests that adolescence is characterized by anxiety, confusion, and, at times, rebellion—but certainly not religion. Yet, are American teens as faithless as many people commonly presume? And what impact, if any, does religion have on the lives of American adolescents? Surprisingly, teens in the United States are more religious than they are typically assumed to be. What's more, religion exerts a strong and generally positive influence on adolescent development.

The Contours of Teen Religiosity—Surveys demonstrate that teens are quite religious.[1] Approximately three-quarters of teens in national surveys reported believing in a personal god and praying at least occasionally. When asked about the role of religion in their lives, about 30% of high school seniors said that religion is very important to them. There are some signs, however, that

teens today are less religious than previous generations. About 40% of high school seniors attended religious services weekly in the late 1970s compared to about one in three who do so today. Moreover, high school seniors reported attending religious services less frequently than adolescents in their early high school years. This decline in attendance among older teens is linked to driving privileges and the increased autonomy that this group enjoys.

Gender, race, and family upbringing are important determinants of youth religiosity. Girls are consistently more religious than boys in both their attendance at worship services and their belief that religion is important in their lives. Black youth are considerably more religious than their White counterparts. About 40% of Black youth reported weekly church attendance, as compared to 29% of Whites. And the proportion of Black youth (55%) who defined religion as very important is more than double the proportion of White youth (24%) who did so.

> **Religion is an important and generally positive force in the lives of American teens.**

Parents are widely considered to have the most profound influence on youth religiosity, although faith traditions are transmitted from one generation to the next with varying degrees of success. As they grow to adulthood, children raised in conservative faith traditions (e.g., Southern Baptists and Latter-Day Saints) are more likely than mainline Protestants to remain active in their parents' denomination. Among parents, mothers seem to exert a stronger influence on the development of faith in children. However, as older teens mature into young adults, it is the religious practices of their peers—rather than their parents—that exhibit the strongest influence on their faith. Nevertheless, as is the case with many dimensions of youth development, parents are crucial in laying the foundation for young people's religious habits.

The Consequences of Teen Religiosity—Given the prominent place of religion in many teens' lives, what effect does religious involvement have on adolescent development? Research reveals that religious teens typically fare better than their

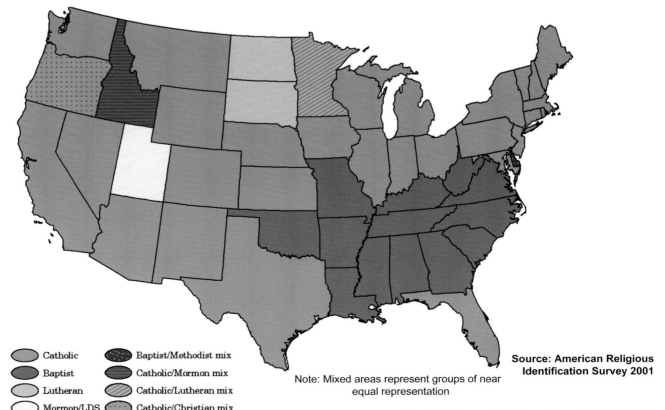

Catholic
Baptist
Lutheran
Mormon/LDS
Baptist/Methodist mix
Catholic/Mormon mix
Catholic/Lutheran mix
Catholic/Christian mix

Note: Mixed areas represent groups of near equal representation

Source: American Religious Identification Survey 2001

Map 36.1: Largest Religious Group by State, 2001

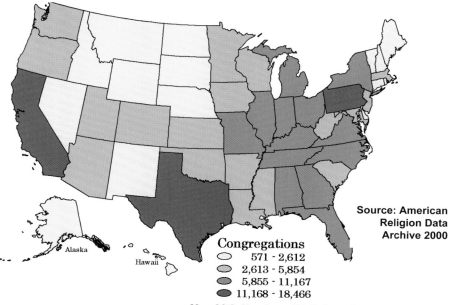

Source: American Religion Data Archive 2000

Congregations
- 571 - 2,612
- 2,613 - 5,854
- 5,855 - 11,167
- 11,168 - 18,466

Map 36.2: Number of Religious Congregations, 2000

aspirations and levels of educational achievement, teens involved with fundamentalist groups are considerably less likely to value and pursue higher education.[4] This finding has led some scholars to suggest that the anti-intellectual orientations of some faith traditions may undermine the life chances of their youth adherents. Thus, religion strongly influences the educational choices of American youth. However, orientations toward education vary considerably by religious tradition.

Other important nuances have also emerged. Religion fosters some sort of academic competence—namely, performance on verbal tests—among teen girls, but is largely ineffectual for boys in this capacity. What's more, attendance at religious services enhances academic progress among youth in low-income areas more so than those from affluent neighborhoods.[5] However, neither theological beliefs nor denominational affiliation bolsters academic achievement among disadvantaged youth. Only regular attendance does so. Researchers surmise that regular attendance at religious services in disadvantaged neighborhoods creates cohesive social networks that reinforce pro-educational values and achievement-minded orientations.

The greatest amount of research on religion and adolescent developmental outcomes has examined juvenile delinquency and risk behavior. In general, religion provides a protective

nonreligious counterparts on a wide range of outcome measures that track adolescent development.[2] Religious adolescents are often found to exercise, diet, and even have higher self-esteem and a sense of self-mastery more than those who do not practice their faith. Those high school seniors who regularly attend religious services and consider religion very important are significantly more likely to report having positive attitudes about themselves, feeling satisfied with their lives, feeling that life is meaningful, and being hopeful about their future. Several positive outcomes are also associated with religious youth group involvement. Teens who have been affiliated with a religious youth group for 6 or more years are significantly more likely to believe that they have something to be proud of than those who have never participated in a religious youth group. As sociologist Mark Regnerus and colleagues conclude, "Religious communities might provide favorable self-images among youth by providing opportunities for positive reflected appraisals (e.g., within youth small groups or activities) and by encouraging cultivation of spiritual resources (e.g., faith and hope, belief in divine grace and benevolence)."[3]

The developmental outcomes associated with religion also have been observed in educational achievement and cognitive development. Here there is a mixture of positive and negative outcomes. While youth in some religious groups (e.g., Catholics and Latter-Day Saints) evince higher educational

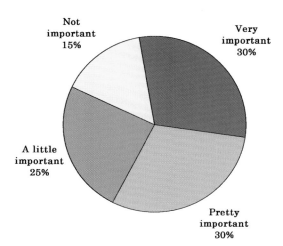

Figure 36.1: Personal Importance of Religion to High School Seniors, 1996

Source: Monitoring the Future 1996

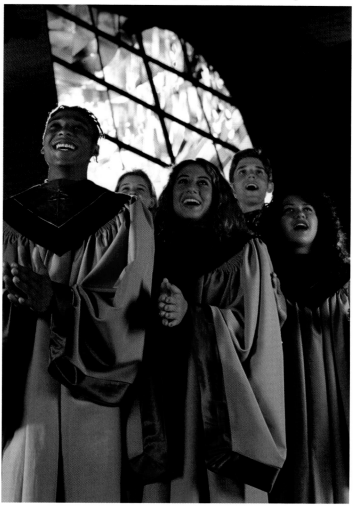

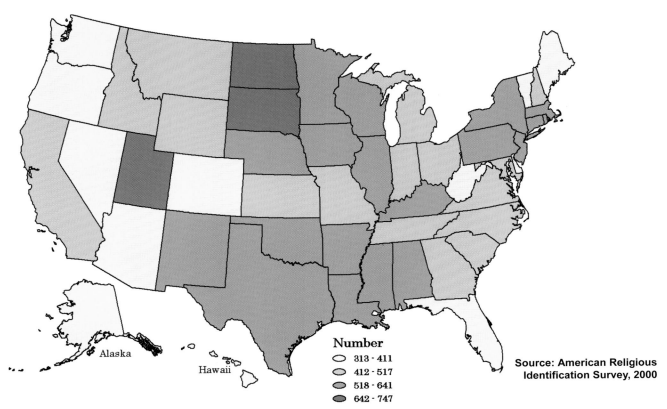

Number

○ 313 - 411
◔ 412 - 517
◑ 518 - 641
● 642 - 747

Source: American Religious
Identification Survey, 2000

Map 36.3: Number of Religious Adherents per 1,000 Population, 2000

barrier against juvenile delinquency and antisocial behavior. Religious high school seniors are considerably less likely to be involved in violent incidents such as getting into fights with peers or assaulting their teachers. They are also significantly less prone to perpetrate crimes such as shoplifting, petty theft, auto theft, vandalism, arson, and armed robbery. Religious 12th-graders seem to be better behaved students. They are less likely to be sent to detention, skip school, and be suspended or expelled than their nonreligious peers.

Religion also seems to inhibit teen involvement in a wide range of youth risk behaviors including the use of tobacco, alcohol, and other drugs while delaying the onset of sexual activity. Only 11.9% of 12th-graders who attend religious services smoke regularly. That number compares to 30% of those who never attend church services. And when asked about the first time they consumed alcohol to get drunk, religious high school seniors reported postponing this event or avoiding it altogether more often than their nonreligious counterparts. Research has shown that religious youth are

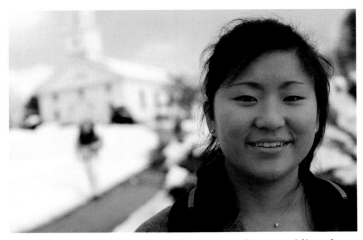

more likely to postpone first intercourse, thus providing them with a broad set of protections against teen pregnancy, sexually transmitted diseases, and the emotional problems that often accompany premature sexual activity.

Despite these positive signs, religion is by no means a panacea for teen drug use or other risk behaviors. Nearly one in three high school seniors who said that religion is very important reported smoking marijuana in the past year. Thus, a significant minority of religious youth are engaged in some illegal or risk-taking behaviors. And yet, by way of comparison, 56% of those for whom religion was not at all important reported smoking marijuana in the last 12 months. In short, religion significantly reduces negative developmental outcomes for American teens, but it does not eliminate them altogether.

In addition, it is worth noting that religion is not the only factor influencing delinquency and risk behavior among American teens. In many studies, peer influence often exerts the most powerful influence over their behavior. Adolescents who associate with juvenile delinquents or risk-taking friends are much more inclined to participate in such activities than those embedded in more pro-social peer groups. In this way,

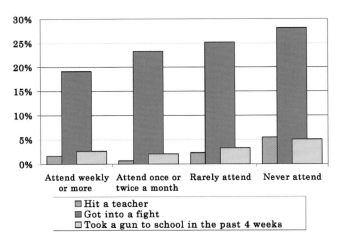

Figure 36.2: Violent Behavior Among High School Seniors by Frequency of Religious Attendance, 1996

Source: Monitoring the Future 1996

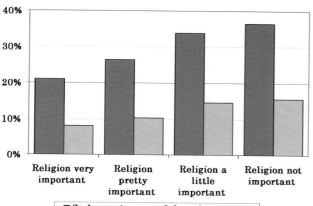

Figure 36.3: Stealing Among High School Seniors and Personal Importance of Religion, 1996

Source: Montioring the Future 1996

■ Stolen an item worth less than $50
□ Stolen an item worth greater than $50

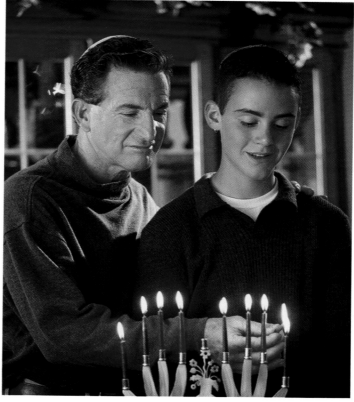

the protective effects of religion must be considered within the broader context of teens' lives. And, make no mistake, the influence of peers in teens' lives—especially during late adolescence—is profound.

Explaining the Influence of Religion in the Lives of American Teens—Although scholars continue to debate the mechanisms through which religion exercises influence on adolescent outcomes, there seems to be a growing appreciation for the power of religious networks in faith communities. Recent research suggests that religion promotes "network closure."[6] Network closure is a process in which "birds of a feather flock together." In the case of youth and religion, faith communities act as conduits through which young people can form tight pro-social relationships—that is, connections with other people who collectively steer youth toward positive developmental outcomes. In religious communities, such pro-social relationships come in various forms—a youth minister who serves as a positive role model, peers who together take a virginity pledge to delay sex until marriage, and a church's reinforcement of family proscriptions against illegal drug use.

> **As older teens mature into young adults, it is the religious practices of their peers—rather than their parents— that exhibit the strongest influence on their faith.**

Network closure creates a coordinated effort among a teen's parents, schoolteachers, ministers, and even parents of those in the teen's friendship circle—all of whom know one another and share common values. The effect of network closure is enhanced when parents and teens share the same faith. Thus sociologist Christian Smith argues that "in religious congregations, adolescents are able to form relationships with youth ministers, Sunday school teachers, choir directors, parents of friends, and other adult acquaintances who can relationally tie back to the adolescents' parents. These ties can operate as extrafamilial sources reinforcing parent influence and oversight."[7]

As the discussion presented here suggests, religious youth reap positive developmental outcomes through the tight social networks cultivated in religious communities. However, it is wise to be mindful that religious networks do not promote uniformly positive outcomes. The undermining of educational achievement in fundamentalist faiths likely has economic ramifications for youth that are far from positive. Moreover, adolescent religious involvement inhibits, but does not fully insulate, youth from participating in negative behaviors such as illegal drug use. On balance, though, it is fair to say that religion is an important and generally positive force in the lives of American teens.

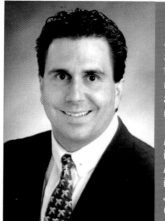

John P. Bartkowski

John P. Bartkowski, PhD, is professor of sociology at Mississippi State University. He is also a research fellow at Mississippi State's Social Science Research Center and at the Center for the Scientific Study of Religion at the University of Texas-Austin. One stream of his research examines the influence of religious involvement on family relationships, while another explores the role of religious institutions in the provision of social welfare. His most recent works include the books *Charitable Choices: Religion, Race, and Poverty in the Post-Welfare Era* (New York University Press, 2003, coauthored with Helen A. Regis) and *The Promise Keepers: Servants, Soldiers, and Godly Men* (Rutgers University Press, 2004). He is also the author of *Remaking the Godly Marriage: Gender Negotiation in Evangelical Families* (Rutgers University Press, 2001). Dr. Bartkowski's published articles have appeared in such outlets as *Social Forces, Sociological Quarterly, Journal of Marriage and Family, Journal for the Scientific Study of Religion, Journal of Family Issues, Gender & Society, Qualitative Sociology, The Responsive Community*, and *Sociology of Religion*.

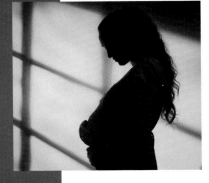

Chapter 37

Paula Duncan
and Emily Kallock

Adolescent Sexuality:
Beyond the Numbers

The decisions youth make related to sexuality in the second decade of life can have dramatic effects on their physical and emotional health. In addition to knowledge of key facts about adolescent sexuality, it is important for parents and other adults to understand and promote strategies that foster healthy decision-making by adolescents.

Data on adolescent sexual activity indicate a decline in teenage pregnancies, births, and abortions across all races and ethnicities.[1] Since 1990, teen pregnancies and birth rates decreased by at least 25%. Teens themselves report less

sexual activity and fewer sexually related health complications.[2] That is the good news. However, worrisome indicators remain.

The most recent U.S. data reveal that "despite declining [pregnancy] rates, more than 4 in 10 teen girls still get pregnant at least once before age 20, which translates into nearly 900,000 teen pregnancies per year."[3] An estimated 18% of 15-year-old girls will give birth before age 20.[3] Sixty percent of Hispanic girls become pregnant before the age of 20, which is twice the percentage of Non-Hispanics.[4] Some of the potential and likely outcomes for teenage parents, particularly teenage mothers, include lower rates of high school completion and higher rates of single parenthood than for people who wait until later to become parents. Children born to teenage parents have been shown to have more health complications, lower cognitive development, and a greater likelihood of becoming teen parents themselves.[5]

Since 1990, teen pregnancies and birth rates decreased by at least 25%. Teens themselves report less sexual activity and fewer sexually related health complications.

Information on sexually transmitted diseases (STDs) indicates that one in four sexually active adolescents becomes infected each year. Syphilis, gonorrhea, and chlamydia are among the most common STDs in the 15- to 19-year-old population.[6] Infections from the human papillomavirus are the most common incurable STD in teenagers.[6] U.S. teenagers have higher STD rates than teenagers in other developed countries such as England, Canada, France, and Sweden, despite the fact that levels of sexual activity and the age at which teenagers become sexually active are similar.[6]

Of special concern is the 20% of youth who become sexually active at age 14 or younger. Among the girls in this group, 81% said they wish they had waited, and 10% said sex was non-voluntary.[5] Sexual pressure, assault, and dating violence are issues of which today's teenagers are acutely aware.[7] Early sexual activity "has been linked to a greater number of sexual partners and an increased risk of teen pregnancy and sexually transmitted diseases."[5] However, only one-half to three-fourths of girls ages 12 to 14 reported contraceptive use the first time they had sexual intercourse, and slightly more than one-half of the girls and two-thirds of the boys used contraception at last intercourse.[5] These young people who have initiated sexual activity are also more likely to smoke, use drugs and alcohol, and participate in delinquent activities than youth who have not had sex. It is

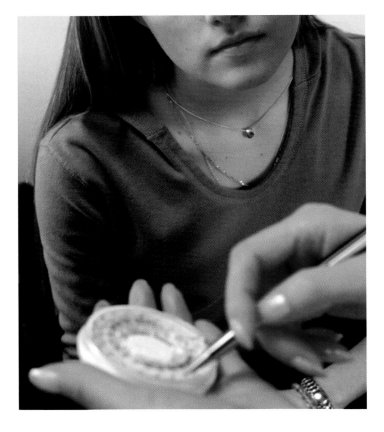

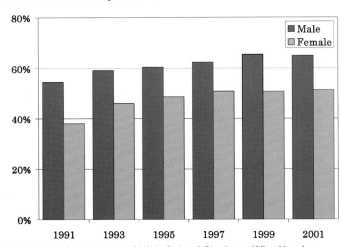

Figure 37.1: Percentage of High School Students Who Used a Condom During Last Sexual Intercourse

Source: Youth Risk Behavior Surveillance Survey 1991-2001

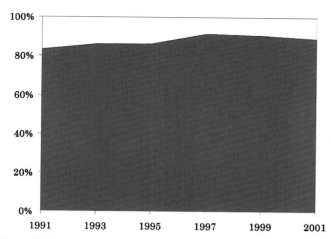

Figure 37.2: Percentage of Students Who Had Ever Been Taught About AIDS or HIV in School

Source: Youth Risk Behavior Surveillance Survey 1991-2001

important to note that of these young adolescents who had experienced sex, 40% had not had sex at all in the preceding 18 months before they were surveyed, and over 50% had only one partner in the same time period.[5]

There is more to the story about youth and sexuality than statistics about pregnancy and disease; decisions about sexual behaviors are part of the larger context of our human needs for respectful and caring relationships. Unlike violence, tobacco use, or drug and alcohol abuse, sexual activity is not something to be avoided for life. Adults should guide teens and provide them with information and opportunities to make healthy, informed decisions about friendships, romantic relationships, and their futures. Sexual activity must be viewed in the context of these larger issues. Teens volunteer, care about world issues, and try to find meaningful

activities in and out of school; adults should recognize the good decisions teens make and give them more chances to demonstrate their abilities.

Using a positive developmental framework, such as the Circle of Courage youth empowerment model with its components of generosity, belonging, mastery, and independence, can help youth and the adults in their lives keep a focus on what youth need to "say yes to" as well as what problems can be avoided.[8]

In *Raising Teens*, A. Rae Simpson provides information to help parents balance opportunities for letting youth make decisions with the need for parents to set limits. Simpson describes "the five basics of parenting adolescents: love and connect, monitor and observe, guide and limit, model and consult, and provide and advocate."[9] Although these principles were written for parents, they speak to all adults about the range of support youth need to pursue activities that drive their well-being and success into adulthood. The need for adults to stay involved with youth from the earliest age into adolescence—not only to stay informed about their needs but also to establish a balance of trust and independent decision-making—is echoed in youth voices with statements like, "We really care what you think even if we don't always act like it."[10]

Overall, parents overestimate the impact media and peers have on youth and underestimate the impact their own care, concern, and understanding can have on youth decision-making, even from an early age. As summarized by Moore and Zaff in the Child Trends brief, *Building a Better Teenager: A Summary of "What Works" in Adolescent Development*, teens who have

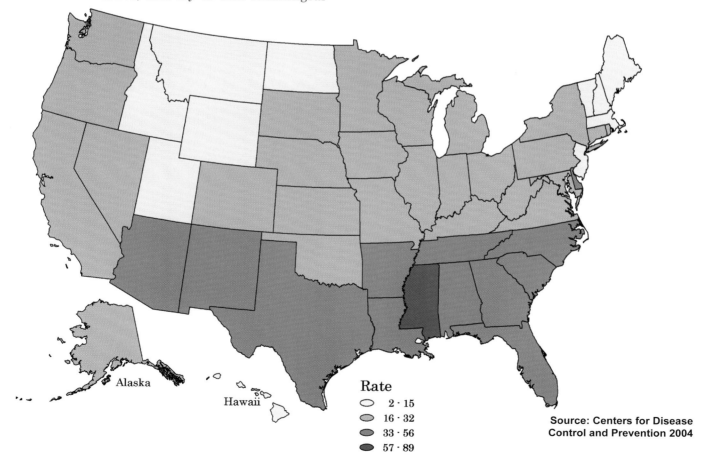

Rate
○ 2 · 15
◔ 16 · 32
◑ 33 · 56
● 57 · 89

Source: Centers for Disease Control and Prevention 2004

Map 37.1: Birth Rate for Women Under Age 15 Per 100,000, 2000

161

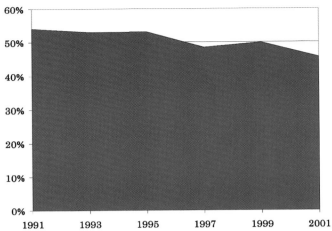

Figure 37.3: Percentage of High School Students Who Have Ever Had Sexual Intercourse

Source: Youth Risk Behavior Surveillance Survey 1991-2001

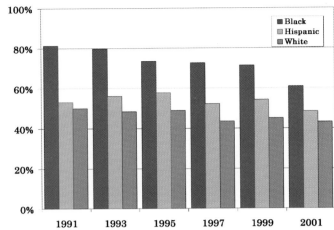

Figure 37.5: Percentage of High School Students Who Have Ever Had Sexual Intercourse by Race and Ethnicity

Source: Youth Risk Behavior Surveillance Survey 1991-2001

warm, involved, and satisfying relationships with their parents are "more likely to do well in school, be academically motivated and engaged, have better social skills, and have lower rates of risky sexual behavior than their peers."[11] Youth whose parents know and monitor their children's activities, friends, and behaviors have less risky behavior.[11] Research by Miller et al. suggests that those same children are less likely to become sexually active.[12]

In Child Trends' *The First Time*, there is an emphasis on communication between parents and teens and among teens in their relationships.[7] Parents can communicate the importance of abstinence and help in their youths' achievement of other goals to further healthy development. Failure in adolescent communication with parents is most pronounced for boys, despite parents' best efforts and belief that the communication is effective. Several studies have shown that parents discuss sexuality-related issues with their daughters more frequently than with their sons.[5] However, boys feel pressured by their peers to engage in sexual activity and do so more often than girls.[13] Boys are also more likely than girls to have multiple partners.[2] This not only raises boys' risk of sexually transmitted disease and teenage fatherhood, but also increases risks for the smaller population of girls engaging in early sexual activity.

There are positive influences other than the parental relationship in an adolescent's world, such as supportive relationships with friends, school success, opportunities to participate in youth development activities, and opportunities to contribute to their community. Youth who have these assets in their lives are less likely to be involved in risky behaviors.[14] "Promising programs to improve reproductive health outcomes include those that focus on early childhood investments, involve teens in school and in outside activities (including youth development in combination with sexuality education and community volunteer learning), and send nurses to visit teenage mothers, which reduces their chance of becoming pregnant again."[15]

Schools are important community-based resources that offer opportunities for healthy youth activities and accomplishments of developmental tasks. The most obvious and important contribution schools can make is the promotion of academic success and eventual graduation from high school for all students.[16] The National Campaign to Prevent Teen Pregnancy cites early school failure as a key risk factor in youth who

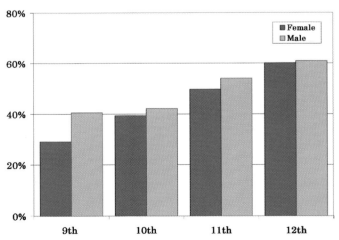

Figure 37.4: Percentage of High School Students Who Have Ever Had Sexual Intercourse by Gender and Grade Level

Source: Youth Risk Behavior Surveillance Survey 1991-2001

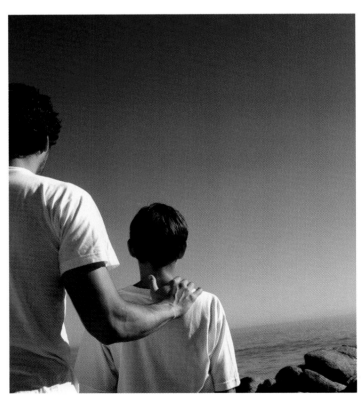

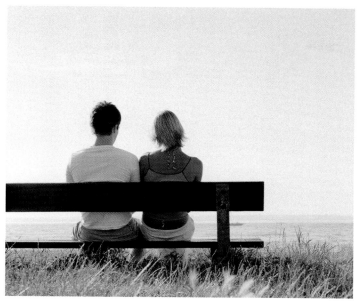

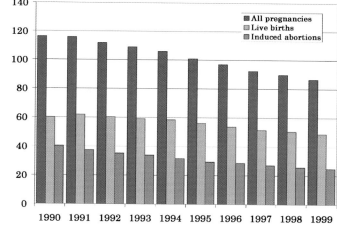

Figure 37.6: Pregnancy, Live Birth, and Induced Abortion Rates for 15- to 19-Year-Old Women per 100,000

Source: National Center for Health Statistics 2003

may become pregnant before graduating from high school.[17] Schools are often a place where youth receive health education—a source of facts critical to healthy decision-making. Child Trends' *Preventing Teenage Pregnancy, Childbearing, and Sexually Transmitted Diseases: What Research Shows* reviews sources of information for the evaluation of health education programs and their impact on teenage sexual activity.[15]

Access to comprehensive and respectful health care and information, as well as community education and support, is particularly important for youth who are gay, lesbian, bisexual, or trans-gendered. Some of these young people are at increased risk for health problems, including STDs, suicide, and physical attack.[18] Similarly, service providers estimate that 25% to 40% of homeless youth may be gay, lesbian, bisexual, or transgendered and that up to 28% of gay or bisexual youth drop out of school due to peer harassment.[19]

> **Parents overestimate the impact media and peers have on youth and underestimate the impact their own care, concern, and understanding can have on youth decision-making, even from an early age.**

Parents and professionals can learn from the successes that other countries are having in sexuality-related adolescent health outcomes. The United States has the highest teen pregnancy and birth rates of western developed nations, and the costs for risky adolescent sexual behaviors, at an individual and societal level, are extremely high. While the Netherlands has a teen (ages 15-19) pregnancy rate of 12 per 1,000 per year and most western European countries have a rate under 40, the United States has a teen pregnancy rate of 70 (along with Belarus, Bulgaria, Romania, and the Russian Federation).[6]

Encouraging trends demonstrate that success is possible. Now is the time to expand promising and proven approaches so that youth in all of our communities have the opportunity and support to complete their education, the knowledge and skills to make healthy decisions related to relationships and sexuality, and the guidance of caring adults.

Paula Duncan and Emily Kallock

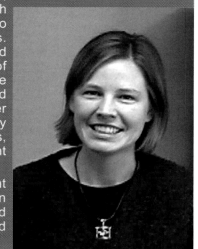

Paula Duncan, MD, is the youth health director at the Vermont Child Health Improvement Program and a professor of pediatrics at the University of Vermont School of Medicine. In partnership with public health, Medicaid, and Vermont health plans, her team works with Vermont pediatric and family medicine practices to improve adolescent preventive health care services. Nationally, she cochairs the Health, Early Care, and Education Consortium of the American Academy of Pediatrics (AAP) Center for Child Health Research. She is the AAP Community Pediatrics Action Group chair and a past chair of the AAP Committee on School Health. Her work has focused on family, state, school, and community partnerships to improve child and youth health outcomes, especially through the use of positive youth development approaches.

Emily Kallock, LICSW, is a project director at the Vermont Child Health Improvement Program. She brings to the program a background in direct-practice social work in schools and with pregnant and parenting teenagers. Ms. Kallock's professional and educational experience also includes work in nonprofit program evaluation and administration.

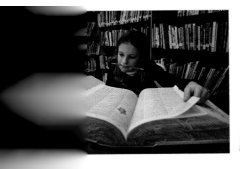

Chapter 38

Karen Hein
and Shannon Flasch

Youth as a Resource

T he first step toward understanding what is meant by "youth as a resource" is to acknowledge the dual nature of this phrase. It may be read as two separate, but complementary statements:

Young people *are* a resource.

Young people *should be treated* as a resource.

These two statements have important implications for young people, youth work, and youth development. If we argue that young people are a resource, then in what way are they valuable? To whom? If we accept that young people are of value, then how can we nurture and sustain this resource?

Young People Are a Resource—As the 21st century begins, the demographics of our country and the world are changing. The United Nations Population Fund reports that nearly half of all people in the world are under 25, and this group constitutes the largest ever generation of young people.[1] In the United States, young people under 25 make up more than one-third of the population, and their numbers are increasing.[2] This group is also demographically notewor-thy because it is more ethnically diverse than the adult population, with 39% of the under-25 population reporting Non-Caucasian status. This figure is up from 25% in 1980. As these young people go to school, take part in community life, and enter the workforce, they experience a more urban and diverse world than their parents, and surveys have found them to be more tolerant than their elders.[3] By growing up with peers of diverse backgrounds, young people are acquiring the worldview that will shape the ethnic and class relations of the future.

Young people are a diverse resource, not only in terms of who they are, but also in terms of what they know. This

> ## In the United States, young people under 25 make up more than one-third of the population, and their numbers are increasing.

generation is technologically astute. Over 57% of American young people have bedrooms equipped with a television, and 20% have bedrooms with a computer. More than half of American households with children own Internet-capable computers, and the family technical expert is likely to be a young person.[4] Additionally, young people are using new media to supplement, not replace, older forms. The Pew Internet and American Life Project found that students use the Internet to research school projects, meet online with study group members, and obtain virtual tutoring for homework.[5] Some students even noted that the Internet was a source of current information at a time when their school textbooks might be a decade old.[6]

How, then, does this growing, diverse, educated, and skilled resource contribute in society? Voter turnout among youth (ages 18-24) has declined from 42% in 1972 to 28% in 2000[7]; in the latter year, this group represented 8% of all voters.[8] Voter participation statistics are an inadequate reflection of youth engagement in civil society because these figures do not indicate the laudable efforts of many youth. Young people's contributions to their communities are better reflected in the range of volunteer and public service roles they play. For example, the proportion of first-year college students who report engaging in volunteer work has increased from 66% in 1989 to 81% in 2000.[9] Some studies have suggested that low levels of voter participation and high levels of

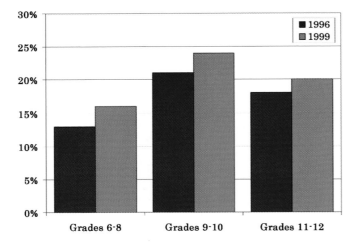

Figure 38.1: Percentage of Students Participating in Community Service Activities by Grade Level

Source: National Center for Education Statistics 1999

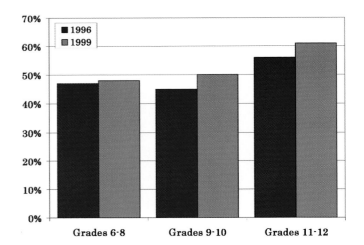

Figure 38.2: Percentage of Schools That Require and Arrange Community Service for Students by Grade Level

Source: National Center for Education Statistics 1999

voluntarism can coexist in this population because of young people's belief in the efficacy of bottom-up, community-based movements.

This combination of civic engagement and grass-roots activism can be seen in youth- and adult-founded organizations. Young people should be, and increasingly are, the staff, consultants, and board members of organizations geared to serve their needs. A national organization, America's Promise, has young people involved through its Youth Partnership Team, made up of students who serve on the boards and leadership teams of constituent, youth-serving organizations.[10] Young people are increasingly involved in philanthropy, serving in youth grant-making organizations.[11] They are also brought into government agencies as advisors in the process of their own care, as in the Massachusetts foster care system, which employs a youth advisory board that meets with the commissioner four times per year to address issues of concern to them.[12] Mass youth organization—such as the popular protests led by young people against the war in Vietnam in the 1960s and 1970s; the World Trade Organization in the 1990s and first part of this century; and, most recently, the war in Iraq—is built upon the idea that young people can affect meaningful change in their communities. Mass youth organization has become another important arena in which young people can wield influence as civic agents.

Young People Should Be Treated as a Resource—
Young people in America are a resource to their peers, their communities, and the nation through their numbers, diversity, tolerance, voluntarism, activism, and familiarity with technology. They also account for a sizable portion of consumer spending ($153 billion annually),[13] a fact many advertisers are exploiting. However, when we accept young people as a resource, we must also acknowledge their need to express their talents, to be encouraged, to be given opportunities, and to be nurtured.

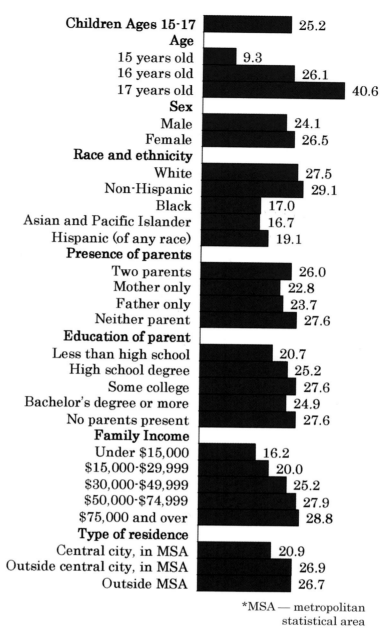

Children Ages 15-17	25.2
Age	
15 years old	9.3
16 years old	26.1
17 years old	40.6
Sex	
Male	24.1
Female	26.5
Race and ethnicity	
White	27.5
Non-Hispanic	29.1
Black	17.0
Asian and Pacific Islander	16.7
Hispanic (of any race)	19.1
Presence of parents	
Two parents	26.0
Mother only	22.8
Father only	23.7
Neither parent	27.6
Education of parent	
Less than high school	20.7
High school degree	25.2
Some college	27.6
Bachelor's degree or more	24.9
No parents present	27.6
Family Income	
Under $15,000	16.2
$15,000-$29,999	20.0
$30,000-$49,999	25.2
$50,000-$74,999	27.9
$75,000 and over	28.8
Type of residence	
Central city, in MSA	20.9
Outside central city, in MSA	26.9
Outside MSA	26.7

*MSA — metropolitan statistical area

Figure 38.3: Children Ages 15 to 17 in Labor Force. Percent Working by Select Characteristics, 2002

Source: U.S. Census Bureau 2003

The National Research Council (NRC), in the 2002 publication *Community Programs to Promote Youth Development*, outlined a positive youth development approach using an asset-based, rather than deficit-based, model. Whereas deficit-based approaches seek to identify and focus on the problems and risks young people face, an asset-based approach is a "broader, more holistic view of helping youth realize their potential."[14] Rather than

focusing on making young people problem-free, the goal becomes making all youth fully prepared to enter adulthood by decreasing risks and increasing supports and opportunities.

The NRC identified eight "features of positive developmental settings" that enable this process. They

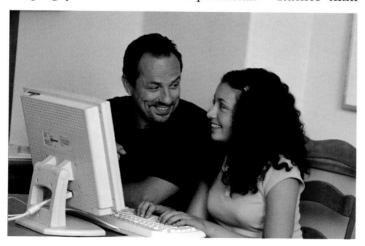

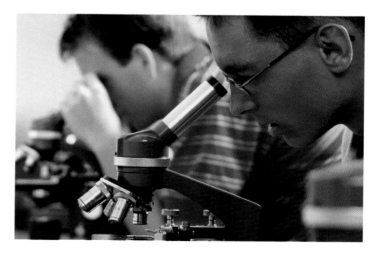

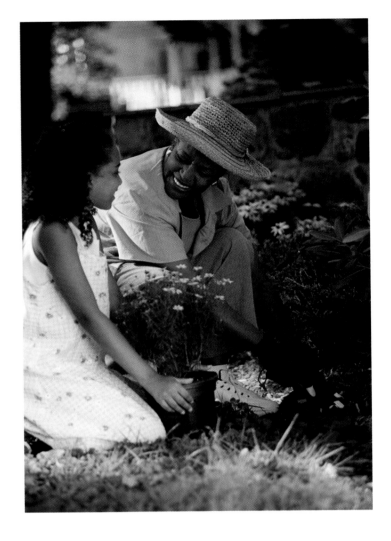

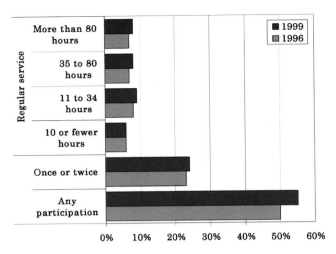

Figure 38.4: Percentage of High School Students Volunteering by Number of Hours Expended, Annually

Source: Forum on Child and Family Statistics 2002

are: physical and psychological safety; appropriate structure; supportive relationships; opportunity to belong; positive social norms; support for efficacy and mattering; opportunities for skill building; and integration of family, school, and community efforts. The NRC argues that by supplying these positive opportunities in the greatest numbers and the greatest variety possible, communities can decrease risk and increase positive development for a greater number of youth. Contrary to a problem-based framework, which might focus on stopping current behaviors, the positive developmental setting framework focuses on improving current behaviors and supporting future well-being and transitions to adulthood.[15]

This approach does not imply ignoring the problems of young people. Rather, by emphasizing the potential of youth and creating opportunities for them, the scope of possible programs is expanded beyond those focused on correction to include those promoting well-being and success. This asset model shifts the loci of interventions away from young people as individuals to the context in which they grow up. If young people are to be nurtured as a resource, then the contexts in which they develop should better reflect the eight features identified by the NRC. Young people exist at the confluence of many societal threads: peer and family groups; youth and educational programs; and the systems and

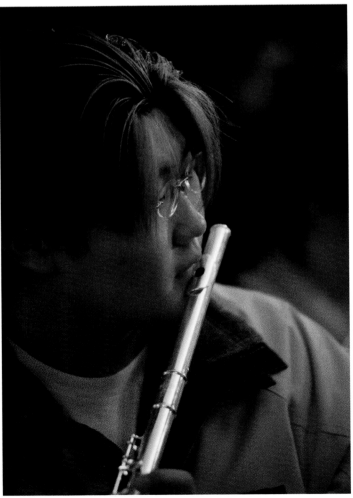

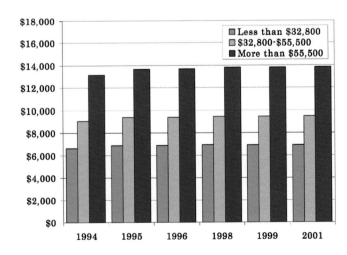

Figure 38.5: Average Annual Expenditure per Child by Two-parent Families by Income Level

Source: U.S. Statistical Abstract 1995-2002

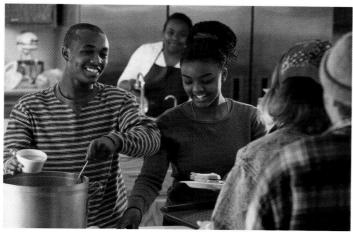

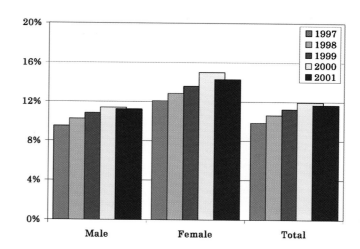

organizations of larger society that include policy decisions, media attention, and many other influential forces that come to bear on young people. Therefore, young people are affected by each of these arenas, and it is through improvements to them that all youth will have the greatest opportunity—not simply to survive, but also to thrive.

Investing in Youth Can Make a Difference—When we identify youth as a resource, we acknowledge many aspects of positive youth development: young people are a significant and talented portion of the population; young people contribute to society and are capable of becoming agents of change in their communities; and, in order to realize this potential, we should adopt an asset-based approach to youth development that seeks to foster and support their growth. The task that we now face is to find the most effective systemic interventions to ensure that more young people will find the opportunities they need to be nurtured as a resource.

In any community, there are many organizations and structures that can help create the developmental environment described by the NRC. Our goal becomes helping the community reorganize to offer more opportunities to youth through schools, social and civic groups, religious organizations, and the business community, among others.

Figure 38.6: The Proportion of Male, Female, and Total Active Military Personnel Who Are Between the Ages of 17-19

Source: U.S. Department of Defense 1999-2003

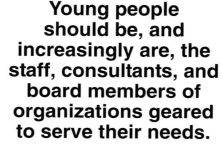

> **Young people should be, and increasingly are, the staff, consultants, and board members of organizations geared to serve their needs.**

At this time, which marks the beginning of a new century, young people are at a crossroads in this country. The current context for their development includes an unstable economy, a high jobless rate, and a high proportion of uninsured—more for this age group than any other. Valued for their military role in the war with Iraq, their needs seem invisible in domestic policy.

However, this generation must also be viewed in a global context. Nearly half of the world's population is under 25, and the proportion of young people is even higher in some developing nations. The number of young people in the world will continue to grow, and the choices we make now will define the context for development for this and future generations. As we look ahead to 2025, when infants born now will enter adulthood—in this country as well as in Afghanistan, Iraq, Africa, and other developing areas—we should ask if they will find a country and a world that will value and nurture them through their adolescence and enable them to fulfill their potential. Young people are a resource. The way we demonstrate their worth today will make all the difference tomorrow.

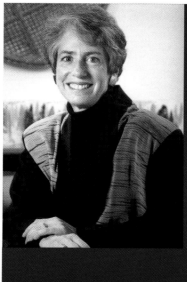

Karen Hein and Shannon Flasch

Karen Hein, MD, is the immediate past president of the William T. Grant Foundation. She served as president from September 1998 to July 2003. As president, she shaped the foundation's efforts to help create a society that values young people and enables them to reach their full potential. The foundation pursues this goal by investing in research and in people and projects that use evidence-based approaches. In addition, Dr. Hein was the executive officer of the Institute of Medicine (National Academy of Sciences) from December 1995 to June 1998. Dr. Hein is clinical professor of pediatrics, epidemiology, and social medicine at Albert Einstein College of Medicine in New York. From 1993 to 1994, she worked on health care reform as a member of the Senate Finance Committee staff in Washington, DC. This chapter was co-written and conceived with Shannon Flasch, assistant to the executive office at the foundation.

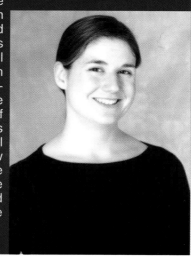

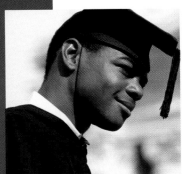

Chapter 39

Access to Postsecondary Education

Kati Haycock and Yun Yi

Postsecondary education has never been more important than it is in today's information society. Businesses are demanding greater skills and more education from their employees. Indeed, without strong skills, new employees do not even make it to the bottom rung of the ladder leading to jobs that pay a family-supporting wage. And it is not just work; it also takes sophisticated skills to participate actively in our democracy. For all these reasons and more, it is as important today for all young people to have at least some postsecondary education as it was for them to have a high school diploma just a generation ago.

Fortunately, students seem to understand this better than anyone else. Among those who graduate from high school, a full 75% enroll in postsecondary education within 2 years after getting their diplomas.[1] And those numbers have been increasing steadily over the past two decades. Unfortunately many of those college freshmen do not make it even to the sophomore year. Only about half of those who begin 4-year colleges eventually earn a degree.[2] Clearly, we must do better.

In fall 2000, there were approximately 13.2 million undergraduate students enrolled in degree-granting public and private postsecondary educational institutions in the United States.[3] Sixty percent attended full-time, while 40% attended part-time. Fifty-five percent were enrolled in 4-year institutions, while 45% attended 2-year institutions. Of the total undergraduate population, 44% were male, and 56% were female. White

Twenty-six percent of freshmen at 4-year colleges and 45% of freshmen at 2-year institutions do not return their sophomore year.

students comprised 68% of the total, followed by Black students at 12%, Hispanics at 10%, and Asians at 6%.

Over the past three decades, college-going rates (that is, the rates of those enrolling in college the year following graduation from high school) have risen for students as a whole, increasing from 47% of high school graduates in 1973 to 63% in 2000.[4]

Race/Ethnicity Differences—Between 1973 and 2000, college attendance grew overall. College-going rates for Whites increased from 48% in 1973 to 66% in 2000, and the rates for Blacks increased from 41% to 56% during the same time period. College-going rates for Hispanic students remained at 49%. Because growth was highest among White students, the gap between White students and Black and Hispanic students widened. Indeed, the gap between White and

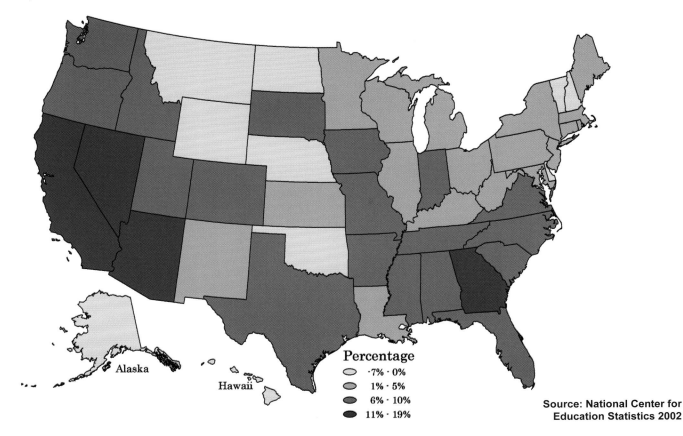

Percentage
- -7% - 0%
- 1% - 5%
- 6% - 10%
- 11% - 19%

Source: National Center for Education Statistics 2002

Map 39.1: Percentage Change in Total Fall Enrollment in Degree-granting Institutions, 1996 to 2000

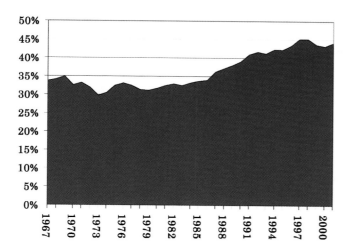

Figure 39.1: Percentage of All 18- to 24-Year-Old High School Completers Currently Enrolled in Postsecondary Institutions

Source: National Center for Education Statistics 2002

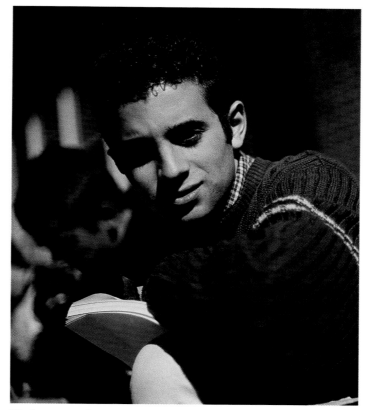

Black students grew from 7% in 1973 to 10% in 2000, while the gap between White and Hispanic students increased by a staggering rate of -1% (in favor of Hispanics) to 17%.

Family Income Differences—Students from every level of family income are attending college in higher numbers today, with the biggest increases among those from middle-class and low-income families. However, there remains a disturbing gap between students at opposite ends of the income spectrum. More than three-quarters of students from high-income families go immediately to college from high school compared to under half of the students from low-income families.

Gender Differences—Thirty years ago, there was a 7% gap in college-going rates between males (50%) and females (43%). Today there is a 6% gap, but now a higher percentage of females (66%) than males (60%) enroll in college immediately after high school.

Although more students are pursuing postsecondary education than ever before, persistence to the second year and degree completion have not kept pace. Twenty-six percent of freshmen at 4-year colleges and 45% of freshmen at 2-year institutions do not return their sophomore year.[5] And even when students do return for the second year, there is no guarantee they will earn a degree. Nationwide, about 52% of students at 4-year institutions graduate within 5 years.[2]

Unfortunately, graduation rates are considerably lower for some groups of students than for others. For example, in NCAA Division I institutions, 59% of students graduate within 6 years. Among White students in these institutions, 6-year graduation rates are 62%, while for Black students they are 41% and for Hispanic students, 50%.[6]

Some higher education officials argue that graduation rates do not tell us much since not all students who go to college intend to graduate. But these claims are not born out by the data. The most recent available data suggest that 99% of freshmen enrolled in 4-year institutions planned to receive a bachelor's degree or higher, most of them from the same institution in which they started.[7]

Because they graduate from high school and enter college at lower rates than their White and Asian counterparts, Black and Hispanic students are far less likely to

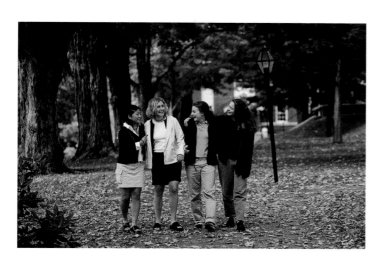

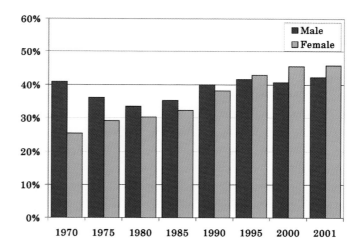

Figure 39.2: Percentage of All 18- to 24-Year-Old High School Completers Currently Enrolled in Postsecondary Institutions by Gender

Source: National Center for Education Statistics 2002

169

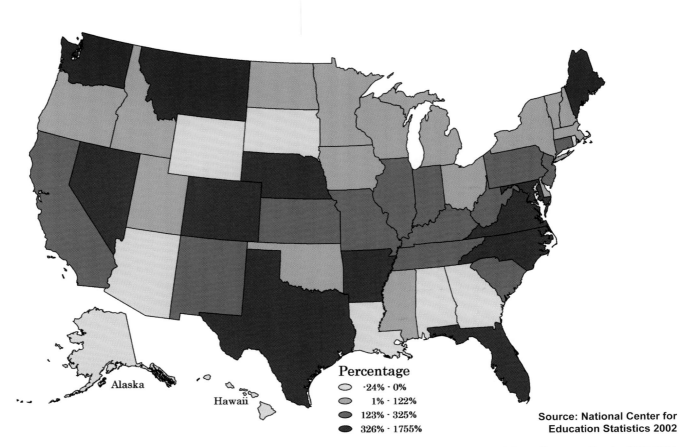

Percentage
- -24% - 0%
- 1% - 122%
- 123% - 325%
- 326% - 1755%

Source: National Center for Education Statistics 2002

Map 39.2: Percentage Change in State Need-based Undergraduate Scholarship and Grant Program Funds, 1987-2001

complete a bachelor's degree. Black students are just over half as likely as White students to obtain a bachelor's degree; Hispanic students are only about one-third as likely.

The picture is even worse for students from low-income families. Children from affluent families are more than 8 times as likely to earn a bachelor's degree by age 26 as those in poor families. By age 26, approximately 7% of young adults from the bottom quartile of family socioeco-

nomic status have earned a BA compared to 60% of young adults in families with socioeconomic status in the top quartile.[8]

One major reason for the disparity between college entrance and degree completion is that students are not being adequately prepared in high school to meet the rigorous demands of postsecondary education. Almost one in three college freshmen must take remedial courses in math, English, or both.[9] Unfortunately, the more remediation students need, the smaller their chances for graduating from college. If our secondary schools and colleges worked together to make sure that students were adequately prepared in high school by taking the appropriate coursework, far more students who begin college would complete a degree.

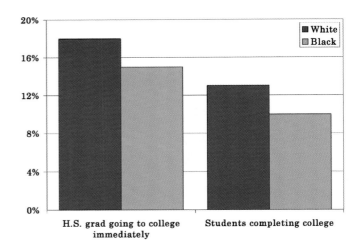

Figure 39.3: Percentage Change in College-going and College Completion from 1973 to 2000

Source: U.S. Department of Education 2002

170

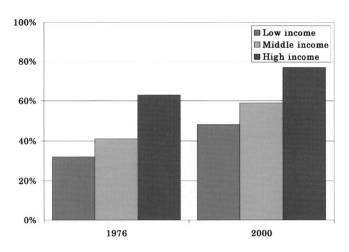

Figure 39.4: Percentage of High School Graduates Going to College Immediately by Family Income

Source: U.S. Department of Education 2002

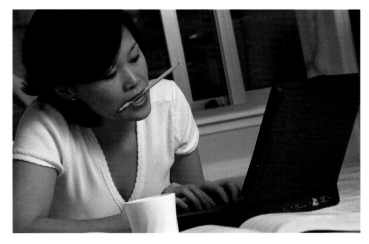

Some students leave college not because they are struggling academically, but because they are struggling financially. Increasingly, states, institutions, and even the federal government are moving away from offering need-based financial aid and going toward assistance based solely on merit. In essence, this moves more money toward those who need it least, leaving less for those who need it most. The federal Pell Grant program, historically a major source of aid for low-income students, is a case in point. Although Pell Grants increased by 23% in inflation-adjusted dollars in 2001 to 2002, the maximum Pell Grant now covers only 42% of the average fixed costs at a public, 4-year institution (tuition, fees, and room and board) compared to 84% 20 years ago.[10] Financial assistance is declining at a time when the cost of a college education is growing exponentially. In the last decade, the price of a college education increased by 21% at public institutions and 26% at private institutions, after adjustment for inflation.[3] This means that students must work harder and borrow more than ever before.

> **In the last decade, the price of a college education increased by 21% at public institutions and 26% at private institutions.**

For years, the United States led the world in high school graduation rates, college entry, and college completion rates. But things are changing. Currently, the United States ranks only 10th among the 30 Organization for Economic Co-operation and Development (OECD) member countries in high school graduation.[11] Because of much steeper increases in college attendance in other countries, we no longer lead the world in college completion rates. Indeed, the United States currently ranks 6th in college completion among 17 OECD countries (behind the United Kingdom, Australia, Finland, Poland, and Iceland).

We must continue to increase the number of American young people who pursue postsecondary education. Their futures depend on it. But it is no longer enough to focus just on increasing access. Educators and policymakers must develop focused policies to ensure that all students are adequately prepared for the rigors of college-level work and that they also have the financial help they need to complete their chosen course of study.

Kati Haycock and Yun Yi

Kati Haycock, MA, is one of the nation's leading child advocates in the field of education. She currently serves as director of The Education Trust in Washington, DC. Established in 1990, The Trust speaks up for what's right for young people, especially those who are poor or members of minority groups. The Trust also provides hands-on assistance to urban school districts and universities that want to work together to improve student achievement. Before coming to The Education Trust, Haycock served as executive vice president of the Children's Defense Fund, the nation's largest child advocacy organization.

A Native Californian, Haycock founded and served as president of The Achievement Council, a statewide organization that provides assistance to teachers and principals in predominantly minority schools for improving student achievement. She has also served as director of the Outreach and Student Affirmative Action programs for the nine-campus University of California system.

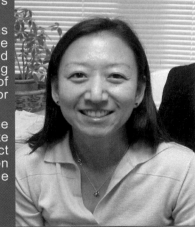

Yun Yi, MA, currently works as a policy associate at The Education Trust. Her primary responsibilities include researching and analyzing state and federal education policies. Prior to joining The Trust, Yi worked as a project manager at the Chicago Panel on School Policy, where she conducted research on Chicago public school programs and policies. Yi's other job experiences include counseling and advocacy work on behalf of disadvantaged youth.

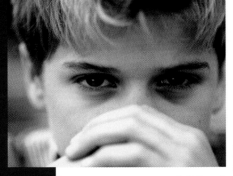

Chapter 40

Shay Bilchik

Children and the Law

I t has been said that how a society treats its children is the best measure of how just it is. Children should be active contributors within any just society and considered essential and worthy of standing in all public settings and of having a right to be heard. Unfortunately for the majority of U.S. history, the phrase "justice for children" has been largely considered a goal that has been unrealized to the degree many would have desired. It has only been over the past 100 years that we have seen a slow but steady march forward in improving children's rights and the status children hold in our nation's legal system. Whether as victims, perpetrators, witnesses in our justice system, or as participants in our systems of care, we have largely relegated them to second-class citizenship. Too little attention has been given to their developmental needs and the investments it would take

to provide a fair and just court system that would attend to those needs.

While this status may be a natural progression from the early days of legal history, as evidenced by such edicts as the Code of Hammurabi ("if a son has struck his father, his hands shall be cut off") or the Hebrew law as reflected in Exodus, Deuteronomy, and Leviticus ("if a man has a stubborn and rebellious son who will not obey his voice...then his father and his mother shall take hold of him and bring him to the elders of his city...and all the men of the city shall stone him to death..."), it is nevertheless disturbing that in today's civilized society, we have not progressed further in acting in our children's best interests.

> **It was not until the late 1800s that the concept of "children's rights" emerged in the public's conscience.**

It was not until the late 1800s that the concept of "children's rights" emerged in the public's conscience. A group of concerned community members in New York went to court to fight for the safety of "Mary Ellen," a young child abused by her parents and left unprotected by the laws of her state. Those community members took the very creative approach of using the laws protecting animals from cruel treatment to petition the court in the interest of Mary Ellen. This bold action raised the country's awareness that our laws did not adequately protect children and brought to light the level of abuse and the unabated maltreatment children suffered as a result. Those caring community members set this country on a path we are still following with mixed results to this day.

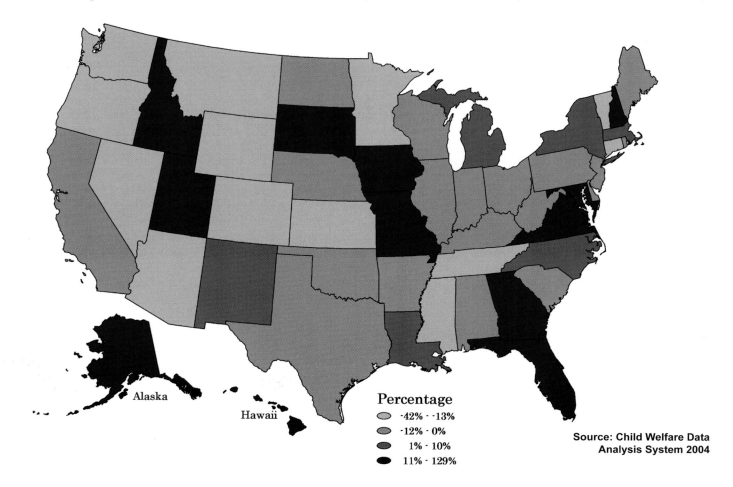

Alaska

Hawaii

Percentage
- -42% - -13%
- -12% - 0%
- 1% - 10%
- 11% - 129%

Source: Child Welfare Data Analysis System 2004

Map 40.1: Percentage Change in Substantiated Child Abuse Cases 2000 to 2001

About Children

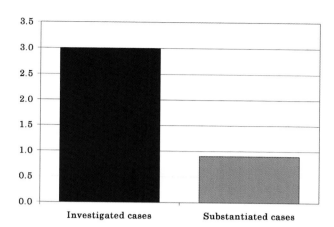

Figure 40.1: Number of Children Referred to Child Welfare Agencies (Millions of Cases), 2001
Source: The Child Welfare League of America 2001

It was also in the late 1800s that we saw action to formalize the treatment of children in the juvenile court who were charged with delinquent offenses. This led to a refining of the doctrine of *parens patriae*, the idea that the state has the right and responsibility to intervene on behalf of its citizens who, by virtue of their youthfulness, require that the state act as a surrogate parent. While to a certain degree limiting a youth's exposure to the full weight of the law, it was also used to deny our youth the right to due process, equal protection, counsel, and a trial by a jury of their peers. Through a number of cases appealed to the U.S. Supreme Court, a greater panoply of rights was granted to our youth, constantly balancing the rehabilitative intent of the law with the denial of constitutional protections.

In virtually each instance, the courts have ruled that the legal protections afforded to our children can be compromised if the law in question is designed to further our society's interests in their protection, nurturance, and overall development. To many child advocates, this balancing has been used to deprive thousands of children many of the rights all other citizens in this country take for granted without the corresponding benefits being realized. Many would argue, for example, that it is neither fair nor just to incarcerate a youth pending trial and then placement, only to fail to provide the treatment indicated in the assessments made of the youth's rehabilitative needs.

There are numerous places that our children's lives cross paths with the law: as victims, as law breakers (delinquents), and as witnesses to crime. In addition, children are the subjects of laws designed to protect their interests such as mandatory school attendance, interventions when they demonstrate behavior indicating their need for services or supervision (e.g., ungovernability), and laws prohibiting their use of alcohol or tobacco. Perhaps the two areas of greatest concern, however, relate to the compromised rights of children charged with violating the law and children "seeking" justice in our family courts as victims of child abuse and neglect.

In 2001, almost 3 million children in the United States were reported as abused or neglected. Approximately 900,000 of those 3 million cases were actually confirmed.

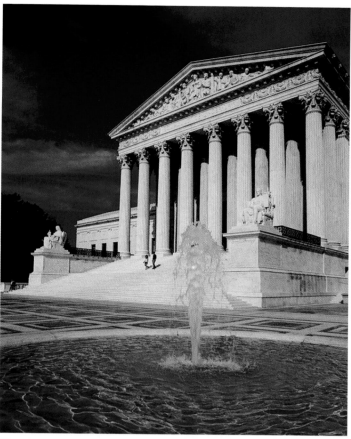

Furthermore, in 2001, over 500,000 children were in out-of-home care as a way of protecting them from further harm. That number was 100,000 more than in 1991. There were also over 1 million delinquency cases referred to our delinquency courts in the year 2001. More than 100,000 youth were placed in residential facilities designed to assist in their rehabilitation that year as well. And there is no reason to believe that these numbers have decreased in the last several years.

One might hear these figures and react with horror at the number of children who, for one reason or the other, were unable to remain in their own homes safe from harm and from harming others. More alarming is the story behind these numbers, a story of courts and related systems of care ill-equipped to act in each and every instance in the best interests of the children that they are charged with serving. It is a story of too many children being removed from their homes to protect them

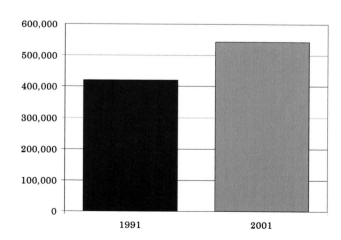

Figure 40.2: Number of Children Placed in Out-of-home Care

Source: The Child Welfare League of America 1991, 2001

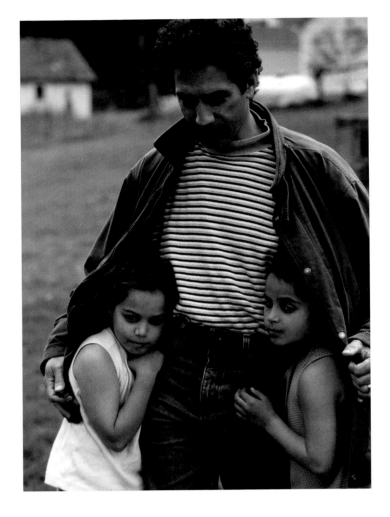

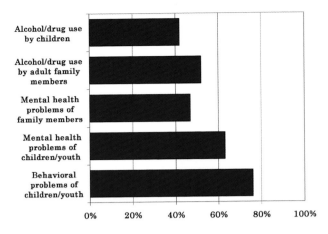

Figure 40.3: Percentage of Child Welfare Agencies Identifying Worsening Situations by Type, 2001
Source: The Child Welfare League of America 2001

from further harm. Yet, they are harmed again as a result of being separated from siblings, forced to change schools because of frequent changes in foster care placement, or denied the basic supports and treatment services they and their families need to ensure their safe and expeditious return home or placement in another safe and permanent home through adoption or guardianship. And it is a story of thousands of children whose lives are frozen in time and end up paying a price for the failure of the state to accurately assess and appropriately address their educational and mental health needs, substance abuse, and increasing levels of aggressive and delinquent behavior.

What is even more alarming than the failures just described are the increases this country has seen in abuse and neglect over the past 20 years. This has occurred without a corresponding increase in an investment in the courts and systems of care that are designed to protect the children. For example, when the states' child welfare systems' performance is measured by the federal government, the states consistently fail to provide full services for these children, performing less than adequately in their Children and Family Service Reviews. These reviews have been implemented by the U.S. Department of Health and Human Services to assess the level of performance by each state in providing safety, a permanent family, and addressing the well-

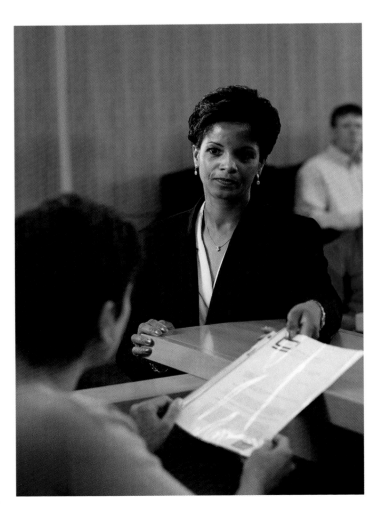

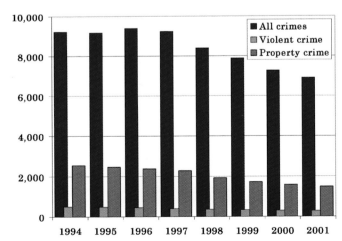

Figure 40.4: Crime Rates for Juveniles Under 18 per 100,000 by Type of Crime
Source: National Center for Juvenile Justice 1994-2001

being of each of the children in their care. Over 40 states have completed their review as of the writing of this chapter, and none have passed more than three of the seven factors being measured.

Starting in the late 1980s and continuing through the early 1990s, there was also a surge in juvenile crime, with a corresponding "get tough" mentality that lead to the building of more juvenile prisons and the increased transfer of youth to the adult criminal justice system. However, these are flawed policies. Research has shown that more community-based interventions and prevention programs located in less restrictive settings are much more effective at reducing juvenile crime and repeat offenses than long-term institutional care in congregate juvenile or adult correctional facilities.

The policies and practices in place in our family and juvenile courts also tend to impact youth of color in a disproportionate fashion, leading to their presence in these two systems of care in percentages that far exceed their overall representation in the population at large. Due in part to societal factors such as poverty, along with systems that are not prepared to provide individualized responses that are culturally appropriate to minority communities, we find deeper penetration into these systems at every stage of decision-making: investigation, intake, initial detention/out-of-home placement, and sentencing/court disposition. Among juvenile offenders, the numbers of children of color who are transferred into the criminal justice system are increasing. In short, children of color fair even worse in this country's legal system than other children.

Unfortunately for the majority of U.S. history, the phrase "justice for children" has been largely considered a goal that has been unrealized to the degree many would have desired.

A recent survey of agencies belonging to the Child Welfare League of America indicated that the level of mental health problems and related alcohol and other drug use was a critically important presenting issue in the families they were asked to serve. Yet, they were only prepared to serve 3 in every 10 of those clients with the service capacity currently in place.

As a society, while we have made progress over the last two centuries, we still are failing to provide justice for

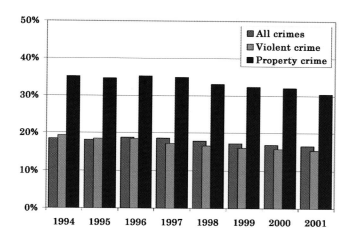

Figure 40.5: Percentage of All Arrests That Were Juveniles Under 18 by Type of Crime
Source: National Center for Juvenile Justice 1994-2001

all. We must provide justice for our children. In carrying out our broader societal role as *parens patriae*, we have failed to achieve the kind of just and fair outcomes our children and youth deserve. In fact, an impartial analysis reveals a flawed system of justice for children, demonstrated by near all-time highs in the number of juveniles arrested and those victimized.[5] A better way must be implemented, one based largely on evidence-based practices that respect the notion of a judicial system that has the capacity to provide individualized justice for each juvenile offender and victim. It should be one that is supported by systems of care that provide appropriate treatment and services that lead to the fair and just outcomes we desire for our children.

Many communities have taken on this difficult but essential challenge by providing counsel in order to ensure fair and competent representation; investing resources to lower case dockets so individualized case reviews and treatment plans may be adopted and implemented by the courts; and giving full credence to the notion of utilizing community-based care and least restrictive options for children and youth in need of services. It is now time for us to adopt these types of approaches nationally as we seek to create the just society our children deserve.

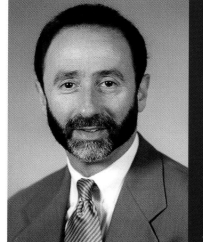

Shay Bilchik

When Shay Bilchik, BS, JD, became president and chief executive officer of the Child Welfare League of America (CWLA) in February 2000, he assumed leadership of the nation's oldest and largest membership-based child welfare organization. Mr. Bilchik has emerged as a leading national spokesperson for children's issues and a top advocate for America's children, youth, and families. His years of experience focusing on children's issues from both a child protection and a public safety perspective, as a prosecutor in Miami and as a U.S. Department of Justice official, in addition to his current role at CWLA, enable him to provide a working knowledge of the most current research, policies, and programs affecting the field. Mr. Bilchik always carries the underlying message that children must be made a top priority in our society. He has received numerous awards for his tireless advocacy on behalf of America's most vulnerable children, youth, and families and was recently named Youth Crime Watch of America's "National Champion of Youth." He is also currently the chair of the National Collaboration for Youth and the Child Protection Advisory Board of the Archdiocese of Washington.

Part Five: About Their Demography and Diversity

Change is a constant. This book is written at a moment in time. The population of this country is in a process of rapid change, with increasing racial and ethnic diversity and growth of minority populations. All components of the lives of children exhibit change. The deep concerns about inequities facing children and youth need to be balanced by significant overall improvements in their health and well-being. Understanding the components and characteristics of change enables a clearer focus on the evolving needs of children and their families for all racial, ethnic, and socioeconomic groups.

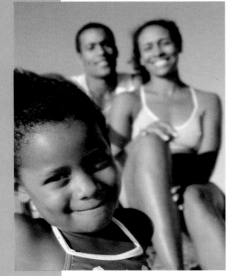

Chapter 41

Daniel T. Lichter

Families:
Diversity and Change

Over one-third of the U.S. population under age 18 is a racial or ethnic minority. This is the highest percentage in U.S. history, and the share of minority children is expected to grow for the foreseeable future.[1] Hispanic children, rather than Black children, make up the largest share of minority children (16%). They also represent the fastest-growing share of American children, reflecting high rates of fertility and immigration among Hispanics. Indeed, 35% of the Hispanic population is under age 18, compared with 26% of the U.S. population.[2]

The economic circumstances and family lives of minority children are as diverse as their racial and ethnic backgrounds. Minority children are no monolith; they face very different living conditions in American society.

The United States continues to have one of the highest child poverty rates in the developed world.[3] Poverty in America is sometimes viewed stereotypically as a minority problem. Indeed, the poverty rate among Black children, for example, was 31.2% in 2000, while Hispanic children had a poverty rate of 28.4%.[4] However, 12.7% of Asian children were poor, a figure lower than that of White children (13.1%). Clearly, minority children's full incorporation into the economic mainstream of American society is uneven across racial and ethnic groups.

The fact that the U.S. poverty rate (16%) among children in 2000 was lower than any time since the late 1970s is

Children's changing economic circumstances, especially among minorities, are inextricably linked to family structure.

encouraging news.[5] In fact, the poverty rate among children declined in the 1990s in 41 of the 50 states.[6] Poverty among female-headed families with children (32.5%) was the lowest on record. Significantly, child poverty declined by about one-third among Black children between 1990 and 2000, and by one-quarter among Hispanics. Such rapid declines are unusual by historical standards, and they far exceed the recent declines experienced by Non-Hispanic White children.

The rise in working mothers played a significant role in this regard.[7] In 2000, more women with children were working and fewer unwed mothers were receiving cash assistance from the government. Fifty percent of children living in a single female-headed family had a full-time, full-year worker in the household.[8] The growth in the number of working parents has been especially rapid for minority children.

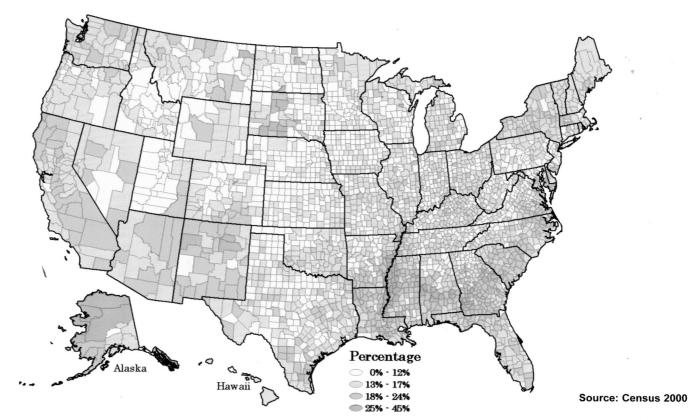

Percentage
- 0% - 12%
- 13% - 17%
- 18% - 24%
- 25% - 45%

Alaska

Hawaii

Source: Census 2000

Map 41.1: Percentage of Households with Children Headed by a Single Parent, 2000

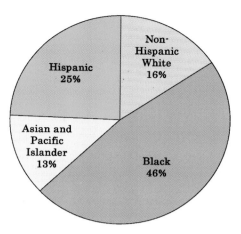

Figure 41.1: Racial Composition of Female-headed Households with Children, 2000

Source: Census 2000

Between 1993 and 2000, the percentage of Black children with a full-time working parent increased from 49% to 69%. It increased from 57% to 72% for Hispanic children.[1] In spite of these trends, poverty rates for many minority children remain high.

Children's changing economic circumstances, especially among minorities, are inextricably linked to family structure. Over 1.3 million children are born each year out-of-wedlock, and another 1 million experience the divorce of their parents. Roughly 11.7 million children live in poor families, most in female-headed families. Only 13% of all married-couple households exhibit the traditional arrangement of a working father and stay-at-home mother.[9] About 70% of children live with two parents. Of these, 12% are living in blended families with a stepparent.

Minority children have been on the front line of family change over the past half-century. Nearly 70% of Black children, for example, are born out-of-wedlock. This compares with one-third among all U.S. children. As a result, only 38% of Black children live with two parents, and only 31% live with their married biological parents. Although Hispanic children share similar economic circumstances to Blacks, 68% live with two parents. One study suggests that a large share of growing racial inequality over the past three decades reflects differences in family structure, especially the rise in female-headed families in the Black community.[10]

Yet, it is important to remember that the post-1960 rise in divorce, unmarried childbearing, single-parent families, and cohabitation has been experienced broadly across America. It has touched virtually every social and economic segment of American society. Family change is not just a "problem" of historically disadvantaged minorities.

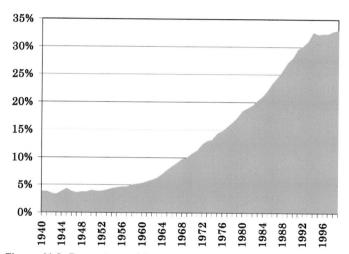

Figure 41.2: Percentage of Births to Unmarried Women

Source: National Center for Heath Statistics 2000

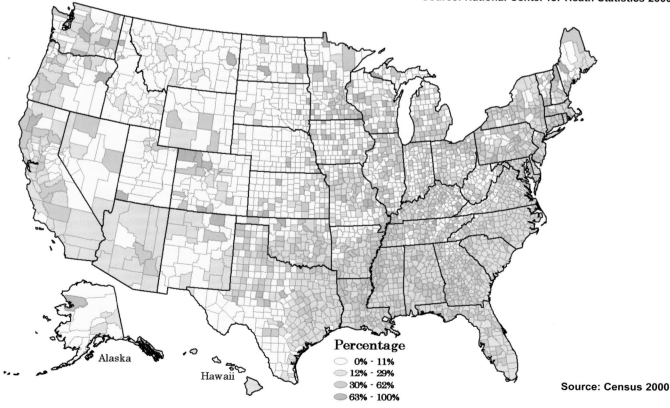

Alaska

Hawaii

Percentage
- 0% - 11%
- 12% - 29%
- 30% - 62%
- 63% - 100%

Source: Census 2000

Map 41.2: Percentage of Black Households with Children Headed by a Female, 2000

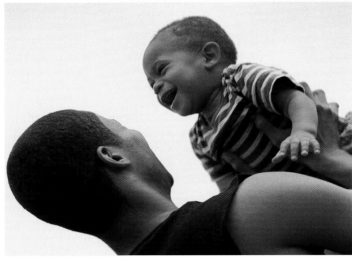

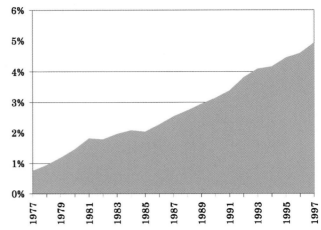

Figure 41.3: Percentage of All Children Under 18 in Cohabiting Households
Source: Demography 2000

Fortunately, the late 1990s and early 2000s have provided reasons for new optimism about the state of America's families. The decline in the share of American children residing in married-couple families finally was halted in the late 1990s. For Blacks, the percentage actually increased slightly, after a free fall during much of the preceding three decades.[11] Moreover, since 1991, the birthrate among adolescents (mostly unmarried) declined by one-third and is now at a record low of 27 births per 1,000. The decline was even more rapid among minority adolescents, dropping by two-fifths for Blacks and by one-fifth for Hispanics since 1994. Racial and ethnic group differences, however, remain large. Hispanic adolescents have the highest birthrate, about 60 births per 1,000 per year, compared with 52 for Blacks and 16 for Whites. Asian adolescents have even lower birthrates.

The growth of female-headed families, especially among Blacks, has attracted much attention from policy makers,

but it should not divert us from other important shifts in American families. Cohabitation, or living together while not married, increased rapidly over the past three decades. Roughly 11% of Hispanic couple households are cohabiting rather than married, compared with 7% for the overall population.[12] Family diversity is the watchword today. For example, recent evidence suggests that 13.3%—about 1 out of 7—of America's children living with single mothers also co-reside with her cohabiting partner.[13,14] The estimates are even higher among some racial and ethnic groups: 17.6% among Mexican American children and 16.2% among Puerto Rican children. Only 1.4% of all Asian children live in a cohabiting-couple family.

At first glance, these figures may seem small, but they underestimate children's experiences in cohabiting-couple families. Current estimates of the share of children who will live with cohabiting parents sometime during their childhoods range from 25% to 40%.[15,16] This

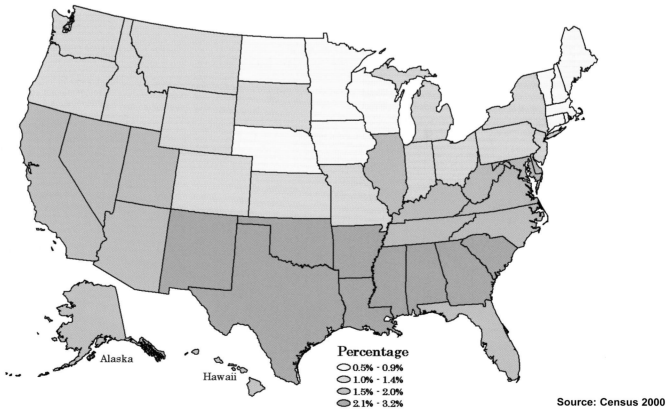

Percentage
- 0.5% - 0.9%
- 1.0% - 1.4%
- 1.5% - 2.0%
- 2.1% - 3.2%

Source: Census 2000

Map 41.3: Percentage of Households with Children Headed by a Grandparent, 2000

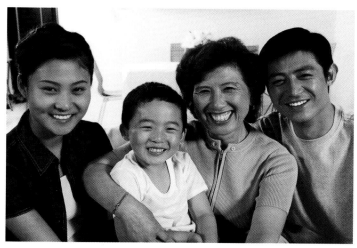

is a significant, but typically understudied, pattern in American family life. Most young adults cohabit before marriage, often more than once, and over 40% of nonmarital fertility occurs among cohabiting couples. Cohabitation is increasingly a context for childbearing and childrearing. Unfortunately, children born into these families often experience instability; most cohabiting couples dissolve. The implications for minority children are unclear, although we know that these children are disproportionately poor.[13]

Fathers have become increasingly involved as caregivers for their children. Yet, only 17% of the children living in a lone-parent family in 2001 were living with the father.[17] This figure grew over the past few decades, thanks to new joint custody arrangements and the efforts of some men's advocacy groups for greater equity in child custody cases.

The share of Black children in lone-parent families living with their fathers is only 9.7%.[18] Most Black children live with single mothers and face high rates of poverty. To compound matters, custodial Black mothers are disproportionately less likely to receive full child support than other groups. They represent 28% of all custodial mothers, but only 16.1% of custodial mothers actually receive full child support.[19] Part of the reason is that most single-parent, Black families result from unwed childbearing rather than from divorce. It is less common for unwed fathers than divorced fathers to seek or gain custody of their out-of-wedlock children, despite new efforts to identify unmarried fathers; enlist

Cohabitation increased rapidly over the past three decades [and] is increasingly a context for childbearing and childrearing.

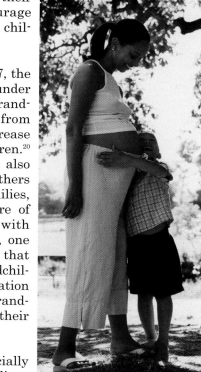

financial support for their children; and encourage involvement in their children's daily lives.

Between 1970 and 1997, the percentage of children under 18 that lived in their grandparent's home rose from about 3% to 5.5%, an increase of nearly 4 million children.[20] Most of these children also co-resided with their mothers in multigenerational families, but an increasing share of these children lived with neither parent. Indeed, one recent study reported that over 1.5 million grandchildren lived in split-generation families headed by grandparents but not with their parents.[21]

Minority children, especially those living in metropolitan central cities, are much more likely than White children to live in multigenerational families or live alone with their grandparents (usually the grandmother). Moreover, 13.5% of Black children lived with their grandparents in multigenerational and split-generation families. Grandparents (usually the grandmother) play a larger child care role in the Black community. Unfortunately, grandchildren living with their grandparents only (i.e., no parent) are more likely to be poor (63%) and receive public assistance (90%) than children in any other family type.[20]

Today's children will be tomorrow's political leaders, voters, employers, workers, neighbors, spouses, and parents. The fact that today's children are disproportionately minority children also means that America's adult population of the future will be much more racially and ethnically diverse than today's. Whether or not this nation and its people support the diverse population of children today will have long-term implications for American society for generations to come.

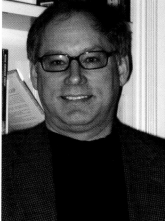

Daniel T. Lichter

Daniel T. Lichter, PhD, is the Robert F. Lazarus Professor in population studies and professor of sociology at The Ohio State University. He also is current director of the University's Initiative in Population Research. Dr. Lichter received his PhD from the University of Wisconsin-Madison in 1981. He spent 18 years on the faculty at Penn State University, where he served as director of the Population Research Institute from 1995 to 1999 before joining the faculty at The Ohio State University. Dr. Lichter is past president of the Association of Population Centers and the current editor of *Demography*, the official journal of the Population Association of America. He sits on advisory boards for the National Center for Children in Poverty, the Campaign to Prevent Teen Pregnancy, and the Census Bureau's Advisory Committee of Professional Associations. Dr. Lichter has published widely on demographic topics related to the family and welfare policy. His recent work has focused on marriage among welfare-dependent, unwed mothers and on pro-social behavior among economically disadvantaged adolescents and young adults.

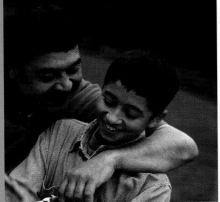

Chapter 42

Steve H. Murdock

Minority Child
Population Growth

Much of the recent growth in the U.S. child population is due to minority children (i.e., children other than Non-Hispanic Whites). However, little is known about the pattern of growth among minority child populations across the country. Substantial differences between rural and urban patterns for minority growth are assumed. On closer examination, it becomes evident that the growth of minority populations is affecting not only urban areas, but rural areas, as well. Equally intriguing are the predictions for future growth in the child population over the next century. A rapidly emerging U.S. minority population will present special needs and require additional resources beyond what is currently available if current socioeconomic disparities are left unaddressed.

The Department of Agriculture has developed a classification system of U.S. counties. The four categories of counties include central city metropolitan counties, commonly referred to as inner-city areas; suburban metropolitan counties; adjacent nonmetropolitan counties, which share a common border with a metropolitan county; and nonadjacent nonmetropolitan, or rural, counties.

There is a common perception that the growth of the minority child population in the United States is a largely metropolitan, inner-city phenomenon, but this is not the case. Whereas the overall number of Non-Hispanic White children increased by 2% during the period from 1990 to 2000, the number of Black children increased by 20.2%, the number of Hispanic children increased by 57.8%, and the number of children from other racial/ethnic groups increased by 39.8%. In metropolitan, inner-city counties, these figures were 1.0%, 23.0%, 56.4%, and 43.6%, respectively. These numbers do not differ dramatically from the numbers for the nation as a whole, indicating that metropolitan, inner-city counties are not the sole sites for minority growth.

In metropolitan suburban areas, the increases were 17.1% for Non-Hispanic White children, 25.0% for Black children, 96.7% for Hispanic children, and 66.3% for children classified as being from other racial/ethnic groups. In nonmetropolitan counties that are adjacent to metropolitan counties (on the outskirts of urban areas), Hispanic children accounted for the largest percentage of net growth (53.6%). In nonmetropolitan, nonadjacent (rural) counties, the number of White children actually decreased while the number of minority children increased. Therefore, contrary to popular belief, minority child population growth is more significant to the growth of rural areas than to the growth of urban areas.

The contribution of minority population growth to the overall U.S. population growth is evident. The net increase in the total number of children in the 1990s attributable to Non-Hispanic White children was only 10.8%, whereas 22.7% of the net increase was attributable to Black children, 54.0% to Hispanic children, and 12.5% to children from other racial/ethnic groups. Only in suburban counties was a majority of the net growth due to Non-Hispanic Whites, and even in such counties, nearly one-third of the net increase was due to minority children.

The particularly pervasive impact of Hispanic population growth is evident in all types of areas. Except in suburban counties, the increase in the number of Hispanic children accounted for more than 50% of the total net increase in the number of children from 1990 to 2000. Even in suburban counties,

> **There is a common perception that the growth of the minority child population in the United States is a largely metropolitan, inner-city phenomenon, but this is not the case.**

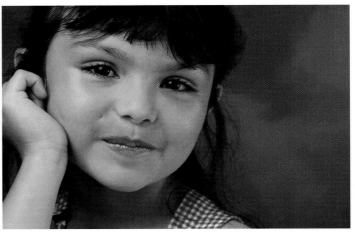

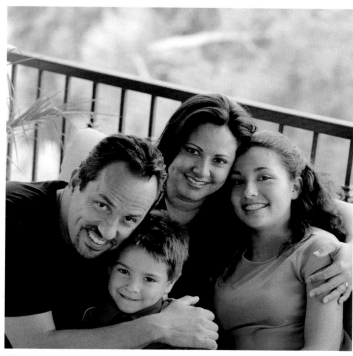

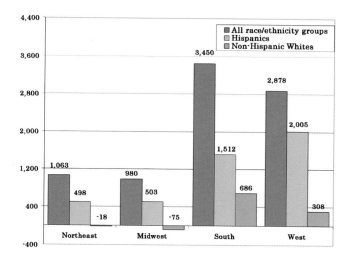

Figure 42.1: Change in Population Less Than 18 Years of Age, 1990-2000 (Numbers in 1,000s)

Source: Calculations by Steve H. Murdock, PhD 2003

Hispanic children accounted for nearly 20% of the net increase in the number of children, although the Hispanic population was only 3.1% of the total population in suburban counties in 1990.

In all four major U.S. census regions, the 1990 to 2000 percentage increases in the child population were greater for minorities than for Non-Hispanic Whites. The national patterns of disproportionate levels of minority, particularly Hispanic, child growth were evident for each of the four county types in each of the regions. Therefore, the rural versus urban geographic

distribution of minority child populations was pervasive throughout the United States.

Future growth in the child population of the United States is projected to be extensive and increasingly diverse. The U.S. Bureau of the Census' most recent projections for the under-18 population point to substantial increases in the future. The number of children in the United States is projected to increase from roughly 70 million in 2000 to nearly 96 million by 2050 and to nearly 130 million by 2100. These changes represent the addition of more than 25 million children (36.1%) between 2000 and 2050 and nearly 59.5 million children (84.5%) between 2000 and 2100.

The growth in the population of children will be largely attributable to the increase in the number of

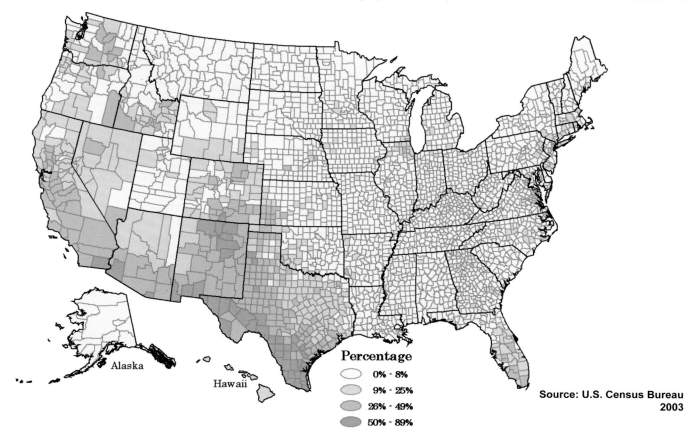

Map 42.1: Percentage of Population 18 and Under That Is Hispanic, 2003

Source: U.S. Census Bureau
2003

Percentage
0% - 8%
9% - 25%
26% - 49%
50% - 89%

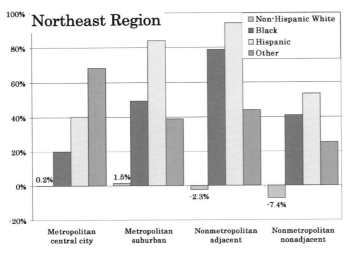

Northeast Region

Legend: Non-Hispanic White, Black, Hispanic, Other

0.2% 1.5% -2.3% -7.4%

Metropolitan central city | Metropolitan suburban | Nonmetropolitan adjacent | Nonmetropolitan nonadjacent

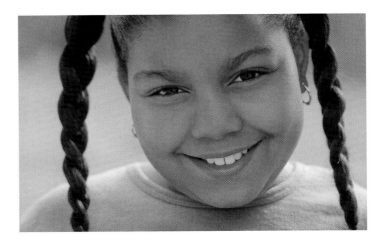

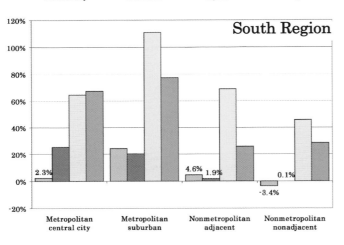

Midwest Region

-1.2% -0.7% -6.0%

Metropolitan central city | Metropolitan suburban | Nonmetropolitan adjacent | Nonmetropolitan nonadjacent

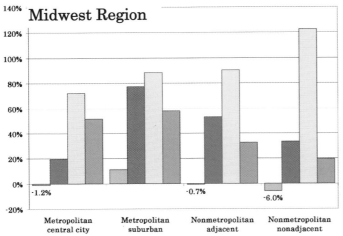

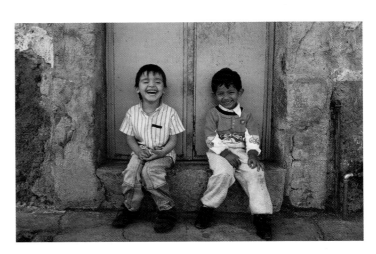

South Region

2.3% 4.6% 1.9% 0.1% -3.4%

Metropolitan central city | Metropolitan suburban | Nonmetropolitan adjacent | Nonmetropolitan nonadjacent

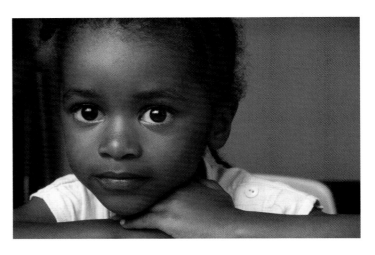

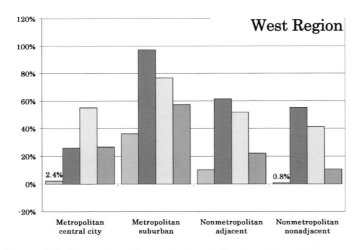

West Region

2.4% 0.8%

Metropolitan central city | Metropolitan suburban | Nonmetropolitan adjacent | Nonmetropolitan nonadjacent

Figure 42.2: Percentage Change in Population Less Than 18 by Race/Ethnicity and Metropolitan Status, 1990-2000
Source: Calculations by Steve H. Murdock, PhD 2003

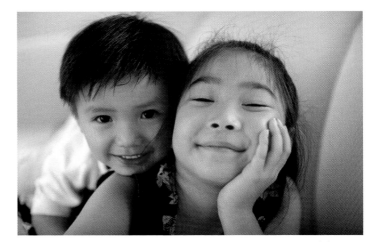

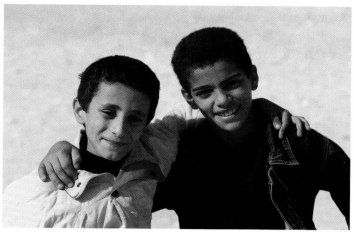

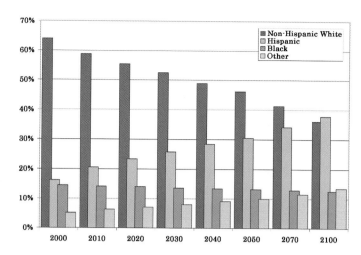

Figure 42.3: Projections of the Percentage of the Population Less Than 18 Years of Age by Race/Ethnicity

Source: Calculations by Steve H. Murdock, PhD 2003

minority children. Whereas the Non-Hispanic White population of children is projected to increase by 4.0% from 2000 to 2100, the number of Black children is projected to increase by 61.1%. The number of Hispanic children is expected to increase by 328.2%, and the number of children from other racial/ethnic groups is expected to increase by 379.6%. Although Non-Hispanic White children accounted for 64% of all children in the United States in 2000, that percentage is expected to drop to less than 50% between 2030 and 2040 and is expected to be 36.1% by the year 2100. It is expected that the United States child population in 2100 will have 12.7% of its make-up from Black children, 37.7% from Hispanic children, and 13.5% from children of other racial/ethnic groups.

What do recent and projected patterns of growth in child populations suggest about the issues that are likely to impact children such as the provision of health, education, and other services? Clearly, programs aimed at providing services to children must be increasingly oriented to minority children. The provision of services in multiple languages and with appropriate sensitivity to cultural differences will be increasingly essential. Even more critical is the need to recognize that, in the absence of change in socioeconomic characteristics among racial/ethnic groups, serving the needs of

A rapidly emerging U.S. minority population will present special needs and require additional resources beyond what is currently available if current socioeconomic disparities are left unaddressed.

children will likely involve serving the needs of a disproportionate number of impoverished children. Whereas 9.3% of Non-Hispanic White children came from poverty households in 2000, 33.1% of Black, 27.8% of Hispanic, and 17.5% of children from other racial/ethnic groups came from impoverished households in the same year. When issues such as those related to health care are examined, the well-documented differences in disease and disorder incidences and the care needs among minority populations— and the clear association of such differences with differences in socioeconomic resources—suggest that serving the needs of future children will likely require additional, per child resources compared to those presently provided.

Overall, the information presented here suggests that the needs of children in the United States will grow with their numbers and changing characteristics. Equally important, such patterns are likely to be geographically pervasive, impacting the populations of both rural and urban children in all regions of the United States.

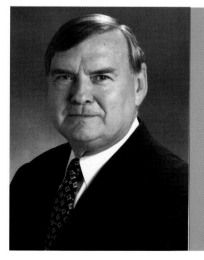

Steve H. Murdock

Steve H. Murdock, PhD, is currently the Lutcher Brown Distinguished Chair in management science and statistics at the University of Texas–San Antonio in the College of Business. He is also the official state demographer of Texas. Formally, he was a Regents Professor, head of the Department of Rural Sociology, and director of the Center for Demographic and Socioeconomic Research and Education at Texas A&M University. He holds a PhD in demography and sociology from the University of Kentucky and is the author of 11 books and more than 150 articles and technical reports on the implications of current and future demographic and socioeconomic change. Dr. Murdock has received the Faculty Distinguished Achievement Award in Research from Texas A&M University, the Excellence in Research Award from the Rural Sociological Society, and the Distinguished Alumni Award from the Department of Sociology at the University of Kentucky.

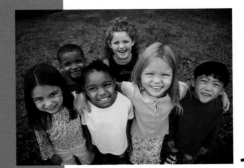

Chapter 43

Changes in the
Well-being of Children

William P. O'Hare

An assessment of America's children is particularly timely because many of the social, economic, demographic, and policy changes that took place in the United States during the 1990s had important implications for children and families. For example:

- Welfare reform ended "welfare as we know it" and ushered in a new relationship between the government and poor families, particularly poor families with children.

- Increased immigration produced a national population in which one-fifth of all children were immigrants or children of foreign-born parents.

- The percentage of mothers in the labor force reached an all-time high, and labor force participation rates for never-married mothers skyrocketed.

- The number of children in the United States grew by nearly 9 million—the largest increase since the 1950s.

There is little doubt that the well-being of American children improved significantly during the 1990s. The 14th annual *KIDS COUNT Report*[1] from the Annie E. Casey Foundation shows that between 1990 and 2000 there was improvement on 8 of the 10 indicators used to track how children are doing. The report also shows that the improvements were widespread. Of the 50 states, 43 had improvement on 6 or more of the 10 indicators. Moreover, Black and Hispanic children experienced significant improvements during the 1990s. Poverty among Black children fell from 45% in 1990 to an all-time low of 30% in 2001, and Hispanic child poverty fell from 38% to 28% during the same period—also an all-time low.[2]

Other reports that focused on the well-being of children reached the same conclusion. A comprehensive index of child well-being developed by Land and Associates showed that child well-being clearly improved during the last half of the 1990s.[3] Also, the Federal Interagency Forum on Child and Family Statistics yearly report, *America's Children*, indicated that there was a lot of improvement in child well-being during the late 1990s.[4] The following specifics help to illustrate the positive trends seen in the 1990s:

- In 2000, the child poverty rate reached its lowest point since the late 1970s.

- The teen birth rate has fallen steadily since 1991.

- The steady decades-long increase in the percentage of children living in single-parent families ended in the mid-1990s.

- The infant mortality rate improved by 25% in the 1990s, with decreases in all but two states.

Although not every measure of well-being improved and not every child experienced improvement, in general, the movement during the 1990s was clearly in a positive direction.

The improvements in child well-being that occurred in the 1990s are somewhat surprising in light of three major demographic trends that also occurred during that period. They are as follows:

- An increase in the total number of children

- An increase in the number of children in racial or ethnic minority groups

- An increase in the number of immigrant children

Any of these trends, by themselves, could depress child well-being. The implications of each trend are examined in more detail below.

The total number of children in the United States increased by 14% during the 1990s as the under-age-18 population grew by 8.7 million. During the 20th century, the 1950s was the only decade that had a bigger numerical increase than the 1990s. The increase in the number of

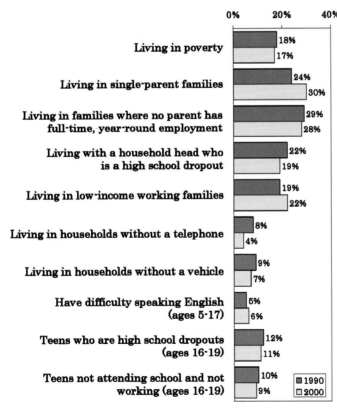

Figure 43.1: Key Indicators of Children Under 18 At Risk Nationally (Percentage of Children)

Source: Children at Risk: State Trends 1990-2000

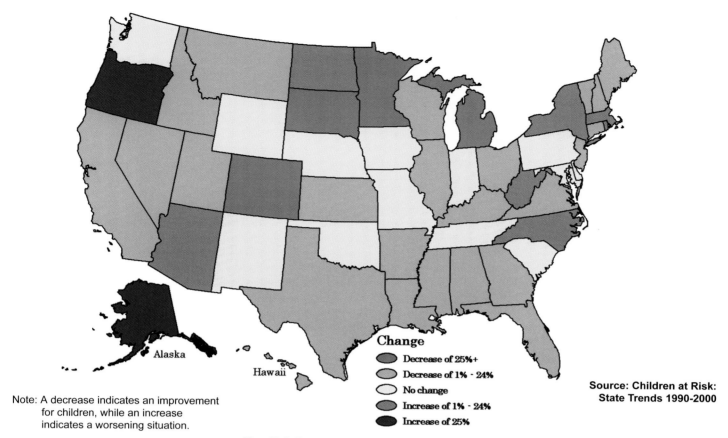

Change

- ⬤ Decrease of 25%+
- ⬤ Decrease of 1% - 24%
- ○ No change
- ⬤ Increase of 1% - 24%
- ⬤ Increase of 25%

Note: A decrease indicates an improvement for children, while an increase indicates a worsening situation.

Source: Children at Risk: State Trends 1990-2000

Map 43.1: Percentage Change in the Share of Children Living in High-risk Families, 1990-2000

children during the 1990s was all the more startling because it stands in stark contrast to the decreases of the 1970s and 1980s.

The recent increase in America's under-18 population has put heavy new demands on our already struggling public education, child care, and family support systems. One specific implication of this demographic trend is the growing number of school children. The U.S. Census Bureau reports that the number of children enrolled in elementary and secondary schools now matches the all-time high, set when the youngest baby boomers were entering first grade in 1970.[5]

The large increase in the number of school-age children during the 1990s exacerbated the existing problems in many struggling school systems. Concerns about public education prompted President George W. Bush to focus on

> **There is little doubt that the well-being of American children improved significantly during the 1990s.**

this issue early in his administration. One of the first major social policy initiatives of the Bush administration was passage of the No Child Left Behind Act of 2001, which was an attempt to address problems in schools.

Another major trend documented in the 2000 Census data was the growing diversity of the U.S. population. Pinpointing the exact size of changes in racial groups is complicated by the fact that the racial categories reported in the 2000 Census were not equivalent to those used in the 1990 census. Still, a dramatic change was evident. Minority children (any group other than Non-Hispanic White) accounted for about 98% of the growth in the child population during the 1990s. Of the 8.7 million children added to the population between 1990 and 2000, 4.6 million were Hispanic. Other racial minorities (Asians, Blacks, and American Indians) accounted for most of the remaining increase. Only

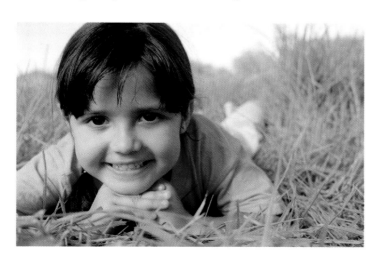

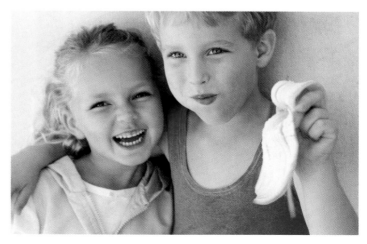

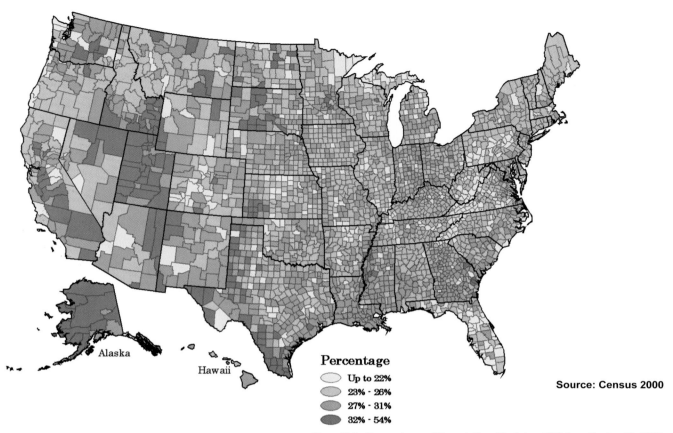

Percentage
- Up to 22%
- 23% - 26%
- 27% - 31%
- 32% - 54%

Map 43.2: Percentage of Population That Are Children Under 18, 2000

200,000 of the 8.7 million children added to the population during the 1990s were Non-Hispanic White children.

Racial diversity is increasing more rapidly among children than it is among adults. Minority children accounted for 39% of the population under age 18 in 2000, compared with 31% in 1990. Analysis of data from the 2000 Census reveals that minorities accounted for only 28% of the adult population, compared to 22% in 1990. Since minority children typically have poorer child outcomes than Non-Hispanic White children, one would expect a growing minority youth population to depress measures of child well-being. However, evidence from the 1990s suggests that our nation can accommodate growing numbers of minority children and still achieve improvements in child well-being at the same time.

The improvements in child well-being that occurred in the 1990s are somewhat surprising in light of [the] major demographic trends that also occurred during that period.

Unlike the 1950s, when the number of children grew because of an increased number of births to mostly Non-Hispanic White parents, much of the increase seen in the 1990s was fueled by immigration. The number of children who had a foreign-born parent increased from 8.7 million in 1990 to 14.2 million in 2000. Immigrant children often have many special needs. The child poverty rate for immigrant children in 2001 was 21% compared to 14% for children with native-born parents.[6] In addition to the sheer numbers of children added to the population, another concern is that a large share of children from immigrant families may not have English as their primary language at home. There were 9.8 million

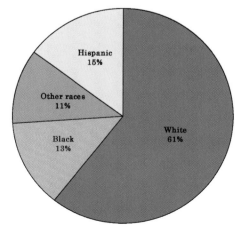

Figure 43.2: Race/Ethnicity of Children Under 18

Hispanic 15%
Other races 11%
Black 13%
White 61%

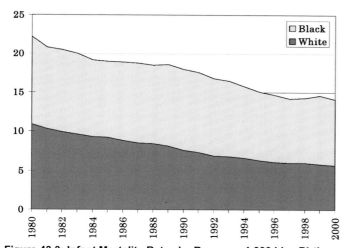

Figure 43.3: Infant Mortality Rates by Race, per 1,000 Live Births

Source: Infant Mortality and Low Birth Rate 2002

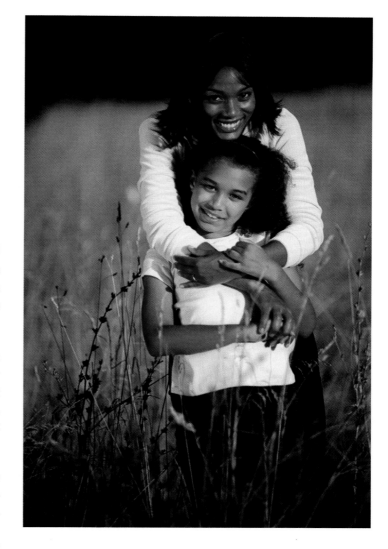

children in 2000 living in households where English was not the primary language. Furthermore, immigrants often adhere to cultural traditions that may be unfamiliar to many educators and service providers.

The increasing racial and ethnic diversity is reflected among children more than adults, due mostly to immigration and fertility trends. Immigrants are typically young adults who are likely to bring children with them when they immigrate or have children soon after arriving. About one-fifth of today's children are children of immigrants.

Why, then, did child well-being improve during the last half of the 1990s when the number of children—particularly minority and immigrant children—was increasing? It is easy to identify some of the likely reasons. First, the robust economy of the late 1990s provided strong

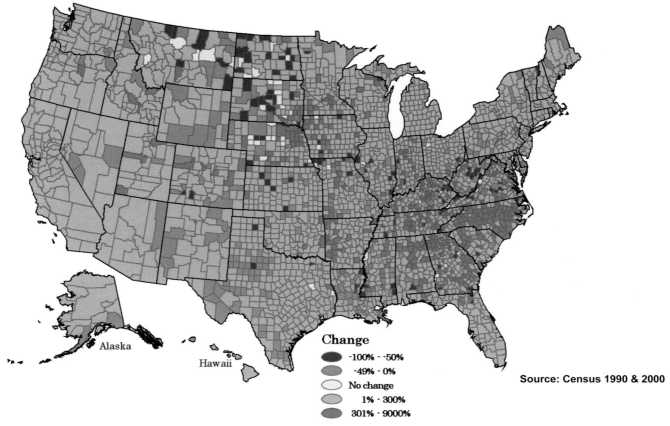

Change

- -100% - -50%
- -49% - 0%
- No change
- 1% - 300%
- 301% - 9000%

Source: Census 1990 & 2000

Map 43.3: Percentage Change in the Number of Hispanic Children Under 18, 1990-2000

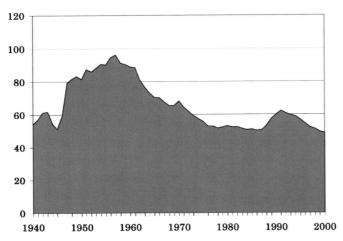

Figure 43.4: Birth Rates per 1,000 Teens Ages 15 to 19
Source: Birth to Teenagers in the United States 2001

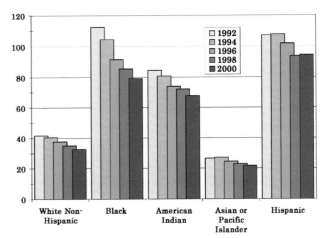

Figure 43.5: Birth Rates per 1,000 Teens Ages 15 to 19 by Race
Source: Birth to Teenagers in the United States 2001

employment opportunities for many low-wage workers. Second, in the wake of welfare reform, numerous public programs were implemented to support low-income working families. Third, there is some evidence that children's issues moved higher on the public agenda during the 1990s.

There is widespread agreement that the improvements in child well-being seen during the 1990s—especially the late 1990s—were due to improvements in the employment situation of low-income families. The unemployment rate fell from 7.3% in January 1993 to 3.8% in April 2000,[7] and real median household income grew from $37,688 in 1993

to $43,162 in 2000.[8] Given the correlation between family income and child well-being, it is not surprising to see an overall improvement in child well-being.

In addition to improvements for individual families, the robust economy of the late 1990s also changed environments for many children. One ramification of the economic improvements is that the number of people living in concentrated poverty neighborhoods (census tracts where the poverty rate was 40% or more) fell by 25% between 1990 and 2000.[9] The demolition of some high-rise public housing complexes and implementation of programs like Moving to Opportunity, a program run by the U.S. Department of Housing and Urban Development designed to disperse public housing residents, also contributed to the deconcentration of poverty. It should be noted, however, that broader measures of neighborhood quality did not show similar improvements over the 1990s.[10]

In addition to the economic expansion during the late 1990s, many programs to support low-income working families were initiated or expanded during this time. Research shows that government investments in programs to support children resulted in better outcomes.[11] Three of

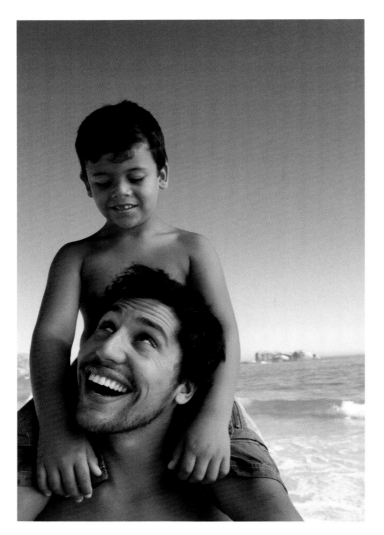

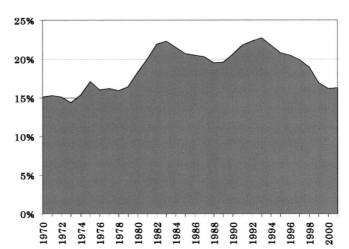

Figure 43.6: Percentage of Children Under 18 Living in Poverty
Source: Historic Poverty Tables 2003

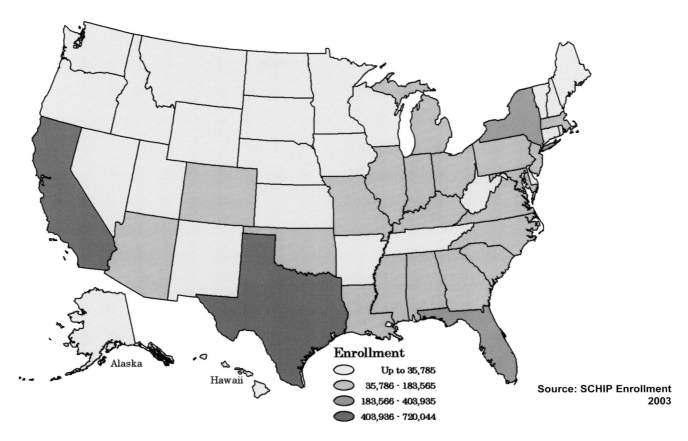

Enrollment

○ Up to 35,785
○ 35,786 - 183,565
◑ 183,566 - 403,935
● 403,936 - 720,044

Alaska

Hawaii

Source: SCHIP Enrollment 2003

Map 43.4: Total SCHIP Enrollment, June 2003

the most important investments in the well-being of children were:

- Expansion of the Earned Income Tax Credit (EITC),

- Growth in child care subsidies, and

- A new health insurance program for low-income children called the State Child Health Insurance Program (SCHIP).

The EITC is a federal program that works through the tax code, allowing low-earning workers to enhance their income. It targets low-income families with children and at least one working parent. The EITC has enjoyed strong bipartisan support since it was first enacted in the early 1970s.

Research shows that government investments in programs [during the late 1990s] to support children resulted in better outcomes.

Since the EITC was expanded in 1993, the number of families receiving the EITC increased by 25%, while the average amount received per recipient family grew by over 50%.[12] In the recent past, the EITC has lifted as many as 2.5 million children out of poverty each year and increased the family income in millions of other families. Research shows that among low-income families, even small increases in income can lead to better child outcomes.[13]

As low-income parents have moved from welfare to work, the need for child care has grown dramatically. Between 1996 and 2000, federal and state spending on child care subsidies for low-income working families tripled, in part, because the Personal Responsibility and Work, Opportunity and Reconciliation Act, often referred to as welfare reform, allowed states to use Temporary Assistance for Needy Families (TANF) dollars for child

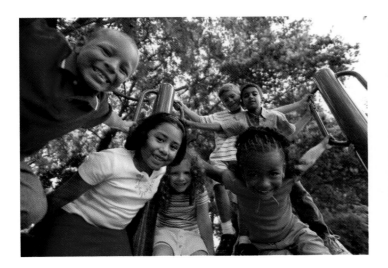

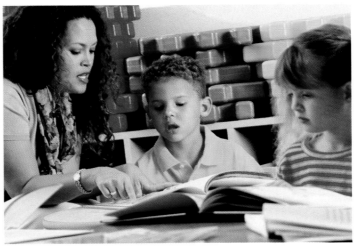

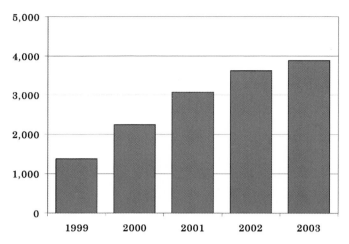

Figure 43.7: National Enrollment Totals for SCHIP in Thousands

Source: SCHIP Enrollment 2003

programs designed to support low-income workers expanded, as well. For example, there was a 20% increase in state funds spent for child welfare services between 1998 and 2000.[16] Nearly every state increased spending during this period.

Given this expansion of programs to help low-income working families, it is not surprising that the well-being of children in low-income families improved. By some measures, the biggest improvements in child well-being during the 1990s were in low-income families. Six of eight indicators related to child well-being for kids revealed that the change from 1990 to 2000 was more positive (or less negative) for low-income children (those below 200% of the poverty line) than for children living in families with income above 200% of the poverty line.[17]

Another factor in the improved welfare of children during the 1990s, increased attention to children's issues, is more difficult to document. Increasing space was allocated to children's issues in print media, and there seemed to be more ads on television promoting reading programs and discouraging child abuse during this time than in the period prior to the 1990s. The SCHIP passed during the Clinton administration and the No Child Left Behind legislation passed during the Bush administration were both examples of national legislation aimed at improving the lives of children. Additionally, much of the discussion about welfare reform (TANF) focused on the well-being of children.

If the improvements in child well-being seen during the last half of the 1990s were driven by a robust economy and expanded supports for low-income working families,

care.[14] States and localities as well as some companies contributed to help many low-income working families find affordable child care. While there were still many low-income workers who did not receive a child care subsidy, the expansion of this support system was undoubtedly helpful.

In the past, one deterrent for leaving welfare for a low-wage job was the prospect of losing health care coverage for children. In response, Congress passed SCHIP in 1997 to provide health care coverage for children in low-income families. By 2003, almost 4 million children were enrolled in SCHIP.[15]

In addition to the expansion of the EITC, child care support, and child health insurance, many other

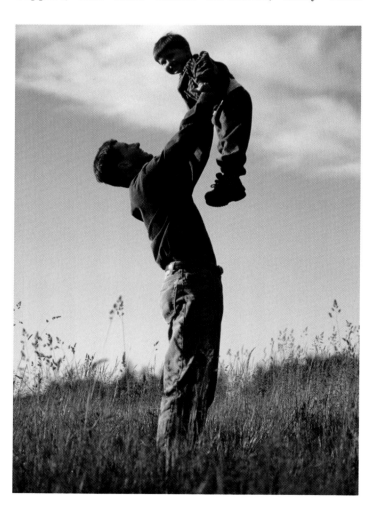

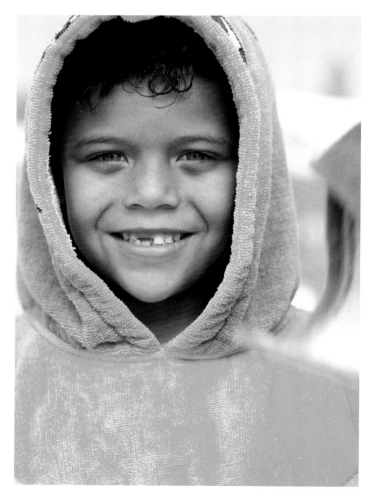

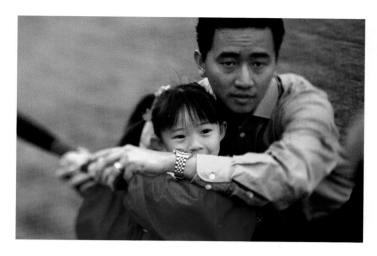

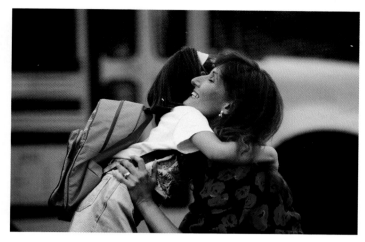

then it is important to look at what has happened since 2000 in these two realms. The unemployment rate rose from 3.8% in April 2000 to 6.0% in April 2003.[7] The real median household income fell by 3% between 2000 and 2002.[8]

In contrast to the nearly uniform improvements in child outcomes between 1995 and 2000, the evidence since 2000 is mixed. Since the economy peaked in April 2000, there have been troubling signs that the momentum established in the late 1990s is dissipating. For example, the child poverty rate, which had fallen steadily between 1993 and 2000, increased slightly between 2000 and 2001 and again between 2001 and 2002.[2] The proportion of children living with at least one parent who has a full-time, year-round job decreased slightly.[4] On the other hand, the teen birth rate and the infant mortality rate continued to fall, as did death rates for children and teens.

> **In contrast to the nearly uniform improvements in child outcomes between 1995 and 2000, the evidence since 2000 is mixed.**

There are also signs that the fiscal stress experienced by federal and state governments since 2000 may lead to cutbacks in support programs. While the EITC has enjoyed strong bipartisan support for many years, there are nagging questions about the level of erroneous payments that have led the Bush administration to consider new EITC rules. The new rules will require participating families to provide a lot more documentation before they can receive the benefit.[18] There is widespread agreement among experts that requiring

more documentation will lower participation rates among eligible families.

Other information on programs supporting low-income families looks discouraging, as well. A recent General Accounting Office report indicates that 26 of the 35 states surveyed have taken steps since January 2001 to decrease the availability of child care assistance.[19] After many years of steady decline, TANF caseloads are now inching upward in many states. During the fourth quarter of the 2002 calendar year, TANF caseloads increased in 38 states, and the national caseload increased by 1.2%.[20]

In summary, data from the 1990s dispel two myths held by many Americans. Survey evidence indicates a large segment of the American public have the perception that children are enduring worsening conditions and that government programs do not help.[21] The evidence presented here shows both perceptions are incorrect. There were widespread improvements in the lives of children during the late 1990s (particularly children in low-income working families), and much of the credit goes to the implementation and expansion of government programs. Moreover, the overall improvements during the 1990s were led by improved outcomes for Black and Hispanic children. Evidence presented here indicates that America can improve the lives of our children, particularly minority children, and that government programs are important in achieving that goal.

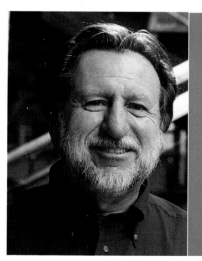

William P. O'Hare

KIDS COUNT coordinator Bill O'Hare, PhD, has worked with the Annie E. Casey Foundation since 1993. He produces the annual *KIDS COUNT Data Book*, which provides comparable data on child well-being for each state. In addition, Dr. O'Hare oversees a growing list of supplementary KIDS COUNT publications. He also represents the foundation's interests with the National Academy of Sciences and other professional statistical/demographic organizations. Just prior to joining the foundation, Dr. O'Hare was director of population and policy research at the Center of Urban and Economic Research at the University of Louisville, where his work included the use of census information to address policy-related issues. Dr. O'Hare received his BS and MA (both in multidisciplinary social science) as well as his PhD in sociology from Michigan State University. He is currently a member of the Population Association of America, the Southern Demographic Association, the American Statistical Association, and the American Sociological Association.

Part Six: Looking Toward Their Future

As one of our primary tenets, our society must accept the responsibility for ushering our children and youth into a future characterized by the realization of individual dreams, collective equity, and recognition of our interconnectedness. The future for children will be influenced by many factors, only some of which might seem subject to our control. The advances in the biological, social, and physical sciences create magnificent opportunities, ones that require a social response to be fully realized. Understanding some of the scientific breakthroughs, their implications for positive change, and their connection to the delivery of health care services occupies the last part of this book. With such understandings, future dreams that we have for our children may be realized.

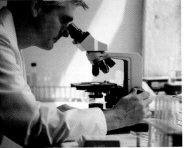

Chapter 44

Paul H. Wise

Medical Progress
and Inequalities in Child Health

The health of children always reflects the nature of the society in which they grow and develop. This fundamental relationship has been documented since the eighteenth century and continues to be as true today as it was back then.[1] Indeed, as recent data suggest deepening social stratification in the United States, an already vast literature continues to grow with studies linking poverty to an elevated risk of child illness, suffering, and death.[2]

However, there can also be no question that child health will increasingly reflect the impact of dramatic advances in preventive and therapeutic interventions. If nothing else, the next decade is likely to be characterized by major discoveries in disease causation and innovations in technical capabilities.

Together, these two fundamental forces—social stratification and medical progress—will increasingly shape patterns of child health in the years to come. However, while the empirical documentation of these two determinants of child health will undoubtedly continue, the central and ultimately most important question remains: How do these two forces interact? Will the impact of social stratification be lessened by new, technical capabilities to improve child health outcomes? Alternatively, will the development of new clinical interventions be overwhelmed by the influences of material deprivation? In other words, what role will medical progress play in shaping and ultimately eliminating social inequalities in child health?

> **Two fundamental forces—social stratification and medical progress—will increasingly shape patterns of child health in the years to come.**

The familiar and tragic portrayal of disparate infant mortality trends in the United States provides some important clues.[3] The first observation is that infant mortality has fallen dramatically for all groups in the United States over the past three decades. These reductions have been shown to be the result of several factors, primarily technical strides in the management of high-risk deliveries and critically ill newborns. However, the second observation is that despite these major reductions in absolute infant mortality rates for both African Americans and Whites, the disparity between the two groups persists. Accordingly, for those concerned with inequalities in child health, the task is less documenting that disparities *exist* than it is explaining why they *persist* in the face of dramatic reductions in absolute mortality.

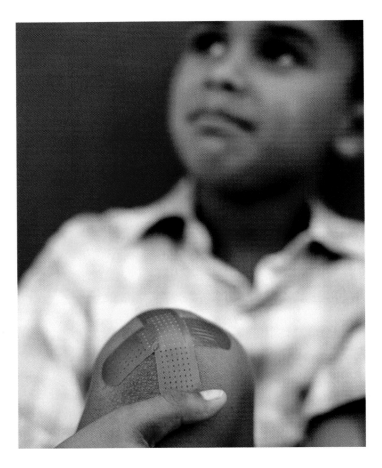

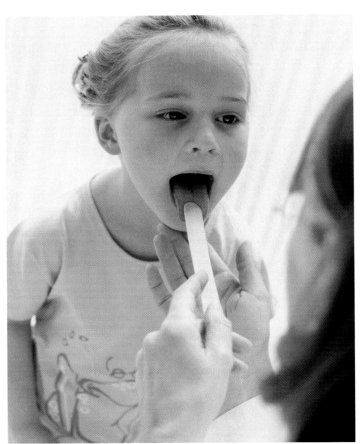

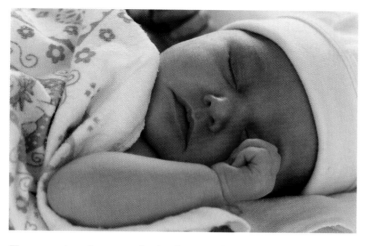

	Number exposed	Number of deaths	Percent mortality
Group I	143	4	3%
Group II	93	15	16%
Group III	179	81	45%

Figure 44.1: Differential Mortality Example

Source: Provided by Paul H. Wise, MD, PhD, 2004

To examine how technical capacity can interact with social forces in creating disparities in outcome, it is useful to examine an illustrative case. Figure 44.1 presents the mortality rates for three groups of people, all of whom experienced the same serious exposure. Three percent of Group I died; 14% of Group II died; and 54% of Group III died. Basically, two things could have happened to result in such a wide difference in mortality. The first possibility is that there were differences in *underlying risk status* among the three groups. For example, Group I, with the lowest mortality rate, could have been comprised of young adults, whereas Group III, with the highest rate, could have been comprised of frail elderly. The second possibility is that, given the existence of an effective intervention, *differences in access* to that intervention somehow occurred. For example, Group I had access to the intervention while Group III did not. Although there are innumerable specific factors that can result in disparate health outcomes, the argument here is that they tend to fall into one of two general categories

of influence—differential underlying risk status and differential access to an effective intervention. Both of course are possible; elevated risk and reduced access, though distinct, often travel together. This example could have been an infectious disease outbreak or any one of a variety of serious, harmful exposures. In reality, however, this case was the sinking of the *Titanic* and the subsequent deaths among the first-, second-, and third-class female passengers. The lifeboats were loaded by deck, by class.[4] This experience not only provides a useful illustration of differential mortality but also serves as a reminder that social class can affect life and death when least expected.

Although the experience of the *Titanic* underscores the potential impact of differential risk and access to disparity creation, there is a third element that provides the essential link between risk and access: the efficacy of

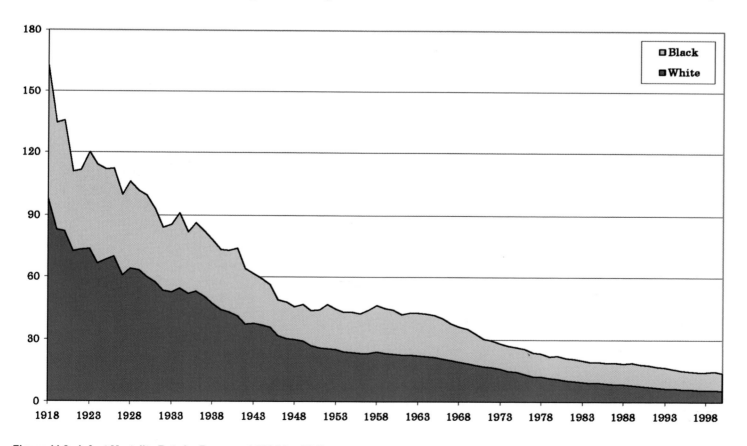

Figure 44.2: Infant Mortality Rate by Race per 1,000 Live Births

Source: National Center for Health Statistics 1996, Murphy 2000, Centers for Disease Control and Prevention 2002

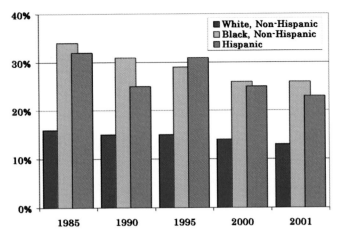

Figure 44.3: Percentage of Children Under 18 Not Ranked in the Very Good or Excellent Health Categories by Race and Ethnicity
Source: Forum of Child and Family Statistics 2002

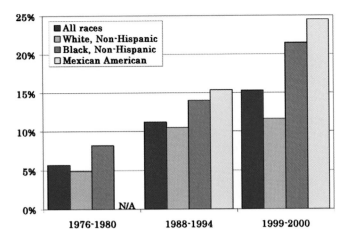

Figure 44.4: Percentage of Children Ages 6 to 18 Who Were Overweight by Race and Ethnicity
Source: Forum of Child and Family Statistics 2002

the intervention in question. When interventions are of high efficacy, then differences in *access* to them will produce disparities in outcome. When interventions are of low efficacy, then differences in *underlying risk* will produce disparities in outcome.

In this manner, the respective impacts of risk and access are mediated by the relative efficacy of the intervention. Examples of this "pivot on efficacy" can emerge whenever new interventions are developed and introduced into wide practice. Surfactant replacement therapy has proven to be a highly efficacious intervention for high-risk newborns with respiratory distress syndrome. However, evidence suggests that the introduction of surfactant, at least initially, widened disparities in neonatal mortality.[5] A similar experience may be emerging with advances in prenatal diagnosis. Traditionally, the birth of infants with lethal congenital anomalies has not been characterized by major social disparities.

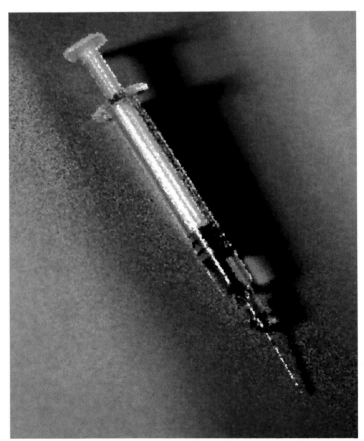

However, with the advent of powerful new tools for the prenatal diagnosis of such anomalies, social differences in access to this clinical capacity could help generate disparities in serious congenital anomalies for the first time.[6]

The importance of clinical efficacy need not be limited to complex, high technology arenas of care. The "Back to Sleep" campaign supporting the adoption of nonprone infant sleep positions to reduce rates of the sudden infant death syndrome (SIDS) has been associated with a dramatic reduction in SIDS mortality rates. However, the social disparity in SIDS mortality may have widened. Although it is difficult to identify the precise cause of this phenomenon, several studies suggest that better educated and wealthier families are more likely to have heard about and adopted the proper sleep position for their infants.[7]

However, when access to a new, efficacious intervention is ensured, disparities in outcome can be reduced. The introduction of a vaccination to prevent many of the most serious forms of *Streptococcus pneumoniae* infection in children has been an important breakthrough in child health. Despite serious financial and administrative problems, extraordinary efforts to ensure that children in greatest need have access to this new immunization have apparently resulted in major reductions in the racial disparity in serious *S. pneumoniae* infection.[8] Likewise, if all premature newborns are ensured equal access to clinical care, there is no indication that there are social differences in neonatal mortality.

These examples emphasize that medical progress does not necessarily guarantee equity in outcome. Rather, medical progress merely provides the substrate for increases or decreases in disparity. The crucial concern is the efficacy of the intervention and the uniformity of access to it across society. For example, if even small delays in transferring critically ill newborns to neonatal intensive care units were to emerge on the basis of differences in insurance coverage or other social characteristics, the impact on disparities in neonatal and infant mortality would be profound. It is worth noting that access to neonatal intensive care, which is among the most highly technological areas of modern medicine, can fuel disparities in infant mortality—the health indicator most widely linked to social conditions.

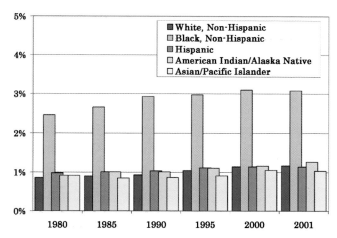

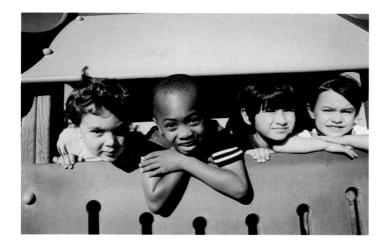

Figure 44.5: Percentage of Infants Born of Very Low Birthweight (Less than 1,500 grams) by Mother's Race and Ethnicity
Source: Forum of Child and Family Statistics 2002

The efficacy of a clinical innovation also erodes clear distinctions between social and medical arenas of causation. Phenylketonuria (PKU) provides an instructive example. PKU is a potentially serious genetic disorder that causes severe neurologic deterioration due to a buildup of the amino acid phenylalanine in the brain. However, with newborn screening and the elimination of phenylalanine from the diet, virtually all disparities in PKU outcome today reflect differential access to these interventions. Here, a completely genetic condition is characterized by disparities in outcome that are largely social in origin.

The policy implications of this logic stem from the acknowledgment that as the clinical efficacy grows, so does the burden on society to provide it equitably to all children in need.[9] This is why pressures for expanded health insurance will continue to grow as clinical efficacy expands. This is also why devaluing the importance of clinical care will always undermine efforts to ensure that it is provided to all those in need.

Poverty is a social phenomenon; disease and mortality are ultimately biologic events. The relationships between medical advances, poverty, and child health

Medical progress does not necessarily guarantee equity in outcome. Rather, medical progress merely provides the substrate for increases or decreases in disparity.

imply a process of transformation by which social phenomena can determine health, illness, and death.[10] At each point along this transformation, one can observe different arenas of interaction and different opportunities for intervention, which dispells the traditional framing of clinical and highly technical arenas as being somehow irrelevant to social inequalities in child health.

All serious child illnesses and deaths are a tragedy. However, all preventable child illnesses and deaths are unjust. At a historical moment when social conditions are becoming increasingly stratified and medical capability is growing at an unprecedented rate, the determinants of inequalities in child health must be seen as intensely dynamic. Inequalities in the social status of children and their families will continue to find expression in the nature and severity of threats to child health. At the same time, the development of new, efficacious technical interventions will continue to improve the opportunity for children to lead full and healthy lives. The coming years, therefore, will witness a deepening interaction between these two forces and, consequently, a growing recognition that the dual struggles, the struggle for efficacy and the struggle for equity, will be increasingly linked.

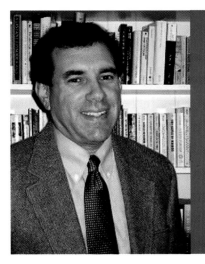

Paul H. Wise

Paul H. Wise, MD, MPH, is vice-chief of the Division of Social Medicine and Health Inequalities in the Department of Medicine, Brigham and Women's Hospital, and professor of pediatrics in the Boston University Schools of Medicine and Public Health. Dr. Wise is director of social and health policy research in the Department of Pediatrics, Boston Medical Center, and associate in medicine at the Children's Hospital, Boston. Dr. Wise earned his AB and MD degrees from Cornell University, did his pediatric training at the Children's Hospital in Boston, and received a master of public health degree from the Harvard School of Public Health. His prior positions include director of Emergency and Primary Care Services at the Children's Hospital, Boston, and director of the Harvard Institute for Reproductive and Child Health at Harvard Medical School. He also served as a special expert at the National Institutes of Health and special assistant to the U.S. Surgeon General. His research focuses on social disparities in child health status and child health policy.

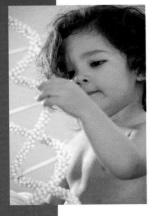

Chapter 45

Edward R. B. McCabe
and Linda L. McCabe

Genetics

The completion of the Human Genome Project, an international research effort to sequence and map all of the genes of Homo sapiens, was celebrated on April 25, 2003, the 50th anniversary of the original description of the double helical structure of DNA by Watson and Crick. April 25th was designated "DNA Day" by both the U.S. House of Representatives and U.S. Senate, and celebrations were carried out in schools throughout the country. By celebrating the completion of defining the structure and sequence of the human genome, the country recognized the excitement engendered among our youth by this project as well as the promise of this knowledge for improving the health and well-being of our children and their

children. Recognized, as well, was the importance of fully understanding the ethical, legal, and social implications of the Human Genome Project.

The Human Genome Project was initiated in 1990 with completion originally planned for 2005. This was a bold initiative since the technology required to complete the project did not actually exist in 1990. The community of genomic scientists from many countries trusted the ingenuity of the participants to develop the necessary tools to complete the sequencing of the human genome and to accomplish this task within an ambitious time frame. Sequencing refers to defining the biochemical structure of DNA and the order in which its components are assembled, a process that describes the hereditary information that is passed from one generation to the next—the genetic code. Spurred by competition from the private sector and facilitated by technological innovation, the sequencing of the human genome was accomplished ahead of schedule and under budget.

Just as this project established the new science of genomics involved in the study of genomes, it also created the new field of genomic medicine. Genomic medicine harnesses the information and technology from the Human Genome Project to benefit the health of individual patients and larger populations. Genomic medicine depends upon identification of sequence variations within our genomes and learning how we can correlate these differences with susceptibility to disease. The DNA sequence of any two persons is 99.9% identical, on the average. While there is little difference in DNA structure between two persons, the difference in DNA structure between people of differing races is actually less than the average difference between two individuals within the same race. The nonidentical part of the DNA sequence may be of immense significance and may markedly affect an individual's risk of developing specific diseases.

Genomic medicine will be significant for each person by predicting future clinical events and preventing the occurrence of disease states. The identification of predisposition to disease will mean that genomic medicine will be predictive, rather than reactive to the acute presentation of disease. By developing approaches to forestall the onset of disease, it will be preventive and

will utilize the strategies of public health and preventive medicine as opposed to approaches that attempt to control a disease once it has become manifest. Because it will individualize preventive strategies to meet our unique genotypes, genomic medicine will be personalized.

The tools of genomic medicine may target specific sequence variants or may utilize new methods to sequence complete genomes. The president of the Institute for Systems Biology, Leroy Hood, is reported to have stated at a meeting of the Biotechnology Industry Organization in 2003, "I think we will have an instrumentation that could well bring sequencing of the human genome...down to a 20-minute process and do it for under $1,000."

The sequencing of entire genomes will create challenges for interpretation. Even if the sequences are 99.9999% accurate, an incredible level of accuracy for any biomedical test, with 3 billion nucleotide base pairs per haploid genome, there will still be 3,000 errors. It will be difficult to know whether the differences that one sees in an individual's sequence are legitimate sequence variants or technological errors. Even for legitimate variants, the importance to the individual's health-related decision-making will be difficult to know. Individuals may differ at a single chemical compound comprising DNA; such sites are called single nucleotide polymorphisms (SNPs), i.e., places where there are alterations in the chemical structure of a single component of DNA. These biochemical alterations are inherited often in association with each other (in a block).

The pattern of SNPs in a block of DNA is referred to as a haplotype. A haplotype map (HapMap) is a map of these haplotype blocks. An international project to develop a HapMap of the human genome was initiated in October 2002 and is anticipated to cost approximately $100 million and to take about 3 years for completion. The International HapMap Project is anticipated to accelerate the identification of genes involved in common, complex diseases like cancer, cardiovascular disease, and diabetes as well as those involved in adverse reactions to medications. As a way of providing perspective on the magnitude of this task, the HapMap will break the genome into haplotype blocks of 10,000

> **The Human Genome Project will result in predictive, preventive, and personalized medicine and will have fundamental influences on the diagnostic tests and therapies available to children.**

base pairs or larger; these blocks are thought to represent 65% to 85% of the total genome. Of the estimated 10 million SNPs, it is thought that only 300,000 to 600,000 will be required to characterize an individual's HapMap. The accuracy requirements, while still a challenge, will not be nearly as daunting as when dealing with the entire genomic sequence that is larger by a factor of 10,000.

How a person looks and functions (phenotype) is not just a result of their genotype. What actually happens to an individual is not just a function of their genetic predispositions, but is also a reflection of environmental influences. The interactions between the environment and genetic factors will be clarified only by using individuals enrolled in large, population-based studies; such studies are required in order to provide the actual information upon which genomic medicine can be accurately practiced.

The Human Genome Project will have a huge impact on children that will span into their adulthood. There will be marked changes in testing technologies and especially in the ability to correlate sequence variations with susceptibility to disease. These changes may seem to be gradual, but when examined over the course of the next 20 to 30 years, they will fundamentally transform the practice of medicine.

The studies that are required to create meaningful insights into the use of genetic information in relation to human disease and wellness all imply the screening of both individuals and populations. Screening programs are currently being routinely conducted during the newborn period (newborn screening) for every newborn child and are being selectively done for certain disorders, primarily to determine frequency of specific sequence variations.

Newborn screening is a model for the practice of genomic medicine. Newborn screening predicts the future health status of the neonate in terms of the specific genetic variants that are tested. It prevents disability and death before signs and symptoms of specific diseases develop, and it personalizes care because we have learned that treatment of the diseases being screened for must be individualized to match the interplay between complex genotypes and the environment, producing individual phenotypes for each patient.

Newborn screening has also addressed issues important to all population-based screening programs. Decisions regarding the inclusion of as many individuals in the population as possible are critical to the success of the screening program and, therefore, to the equity of the program. For newborn screening, the strategy is to target all neonates, and the goal is to detect diseases that affect the newborn and/or the infant. However, if newborn screening is extended to detect disorders that only appear when the newborn becomes an adult, new challenges will emerge. The recognition that newborn screening really represents a system and not just a collection of individual tests for specific disorders is a concept that took several decades to develop.

Currently, newborn screening is the most common genetic testing, with 4,000,000 newborns in the United States tested each year for three or more disorders.

Many more disorders can be detected; indeed, some states test for more than 30 disorders. Due to the variety of mutations for each disorder, molecular genetic testing has not been adopted as a primary method for newborn screening; rather, some aspect of the dysfunction produced by a genetic abnormality is tested for, with molecular genetic testing used as a follow-up test for a number of disorders. The reason that newborn screening is not totally done by analysis of DNA structure is that the same disease can be caused by a variety of mutations. Obviously, if multiple sequence variations led to the same disease, the frequency of a given sequence variation would be much less than the disease for which it is only one of many potential genetic causes. Hemoglobinopathies, cystic fibrosis, medium chain acylCoA dehydrogenase deficiency, and deafness are among the disorders currently being detected by newborn screening.

Hemoglobinopathies—A hemoglobinopathy is a disorder in which a sequence variation leads to an abnormal hemoglobin, the substance in red blood cells that carries oxygen from the lungs to all tissues. Hemoglobinopathies were added to the newborn screening program after it was demonstrated that the routine administration of penicillin to an infant with sickle cell disease, a hemoglobinopathy disorder, would prevent overwhelming infections.

Cystic fibrosis—Cystic fibrosis is a disorder associated with the development of chronic lung disease and dysfunction of the pancreas, leading to poor absorption of foodstuff by the intestine and resulting in malnutrition. Cystic fibrosis was added to the newborn screening program in Colorado when it was demonstrated that malnutrition could occur prior to the development of any lung disease and was amenable to treatment.

Medium chain acylCoA dehydrogenase deficiency—This disease, a disturbance in how the cells handle fatty acids, is a genetically transmitted disorder that may lead to significant developmental retardation as well as behavioral and neurological problems if there is no detection or intervention. It was formerly thought that the disease was due to one particular mutation; indeed, one mutation accounts for 90% of patients with this disorder. However, new mutations are being discovered all of the time.

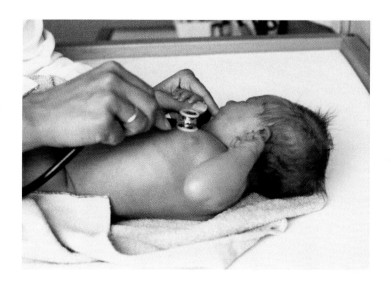

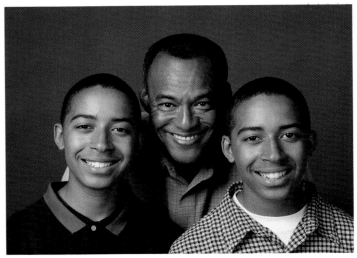

Deafness—Deafness is caused by many known genetic and environmental factors. Genetic factors account for at least half of all cases of profound deafness present at birth. There have been over 120 independent genes associated with deafness, enabling new insights into factors that disturb hearing. The newborn screening program is initially directed towards the use of hearing tests as the primary method of detecting deafness. DNA testing can be used as a second tier to follow up an initial positive newborn screen hearing test.

Application of screening depends upon available technology and the nature of the underlying genetic abnormalities that predispose an individual to a given disease. When a clinical disorder, such as cystic fibrosis, can be caused by a huge number of different mutations, application of screening must be carefully analyzed to determine how, when, and whether such screening can be most effectively implemented. In addition, as time passes, decisions will have to be made on whether direct DNA testing will be the most logical way to detect disorders in which new mutations are being discovered frequently, such as with medium chain acylCoA dehydrogenase deficiency.

More disorders are soon to be included in the newborn screening system. Navajo people have a high incidence, 1 in 2,000 live births, of severe combined immunodeficiency (SCID). This condition is fatal if untreated, and affected infants usually die due to severe infection by 6 months of age. The only effective treatment is bone marrow transplantation.

The Dine, another Athebascan group living in northwestern Canada, have the same haplotype as the Navajos. The high frequency of SCID among the Athabascan tribes, the high mortality rate, and the potential cure via bone marrow transplantation argue that newborn screening would be beneficial, at least among affected Native American tribes. Screening methodologies for SCID are under development.

Multiple problems and uncertainties face both current and projected screening programs. We do not yet have the tools for broad population-based screening for the most common, complex disorders like cancer, cardiovascular disease, and diabetes. Even with more clearly defined genetic disorders, however, problems in developing screening programs abound.

Two genetic disorders exemplify some of the problems: hereditary hemochromatosis, a disorder in which excessive storage of iron in the body may lead to disease and dysfunction of many organs, and factor V Leiden thrombophilia, the most common cause of primary and recurrent blood clots in the veins of women. Both of these disorders include significant proportions of the population who are genetically predisposed to the diseases. Predisposition to hereditary hemochromatosis has a prevalence among people of northern European descent. Five in every 1,000 are at risk. Factor V Leiden has a prevalence among the same population with 50 in every 1,000 at risk. Despite the relatively high prevalence of those at risk for both of these disorders, the penetrance (proportion of those with at-risk genotype who manifest the disease) is quite low. In addition, questions remain regarding whom to screen, the correct timing of screening, and risks versus benefits of currently available interventions. For all of these reasons, screening for these disorders remains a matter of active discussion.

These disorders illustrate the variability in prevalence among those of different ethnocultural backgrounds. The frequency of the genotype that is responsible for the majority of people with hereditary hemochromatosis is much lower in individuals of Italian, Greek, and Ashkenazi Jewish descent than in people from northern European descent. Similarly, factor V Leiden is much more frequent in Sweden and certain Middle Eastern countries and is virtually nonexistent in African and Asian populations.

As seen with the variations among different ethnocultural groups, patterns of migration and isolation are reflected in our genomes. As a developing species with worldwide migration, humans have tended to remain in groups isolated by geography, language, and/or ethnocultural practices. The more ancient the sequence variation or mutation, the more likely it is that it will be carried by a larger proportion of individuals. At one extreme would be a change that occurred in the original, small family-band of our species, Homo sapiens. Such a sequence variation would be anticipated to be identical among all subsequent human groups. If, on the other hand, a genetic alteration is very recent, then it might be unique to a specific group or even a single family.

Some small groups have been isolated due to cultural, geographic, linguistic, or religious barriers. If a genetic change results in a recessive genetic disorder, the members of these small groups may have a high incidence of the disorder due to their isolation. An example would be the neurodegenerative disorder, Tay Sachs disease, which occurs primarily among Ashkenazi Jews. In the Ashkenazi Jewish population, three mutations account for about 93% of the carriers for Tay Sachs disease. A different mutation occurs among Non-Jewish carriers of Celtic origin. The frequency of Tay Sachs disease among the Ashkenazim is estimated to be 1 in 4,100 births, while the frequency for Non-Jewish infants is estimated to be only 1 in 320,000 births.

Genetic bottlenecks are observed when the size of a group decreases suddenly and then expands rapidly. Any genetic changes that are present in the downsized group are seen in the rapidly expanding group. However, frequencies of these gene changes in the rapidly expanded group are higher than in the original group, prior to its decrease in size. The high frequency of a disease associated with progressive degeneration of the central nervous system (metachromatic leukodystrophy [MLD]) among the Navajo is an example of a genetic bottleneck. When the Navajo were forced by the U.S. Army to leave their homeland near the Arizona-New Mexico border for Fort Sumner in eastern New Mexico, 1,000 Navajo remained in what is now the western Navajo reservation in Arizona. This area was very rugged and has remained geographically isolated until recently. Subsequent to this genetic bottleneck, there was a rapid increase in the Navajo population. The observed incidence of MLD in the western reservation is 1 in every 2,250 live births, while in the eastern reservation there are no cases of MLD in the Navajos who live there.

These variations illustrate the importance of and challenges to genomic medicine, as humans are ever-evolving. The practice of medicine will change fundamentally if it is to achieve the promise of the Human Genome Project. Success will not be equated with the effectiveness of acute intervention after disease becomes apparent, but rather with the effectiveness of disease prevention by identification of a disease before symptoms appear and by the development of personalized interventional strategies matched to the unique genetic requirements of each individual.

There should be no fear that these technological advances will dehumanize medicine. The practice of the art of medicine, in which the needs and concerns of children and their families are understood and considered, will be even more demanding as we adjust to the changes. If we are to prevent common, complex disorders like diabetes, cancer, and cardiovascular disease, we will rarely have a "magic pill"; instead, we will rely on individuals to change their lifestyles. Successfully assisting individuals in changing their behaviors and with very specific recommendations (such as exercise, diet, habits) throughout their lives will be challenges that we must meet. To be successful, healthcare professionals will need to become more skilled in the art of medicine than we have been in the past.

The Human Genome Project will result in predictive, preventive, and personalized medicine and will have fundamental influences on the diagnostic tests and therapies available to children. Genomic medicine will increasingly make it possible to utilize knowledge of both individual and group genetic constitutions to improve health. These advances will impact newborn screening in terms of the disorders screened and the technologies utilized.

The promise of the Human Genome Project, however, will only be achieved if we have full knowledge of the frequencies of alterations in the human genome that lead to disease among the individual ethnic and cultural groups that make up our diverse population. Any individual group for whom this knowledge of alterations in their genome is not available will be disadvantaged in the era of genomic medicine. Therefore, it is extremely important that we understand the changing demography of our country and learn how to anticipate population trends. It will be essential to include all segments of our population so that no group is marginalized and, as a result, denied access to genomic technologies and the potential benefits of genomic medicine. As with all aspects of our civic lives and our healthcare system, creating equity among all peoples in terms of access to genomic medicine and healthcare resources presents an urgent and ongoing task.

> **It will be essential to include all segments of our population so that no group is marginalized and, as a result, denied access to genomic technologies and the potential benefits of genomic medicine.**

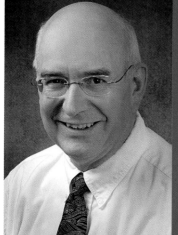

Edward R. B. McCabe and Linda L. McCabe

Edward R. B. McCabe, MD, PhD, is professor and executive chair of the UCLA Department of Pediatrics and physician-in-chief of the Mattel Children's Hospital at UCLA. Dr. McCabe directs the Pediatric Research, Innovation and Mentoring Experience (PRIME) Program, the UCLA Child Health Research Career Development Award Program, the Human and Molecular Development Postdoctoral Training Program, and the UCLA Center for Society, the Individual and Genetics. Dr. McCabe was elected to the Institute of Medicine in 2001 and became a fellow of the American Association for the Advancement of Science in 2003. He has served on numerous committees including the Committee on Genetics of the American Academy of Pediatrics and the Medical Genetics Residency Review Committee for the Accreditation Council for Graduate Medical Education. Dr. McCabe was president of the American Board of Medical Genetics.

Linda L. McCabe, PhD, is an adjunct associate professor at the UCLA Departments of Human Genetics and Pediatrics. She is the coordinator of the PRIME Program, recruiter for the UCLA Child Health Research Career Development Award Program, and coordinator of the Human and Molecular Development Training Grant. She is a member of the advisory board of the UCLA Center for Society, the Individual and Genetics. She serves as a member of the UCLA Institutional Review Board. She is managing editor of the journal *Molecular Genetics and Metabolism*.

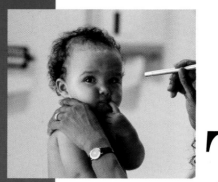

Chapter 46

*Judith S. Palfrey and
Julius B. Richmond*

Health Services:
Past, Present, and Future

The health and well-being of a nation's children and youth are measures of that country's ability to care for its citizens. A review of past and present child health care services helps put the present situation for children of the United States into perspective. The past century brought about a transformation in the scientific understanding of children's health. Major advances in biomedical knowledge as well as changing social policies have intertwined, often unwittingly, frequently at cross-purposes, and only occasionally in direct collaboration. In this chapter, we will review child health and health service trends, briefly outline the current state of children's health, and discuss future needs. We will suggest ways that a child health system can take advantage of the stunning scientific advances of the near past and explicitly blend what we know about biology, genetics, engineering, and pharmacology with what we know about the context of children's lives in the larger community.

Trends in Child Health at the Millennium

Each chronological period poses its own challenges for children and families. The circumstances of one particular time shape the environment and its influence on child health outcomes. The events of one age serve as a backdrop for the next. Figure 46.1 shows the rapid and dynamic emergence of bodies of knowledge that have informed and transformed child health since 1900.[1] This child health science has emerged in a sociopolitical milieu with its own tempo and sequence. Using the notion of a series of interconnected eras, let us review how the experiences and accomplishments of the past 100 years have contributed to the present status of child health and well-being.

The Early Years: 1900s to 1930s

At the dawn of the 20th century, child health practitioners confronted a high incidence of contagious illness, high infant mortality rates, poor nutrition, few cures for chronic disease, many diseases of overcrowding, and infectious disease epidemics. The rates of infant mortality in 1900 were as great as 140 per 1,000 live births per year.[2] Physicians and nurses were limited in what they could offer sick children because there was little basic understanding of pathologic processes, and there were very few effective therapies. Medical schools were so primitive that Isaac Abt reported that the full-time staff of the University of Chicago consisted of a janitor, a registrar, and a professor of chemistry.[3] Often, the best a doctor could do was to document what he or she saw and hope that the natural healing process would ensue. During this *era of pediatric nosology*, the pioneering child health leaders wrote elegant descriptions of diseases and created the necessary categorization that formed the bedrock on which all further clinical investigation could rest.[1]

Fortunately, the scientific breakthroughs of the late 19th century offered a new direction for child health. In the 20th century, physicians began to appreciate the importance of the discoveries of the last quarter of the previous century (in particular Joseph Lister and Louis Pasteur's germ theory, Robert Koch's identification of the tubercle bacillus, and Rudolph Virchow's delineation of cellular reactions and the basics of immunology). The early pediatric pioneers, including Abraham Jacobi and Job Lewis Smith, began to apply these theories to public health.[4] The sanitary revolution accompanied a general realization that the provision of clean water could improve the health of mothers, infants, and children. The social reformers of the early decades—especially the great women of Hull House in Chicago—were particularly effective in translating the new scientific knowledge into specific services for children.[5] They successfully organized infant health stations for better nutrition and sanitation and promoted the pasteurization of milk. These interventions contributed substantially to the decline in infant and early childhood mortality.[4]

> **The 1920s and 1930s ushered in the period of major basic discovery in nutrition, microbiology, immunology, physiology, pathology, and pharmacology.**

The 1920s and 1930s ushered in the period of major basic discovery in nutrition, microbiology, immunology, physiology, pathology, and pharmacology.[1] Then, scientists and physicians understood that large quantities of orange juice cured the one-sided bulging eye associated with scurvy and that cod liver oil prevented rickets among children in colder climates where the absence of sunlight meant the absence of vitamin D.[6] Pediatrics as a science came into its own with recognition (if sometimes grudgingly given by adult-oriented physicians) of the unique aspects of children's growth and physical and psychological development.

Pediatric practice in these early years was largely a private enterprise. Physicians set their own fees for office consultation, home visits, and hospital stays. There were no insurance programs.[7] Wealthy patients had access to "fashionable" pediatric practices. Poor patients depended on charity care delivered most often in dispensaries associated with the fledgling medical training programs that were springing up in association with universities. Advocates for children began to call for a more systematic approach to the delivery of child health and welfare services. By 1909, the advocates persuaded President Theodore Roosevelt to call a White House conference on children that resulted in the 1912 establishment of the U.S. Children's Bureau.[5] Because many medical practitioners and others distrusted the incursion of government into the business of health care, it would not be until the Great Depression and the presidency of Franklin Roosevelt that there was the cementing of a federal policy delineating a systematic approach to ensuring health care service for children. The 1935 Social Security Act included Title V that had provisions for maternal and child health and crippled children's programs. There was then an impetus for the states to establish programs for the continuing improvement of maternal and child health as well as services for children with physical disabilities.[8]

Midcentury: 1940s to 1970s

With the new scientific discoveries, universities began to establish pediatric research centers for the elucidation of children's metabolic and nutritional needs. As new knowledge of nutrients, vitamins, and other basic requirements emerged, this information was rapidly integrated into child health practice. Studies at the pediatric research centers led, over time, to the development of modern parenteral therapy, such as intravenous feeding for children with severe diarrheal disease. With the major discoveries in microbiology, basic scientists and clinicians began to understand the underlying mechanisms of many common conditions such as diphtheria, pertussis, and measles as well as streptococcal, staphylococcal, and pneumococcal illnesses. The new use of antibiotics and the

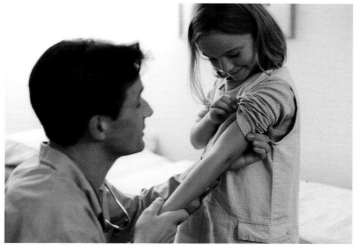

early development of immunizations brought much of the infectious disease mortality and morbidity under control.

Because of the tremendous innovations in pediatric health care, the 1940s and 1950s can be thought of as an *era of laboratory investigation: specific etiology and therapy*. It was during the 1950s that a number of discoveries about chronic disease helped form a better understanding of childhood illness. For example, Helen Taussig's publishing of her classic descriptions of cardiac anomalies provided a solid foundation for the newly emerging subspecialty field of pediatric cardiology.[9] Similar fundamental anatomic and pathophysiologic work contributed to the

---

The Era of Pediatric Nosology (1900-1920s)
    Infectious diseases
    High infant mortality rates
    Poor nutrition
    Few cures for chronic disease
    Epidemics (e.g., influenza, polio)
The Era of Laboratory Investigation (1920s-1940s)
    Studies of nutrition
    Early delineation of fluid and electrolyte balance
    Elucidation of the mechanism of vitamins' effects
    Discovery of sulfonamides
The Era of Pediatric Therapy (1950s-1960s)
    Burgeoning of subspecialty knowledge
    Vaccine development
    Antibiotic use
    Intensive care
The Era of Child Development (1970s-1990s)
    Guiding healthy social and psychological development
    Family dysfunction
    Learning disabilities
    Emotional disorders
    Functional distress
    Educational needs
    Social morbidities
    High technology care
The Era of Bioenvironmental Interface (2000s-   )
    Disorders of lifestyle (obesity, eating disorders, substance abuse)
    Family stress
    Child behavioral disorders and mental illnesses
    Global community concerns
    Cycle of chronic conditions
    Health disparities

Figure 46.1: Trends in Pediatric Morbidity

Source: Provided by Richmond 2004

founding of the other pediatric subspecialties. By the mid 1970s, the American Board of Pediatrics recognized the fields of cardiology, hematology, nephrology, and newborn medicine and offered subspecialty certifying exams.[10] The midcentury heralded the birth of pediatric intensive care with neonatal intensive care coming into its own in the 1960s and 1970s. The highly effective technologies of respiratory support, blood exchange, and meticulous fluid and electrolyte balance contributed to further improvements in infant survival rates.[11]

The new developments in health care meant that a great deal was available that physicians, surgeons, intensivists, and hospitals could offer to fight illness and to address chronic conditions in children. The therapies were increasingly expensive. New mechanisms of employer-based insurance largely replaced out-of-pocket, fee-for-service payment for health care. Such proprietary insurance plans grew up as a uniquely American response to the increasing availability of medical technology. As care became more available, it also became more expensive. The difficulty with employer-based insurance was that it did not help those who were unemployed, namely the elderly, the poor, nonworking mothers, and children. The health insurance dramas of the 1960s were filled with *Sturm und Drang*, heroes and villains, and battles and counterbattles. The outcome was the 1965 passage of both Medicare, which provides federally funded health insurance for the elderly, and of Medicaid, which delineates a federal-state financing program for health insurance for the poor with special provisions for poor mothers and children.[7]

The Later Years: 1970s to 1990s

The innovations of the midcentury made significant impacts on the epidemiology and disease burden borne by children and adolescents. In consideration of the major changes in public health and in pediatric approaches to acute and chronic illness, Robert Haggerty coined the phrase "the new morbidity" in the 1970s. This phrase pointed to new approaches for child health resulting from the reduction in infectious diseases.[12] He and others felt that there was now the capability of addressing problems such as family dysfunction, learning disabilities, coordination of care, emotional disorders, functional distress, and educational needs. The science of child development was also advancing, and the advancement offered the theory and rigor necessary for the establishment of a new branch of child health that would focus on the development and behavior of children and youth.

This *era of child development* benefited from a number of factors. From 1965 to 1976, the nation experienced a "baby bust." Between 1957 and 1970, the birthrate dropped among women 15 to 44 years old from the baby boom high of 123 births per 1,000 women to 88 births per 1,000 women. This trend was to continue until the rate settled at roughly 70 births per 1,000 women in 1980.[13,14] Not only were there fewer children in the population (50 million children under 15 years old in 1980 vs. 60 million in 1970),[15] there was increased capacity in the child health and educational arena. Services had expanded to meet the onslaught of the baby boom, and now the baby boomers themselves were in the workforce as potential doctors,

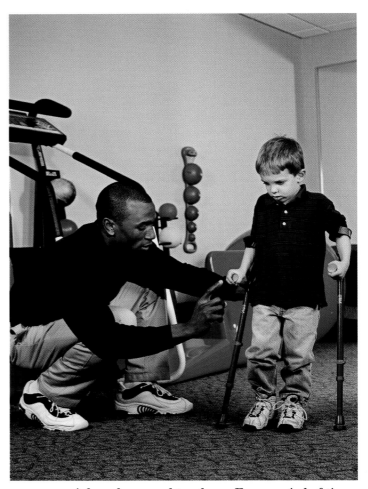

nurses, social workers, and teachers. For a period of time, it was possible for society in general and child health providers in particular to pay attention to both the needs and the capabilities of children with a variety of handicapping conditions, including both learning problems and physical disabilities. There was a burgeoning of new investigation, new services, and new teaching in child development, developmental biology, and the notions of prevention.[1] Major attitudinal shifts included systematic emphasis on function, family, and community.

One of the biggest opportunities in child health and development came with the launch of Project Head Start in 1965.[16] This federally funded program was a strategic weapon in President Lyndon Johnson's War on Poverty. From the inception of the program, Head Start centers provided coordinated child health and development services. With the emphasis on screening for language and educational risks, Head Start programs identified children in need of early intervention and ensured the availability of those services. Another key feature of the Head Start design was the emphasis on family involvement. Head Start was one of the first major ventures to emphasize the importance of comprehensive service provision to children in the context of their family and community. The lessons learned from this aspect of Head Start have continued to inform child health service providers to this day. During the first summer of operation, 500,000 children participated in Head Start; 10 years later, there were 5.3 million Head Start graduates, and the program was well established as a valuable national asset for poor children and families. When Head Start celebrated its 35th anniversary in 2000, 21 million children had benefited from the health and developmental services.

In 1975, the U.S. Congress passed landmark federal special education legislation, the Education for All Handicapped Children Act (PL 94-142).[17] As a result of this law, children with disabilities were promised the right to a free, appropriate public education no matter how severe their handicap. The Education for All Handicapped Children Act also embraced a family approach and gave families the final say in the development of an individualized education program. With the right to due process, families could actually bring their case all the way to the Supreme Court if they felt that their children were not receiving appropriate educational services. The related services provisions of PL 94-142 are of great importance to child health providers. As a result of these provisions, schools became the service agencies for children who needed physical and occupational therapy, speech/language services, and counseling. Moreover, school nurses and their designated staff were authorized to provide health services (such as clean intermittent catheterization, respiratory suctioning, and gastrostomy feeding) so that children with a wide variety of serious medical conditions could attend school alongside their peers.[18]

The midcentury heralded the birth of pediatric intensive care with neonatal intensive care coming into its own in the 1960s and 1970s.

A number of social upheavals in the 1980s brought new challenges to child health. The massive social disarray and political ennui of the time placed many children at risk of disorders with roots that lay deeply in the society. Many families were unable to support their children because of the new epidemics of drug use (particularly crack cocaine),[19] violence,[20] HIV/AIDS,[21,22] and homelessness.[23] These complex social issues created a number of very serious health problems among children, particularly children in poverty.[24] Child health clinicians saw their role expanding to meet the demands of the time. As a result, there was a burgeoning of knowledge and techniques in child development, adolescent medicine, infectious diseases, and emergency medicine. Recognizing the importance of population-based patterns of disease and dysfunction, pediatricians began to seek partnership with statisticians and epidemiologists. New sources of data, such as the Youth Risk Behavior Survey by the Centers for Disease Control and Prevention (CDC), and new computer technologies expanded the capacity of these teams to monitor trends and real-time events for large groups of children. With these new data sets, researchers could create sufficient statistical power to draw definitive conclusions about correlation and cause and effect. Many studies confirmed how important social factors are as determinants of the health of children and youth.

Biomedical breakthroughs and technological innovations continued in the later decades of the 20th century. New medical and surgical interventions increased the survivorship in children with serious disorders. For instance, the number of children assisted by highly technological care had increased substantially. By 1990, 1 in 1,000 children was assisted by some form of technology (e.g., gastrostomy feeding, oxygen use, or intravenous feeding).[25] Physicians and nurses in the 1980s and 1990s were challenged to learn both the language and interventions of socially induced health problems as well as deal with the prevention, care, and cure of children with a wide array of very complex, chronic diseases and disabilities.

In the late 1980s and early 1990s, the costs of medical care escalated at an alarming rate. By 1998, the nation was spending $1 trillion per year on medical care (a full 14% of the gross national product). The skyrocketing costs of medical care were a concern for employers, insurers, providers, and the government. The problem of health care financing for children became an important consideration in all aspects of service with cost and quality consciousness stimulating the creation of the field of pediatric health services research.

Millennial Morbidity

As we move into the 21st century, we see the emergence of a new era, one in which there is a deepening appreciation of the interaction of biology with the environment. Child health providers recognize a new set of opportunities and a new set of challenges, many of which emanate from the scientific and technological breakthroughs of the 20th century. The February 2001 publication of the human genome sequence culminated a 20-year exploration and began an exciting new chapter in child health.[26] This stunning achievement crowned the advances in science and technology that have radically changed daily living for most families. The major lifestyle shifts brought about by the incorporation of various devices are having significant impact on the health of children, some for good and others for ill. The virulent agents are no longer only microbial. Increasingly it is recognized that the television, the computer, mass media, the automobile, and other wonderful innovations of the 20th century have caused new health risks for children. The relationships between television watching and obesity,[27] between media ads and eating disorders,[28] and between high-risk driving and automobile deaths[29] are well established.

The rapidly changing society has placed new stresses on families and communities. Families in dynamically

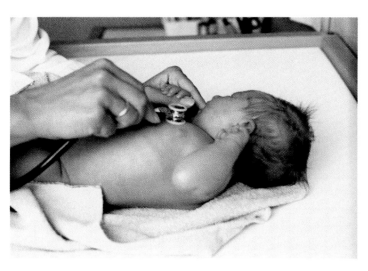

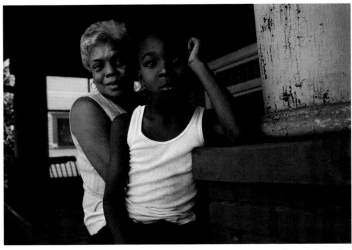

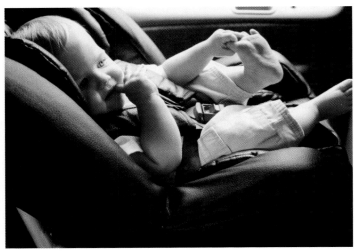

changing configurations are trying to deal with the millennial reordering. Increasing numbers of single parents do their best to support young children. Moreover, grandparents and single-parent fathers are becoming more prominent in the ranks of family providers.[30] Of great concern at the turn of the 21st century is the increase in number and severity of child and adolescent mental illness concerns. The Institute of Medicine has documented a lowering in the age of onset of many serious mental health conditions.[31]

The 20th century innovations in communication and transportation have transformed the global community. The world is more closely knit than ever in history. There were almost as many new immigrants entering the United States in the last decade of the century as there were in the massive immigration of the first decade of the century (9.09 million in 1991-2000 as compared with 8.79 million in 1900-1910).[32] The appearance of many new families from all over the world has led to a call for improved understanding of languages and cultures and of customs and beliefs among people from different racial and ethnic backgrounds.

The appearance of many new families from all over the world has led to a call for improved understanding of languages and cultures and of customs and beliefs among people from different racial and ethnic backgrounds.

While the emergence of the global community brings many good aspects for children and families, there are also inherent risks and concerns. As the world shrinks and there is increased international travel, the spread of infectious illness[33] is enhanced, and there are increased risks of emerging infections (such as severe acute respiratory syndrome, or SARS).[34] The mental health disabilities of children who have experienced war and violence in their native countries present challenges to policymakers and clinicians.[35] Finally, continued world-wide unrest has posed the new potential risks of bioterrorism.[36] All of these international factors have raised new awareness of how critical it is for a nation to have an alert and fully prepared public health infrastructure.

At this turn of the millennium, it is readily apparent that medical and surgical innovations have had a major impact on children's health and health care. Children with rare and complex illnesses and conditions now have much

improved survival rates and opportunities for community life. The increased survival of these children provides new experience and knowledge of the natural history of their chronic illnesses and disabilities.

The interplay between social considerations and physical health problems is nowhere more apparent than in the health disparities that are evident between poor and nonpoor children and between White and Non-White children.[37] The new epidemiologic capabilities that allow careful trending of information by economic status and racial status allow a clearer look at these disparities than has been available in the past. In delineating the health status of children at the dawn of the 21st century, the availability of the 2000 census data and the information from the National Health Interview Survey are allowing a timely look at these issues. In the following sections, we present a quantitative picture of the current health of children and adolescents in the United States.

Current Health Status of Children and Youth

<u>Causes of Death in Children and Youth in the 21st Century</u>
Figure 46.2 is the depiction of the leading causes of death for children and youth compiled by the Centers for Disease Control and Prevention.[38] The early time period from ages 0 to 1 is strikingly different from all of the others. The rate of child death during the first year of life is generally discussed in terms of 1 death for 1,000 infants, whereas the rate is 1 death per 10,000 children for subsequent years of life.

Infant mortality—The U. S. infant mortality rate for 1998 was 7.2 infant deaths per 1,000 live births, placing the United States 28th among 38 countries that reported infant mortality rates to the World Health Organization.[39] The major causes of infant mortality in the United States in 2001 were congenital anomalies (5,513); preterm/low birth weight (4,410); sudden infant death syndrome (SIDS) (2,234); problems related to complications of pregnancy (1,499); complications of placenta, cord, and membranes (1,018); and respiratory distress syndrome (1,011).[40] Almost two-thirds of infant deaths occurred within the first 28 days (neonatal mortality) and one-third occurred during the remainder of the first year of life (postneonatal mortality).

The rates of low birth weight (<5.5 pounds or <2,500 grams) and prematurity (<37 weeks' gestation) in the United States are 7.6% and 11.6%, respectively. The rate of very low birth weight (<3 pounds 4 ounces or <1500 grams) is 1.4%, and the rate of very premature babies (<32 weeks' gestation) is 1.9%.[41,42] The ability to save very small babies has increased markedly over the past century. However, there is still significant morbidity and mortality for very small babies (under 1,000 grams). One of the newest millennial challenges is the increasing rate of multiple births (twins, triplets, and quadruplets).[42] Many of these babies are born as the result of new reproductive technologies.

The capacity to save children with significant congenital defects has improved continuously over the past quarter century. While intervention completely cures many of these babies, some live only a short time, and others survive with significant dependency on the medical and surgical health care system. Many heart, kidney, and bladder anomalies are now potentially treatable with surgical interventions carried out on the fetus in the womb. A number of highly specialized care centers are developing maternal-fetal surgical units.

SIDS accounts for a large part of postneonatal mortality. The death rate from SIDS has actually declined substantially since the institution of the "back to sleep" campaign by the National Institute of Child Health and Human Development and the American Academy of

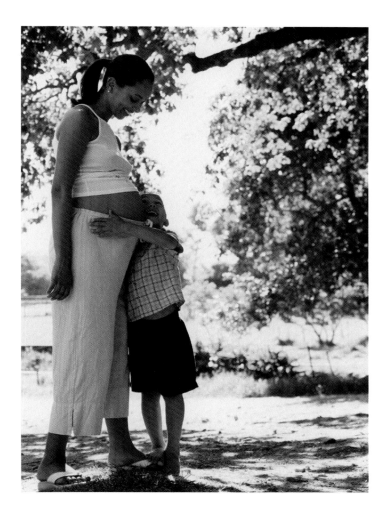

Cause of death ranking	Less than 1 year old	Ages 1-4	Ages 5-14	Ages 15-24
1	Congenital anomalies	Unintentional injury	Unintentional injury	Unintentional injury
2	Short gestation and low birth weight	Congenital anomalies	Malignant neoplasms	Assault (homicide)
3	Sudden infant death syndrome (SIDS)	Malignant neoplasms	Congenital anomalies	Suicide
4	Maternal complications	Assault (homicide)	Assault (homicide)	Malignant neoplasms
5	Placenta, cord, and membrane complications	Heart disease	Suicide	Heart disease
6	Respiratory distress	Influenza & pneumonia	Heart disease	Congenital anomalies
7	Unintentional injury	Septicemia	Benign neoplasms	Human immunodeficiency virus (HIV)
8	Bacterial sepsis	Perinatal period	Chronic lower respiratory disease	Cerebrovascular diseases

Figure 46.2: Leading Causes of Death by Age, 2000

Source: Centers for Disease Control and Prevention 2001

209

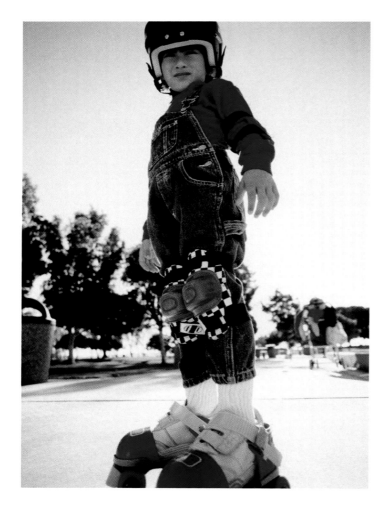

Pediatrics.[43] The other major causes of postneonatal infant mortality are infectious diseases and injuries.

Analyses of the U.S. infant mortality rate and the rates of other industrialized nations point to a number of complex issues.[44] In the absence of a universal methodology for reporting *infant deaths, fetal deaths, and stillborns*, there is some variability in the reports with the United States tending to call many situations *live birth followed by infant death* that would be reported as fetal death or stillbirth in other countries (notably Japan). Nonetheless, after adjustments for these measurement artifacts, the United States still has a higher overall infant mortality rate than that found in other industrialized nations. The factors that contribute to this are (a) higher mortality related to birth weight among some groups of the population (with the worst rates occurring among Black infants), (b) relatively more mothers in the under-20 and over-39 age ranges, and (c) the tendency of U.S. mothers to have a different pattern of prenatal care.

Toddler, preschool, and child deaths—Injuries are the predominant cause of death for both 1- to 4-year-olds and 5- to 14-year-olds. Children are at risk for falls, pedestrian accidents, and bicycle injuries. They also can be the occupant victims of car crashes. The institution of safety seats and bicycle helmets as well as the installation of window guards in high buildings have made significant inroads in the prevention of these types of injuries.[45] Young children also can succumb to chronic illnesses and infectious diseases. Since 1996, death from HIV/AIDS is no longer on the list of leading causes of death for young children in the United States. Prenatal and perinatal treatment of HIV-infected mothers with AZT (azidothymidine) has changed the epidemiology of HIV disease dramatically.[46]

Youth deaths—Mortality for teenagers and young adults reflects many lifestyle issues. Injuries from automobile accidents are predominant among 15- to 24-year-olds, accounting for nearly a third of the deaths in this age group. In 1998, 32.8% of adolescent deaths were automobile-related. Other unintentional injuries accounted for 10.8% of deaths, homicide for 18.0%, and suicide for 13.4%. Causes including malignant neoplasms (tumors), diseases of the heart, congenital anomalies, and cerebrovascular disease comprised 24.9%.[47] The good news is that the rates of adolescent mortality have been declining over the past decade with much of the decline referable to interventions in youth risk taking and violence.[48]

<u>Child Illness and Morbidity</u>

Acute illness—Vaccines and new antibiotic regimens have had a great impact on the pattern of childhood acute illness. The last quarter of the 20th century witnessed the near disappearance of a number of common childhood illnesses including measles, mumps, rubella, and *Haemophilus influenzae* infections.[49] In the past decade, the introduction of varicella and pneumococcal vaccines has improved the preventive arsenal available to child health clinicians even further. In addition, the prompt use of appropriate treatment (intramuscular cephalosporin) for potential sepsis in small babies[50] and the availability of home care (including administration of intravenous medications for conditions such as osteomyelitis, a type of

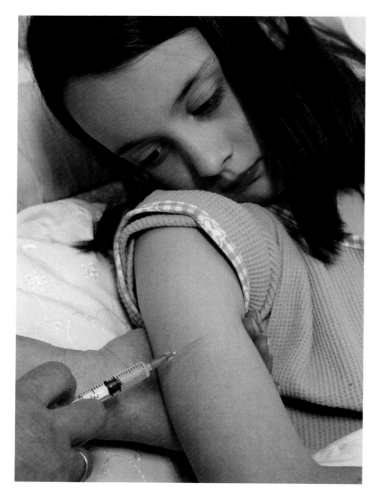

bone infection) have allowed the outpatient surveillance and care for many children who would previously have required extensive inpatient stays. The rate of hospitalization for children has dropped from 715 hospital admissions per 10,000 children in 1962 to 209 per 10,000 children in 2000; only 26% of admissions in 2000 were for acute illness compared to 62% in 1962.[51]

The availability of potent new antibiotics has been a major boon for children in the early 21st century, but the widespread use of these drugs has had a serious consequence: the emergence of new strains of bacteria that are resistant to multiple drugs. A 1998 national study indicated that over 30% of the *Streptococcus pneumoniae* isolates analyzed from Georgia and Tennessee were resistant to penicillin.[52] The problem of antibiotic resistance has led to serious reevaluation by pediatricians about the treatment of common infections such as otitis media (inflammation of the middle ear). This rethinking comes at a time when group child care arrangements have led to higher rates of infectious diseases (particularly otitis media) among young children.[53] Resolution of this dilemma will necessarily involve the careful assessment of multiple group and individual factors. At this point, the general medical consensus is to urge practitioners to be increasingly judicious in their use of antibiotics[54] and to err on the side of watchful waiting in cases when the children are not obviously very sick and their physical findings are equivocal.

Chronic Illness and Disability—At the advent of the 21st century, childhood chronic illness and disability are of particular relevance. Despite enormous expenditures on health care and the highest standard of living in the world, the latest estimate from the State and Local Area Integrated Telephone Survey by the National Center for Health Statistics[55] is that 13% of U.S. children are "those who have or are at increased risk for chronic physical, developmental, behavioral, or emotional conditions and who require health and related services of a type or amount beyond that required by children generally."[56-58] These new data confirm a growing recognition by clinicians and epidemiologists that while the majority of the children of the millennium enjoy a high level of health, a substantial subgroup of children and youth—now identified as children with special health care needs—have serious health concerns and rely heavily on the health care system. Approximately one-half of these children (6.5% of the nation's total child and youth population or nearly 6 million children and youth) are impaired in their functions of daily living.[59] Children with special health care needs have 3 times as many bed days and school absences as other children.[60] The money expended on their care annually is greater than that for other children.[59,61] For example, Henry Ireys and colleagues found that children with chronic conditions who were Washington state Medicaid recipients incurred costs ranging from 2.5 to 20 times more than children without chronic conditions.[62]

> **The availability of potent new antibiotics has been a major boon for children in the early 21st century, but the widespread use of these drugs has had a serious consequence: the emergence of new strains of bacteria that are resistant to multiple drugs.**

Among the children with chronic illnesses and disabilities are children with severe disorders who have survived longer than was previously possible as a result of the enormous advances in medical and surgical technology. For instance, the mean age of death from cystic fibrosis was 6 months in 1938; in 1998, it was 32 years.[63] This dramatically improved life expectancy is the result of advanced pharmacotherapy, vigilant medical care, and the advent of interventions such as lung transplantation. Many chronic illness cohort survivors live full and healthy lives, but others shuttle between home and hospital and are constantly teetering on the edge, depending on multiple medications, nursing interventions, and the availability of rapid response teams in the event of serious emergencies. As children with chronic conditions and disabilities continue to survive, new health conditions are becoming apparent. Children are developing additional manifestations and secondary difficulties such as diabetes in young people with cystic fibrosis,[64] cancer among young people who have survived renal transplant,[65] and second leukemias among cancer survivors.[66] Each of these complex conditions helps us to learn more about the natural history of disease entities but also places a stress on the children, their families, and the health care system.

The majority of the children with chronic illness and disability have moderately severe disorders such as asthma, autism, diabetes, significant obesity, and behavioral concerns such as attention deficit hyperactivity disorder (ADHD). There is a general consensus that this group of children with moderately severe conditions is increasing at a rapid rate. The growth is of "epidemic proportions" for several of these conditions. In 1971 to 1974, 6.1% of 12- to 19-year-olds were overweight. Their body mass index, or BMI (weight in kilograms divided by height in meters squared), was greater than or equal to the age- and sex-specific 95th percentile in a U.S. reference population. In 1988 to 1994, the comparable group had a 10.5% rate of overweight, and by 1999 and 2000, 15.5% of 12- to 19-year olds were in the overweight category.[67] Children and youth who are overweight are at high risk of lifelong obesity with all the attendant health consequences. The cause of the extraordinarily fast increase in overweight and obesity among children and adolescents is unclear but seems to be attributable at least in part to lifestyle issues, including high-fat, high-calorie diets, lack of regular exercise, and long hours of television watching. The high prevalence of obesity is particularly marked among Black children and youth. A concomitant to the rise in obesity is the emergence of type 2 diabetes.[68] Generally considered an adult-onset disorder, insulin-resistant diabetes is now diagnosed on a regular basis in adolescent and school-age children; most of these children with diabetes also meet the criteria for obesity. The long-term health sequelae of overweight and diabetes include pregnancy complications, heart disease, hypertension, and early death.

Pediatric involvement in the diagnosis and management of ADHD has been increasing over the past 10 to 20 years,[69] and there has been a massive (140-fold) increase in visits to physicians for the monthly prescription of stimulant medication.[70] It is unlikely that the explosive increase in pediatric visits is a function of an acute increase in the prevalence of the disorder.[71] It is far more likely that the threshold for making the diagnosis and providing therapy has been lowered. In fact, Mark Wolraich and colleagues have shown that the incorporation of attention deficit disorder (ADD), the inattentive disorder rather than the inattentive and hyperactivity disorder (ADHD), in the latest edition of the *Diagnostic and Statistical Manual of Mental Disorders-Fourth Edition* contributed to a substantial amount of the increase in the number of children being diagnosed.[72] The new definition makes it more likely that girls will be diagnosed[73] since the hyperactivity feature is not as frequent among girls as it is among boys. Another possible explanation is a greater mismatch between children's makeup (temperament) and school and parental expectations. If there actually is an increase in prevalence, what might be the causative agent? Some have postulated food additives; others blame the television and the computer. Low-level lead poisoning is associated with attention problems.[74] Is it possible that there are other chemical compounds that have yet to be identified as associated or causative agents? Certainly this is the thesis of a number of investigators in the new field of environmental toxicology.[75]

Another condition that seems to be on the rise is childhood autism. In the 1980s, autism was found in 4 to 5 per 10,000 children. More recent studies put the prevalence at 4 to 6 per 1,000 children.[76,77] There are no clear explanations for this 10-fold increase, but doubtless some part of the change reflects more precision in the diagnosis of children with developmental delay and mental retardation. The search for a unitary cause for autism has not yet proved fruitful, although there are some promising leads toward a genetic explanation. There is no evidence of an association of autism with immunization for measles, mumps, and rubella, although there has been a scare campaign in the lay press alleging such a causal relationship.[78]

Many scholars, political analysts, and child health advocates contend that without progress on this fundamental problem [universal access to health care], few other child health issues will be resolved.

Disparities in Child Health

Social factors such as poverty, environment, geography, and race help determine children's health. The profound effects of poverty are shown by 2- to 4-fold differences in child and adolescent morbidity and mortality between children in poverty and children of greater means. Health outcomes are not equally distributed for children in the United States. Infant mortality rates are much higher for Black children (13.6 deaths for every 1,000 births) than for either White (5.7 deaths for every 1,000 births) or Hispanic children (5.6 deaths for every 1,000 births).[79] Black children are at higher risk of neonatal mortality than White children because of a significantly higher proportion of Black children being born at low birth weight (13.1% vs. 6.6%). Somewhat surprisingly, children of Hispanic and Native American backgrounds are not at increased risk of neonatal mortality, suggesting certain protective factors that account for healthy pregnancies even in the face of poverty.

There are marked racial disparities in conditions that affect adolescents and young adult men and women. Even though Black youth ages 15 to 24 years constitute only 14% of the U.S. population, 56% of HIV/AIDS cases for youth 13 to 24 years old are among Black young people.[80]

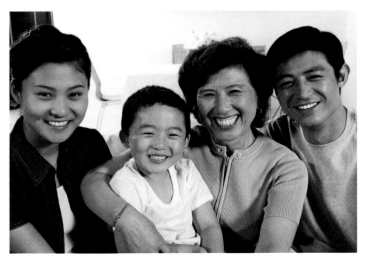

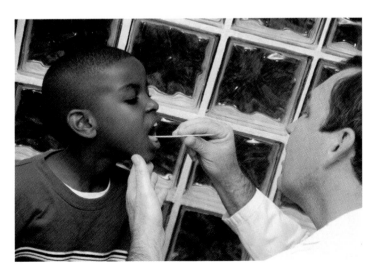

Black male adolescents and young adults have a 15 times greater chance of dying from homicide than White males of the same ages. The rate for homicide death is 6 times greater among Black female adolescents and young adults than among White female adolescents and young adults.[81] Black male life expectancy is significantly less than that for any other racial or gender group at 68.6 years compared to 77.2 for all groups.[82]

The Future

Addressing the future health needs of children requires serious attention to three issues: (a) acknowledging the social, community, and behavioral contributors to child health outcomes; (b) fulfilling the promises made to children and youth with chronic illnesses and disabilities, and (c) addressing inequities.

Integrating Social, Community, and Behavioral Interventions into Health Care Delivery

To come to grips with the pressing and increasing needs of children and youth (such as needs that arise as a result of obesity, asthma, injuries, violence, and mental health concerns), new models of intervention are required. Many of these models have been outlined in the Healthy People 2010 goals for the nation issued by the U.S. Department of Health and Human Services.[83] The public health agenda takes into consideration the importance of interweaving healthy lifestyles, community health initiatives, health education, and private health care delivery. Models for community-based integrated efforts have demonstrated the success of comprehensive, preventive health promotion strategies.[84-90] The real challenge for the nation is to move the knowledge gleaned from these successful demonstration projects to widespread use and state- and national-level adoption.

To effect such integration at the state and federal levels requires the commitment of funding, personnel, and energy. Such commitment will not occur until there is sufficient political will and general acceptance that the health of children and youth is directly contingent on the health of families, the community, and society. It is incumbent on health care providers, policymakers, and educators to keep articulating the linkages between social determinants and child health outcomes in the clearest possible terms. Statements like the following do wake the public to the concerning realities: "Poor children are 4 times more likely to die than nonpoor children"; "Parents' smoking causes prematurity, infant death, SIDS, asthma, and lung cancer"; "Adolescent drinking and driving is responsible for more teenage deaths than cancer and infectious diseases combined." Plain speaking about the linkage between social determinants and health outcomes is not enough, however. Policymakers, legislators, and insurers need concrete, creative solutions. They want to hear what can be done about the high rates of health problems in poor children and what are the effective strategies for reducing smoking and alcohol use in teenagers.

Universal access to health care is one such strategy. Many scholars, political analysts, and child health advocates contend that without progress on this fundamental problem, few other child health issues will be resolved.

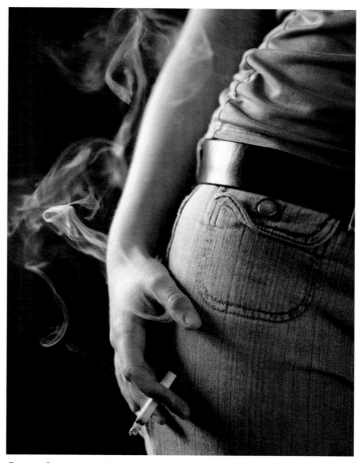

Over the past 20 years, great strides toward achieving universal health care have occurred only to suffer serious erosion in the past 5 years.[91] With 9.7 million (13.6%) of 0- to 17-year-old children uninsured, a simple calculation suggests that ensuring full coverage for children would be no more than $10 to $15 billion per year, which is less than 1% of the $1.7 trillion expended on health care annually in the United States.[92] Raising such money from a combination of state and federal taxes is not out of the realm of possibility, particularly if states add the taxation of items like tobacco, alcohol, firearms, automobiles, televisions, and movies into the mix.

Beyond financial access is the question of the content of pediatric services. A crucial step to expand the scope of child health care is the coordination of the Healthy People 2010 goals and objectives with primary care practice guidelines. This is the approach that the Bright Futures[93] project of the American Academy of Pediatrics is taking. As the Bright Futures recommendations move forward, they are becoming increasingly specific and targeted, using quality improvement strategies so that the investment of time and energy by clinicians can be monitored and compensated. As pediatricians, nurses, families, policymakers, and insurers see preventive strategies (such as injury risk reduction, parental smoking cessation programs, developmental screening, home visits for new parents, school interventions for children with asthma, etc.) paying off with fewer emergency department visits, fewer hospitalizations, and less loss of parental work time, the general presumption can shift more toward prevention. This is already happening with some successful disease prevention/health promotion strategies.[84-90] A future direction that would hold increased adoption of these integrated strategies could benefit many children and youth.

<u>Fulfilling the Promise to Children and Youth with Chronic Illness and Disability</u>

The remarkable accomplishments in medical and surgical science of the 20th century have revolutionized the life chances for children with serious chronic illnesses and disabilities. The challenge for the future is to match these triumphs with health and social care innovations that ensure the saved lives are free from pain and suffering and that the children achieve their full potential physically, intellectually, socially, and emotionally.

To alleviate the stress and discomfort that comes with chronic conditions, health care services need to be expanded. It is not enough for children and youth to have access to operations and inpatient hospital care. Families of children with chronic conditions and disabilities deserve help with home care, transportation, physical and occupational therapy, speech and language intervention, mental health care, and behavioral counseling. Children with chronic conditions and disabilities should receive the same (if not enhanced) primary care and preventive services as all other children. Too often families have to fight for each of these aspects of care.

The Healthy People 2010 objectives for the nation spell out important steps that can be taken to improve health care for children with special health care needs.[94] These objectives are as follows:

- "All children with special health care needs will receive coordinated, ongoing, comprehensive care within a medical home.

- All families of children with special health care needs will have adequate private and/or public insurance to pay for the services they need.

- All children will be screened early and continuously for special health care needs.

- Families of children with special health care needs will partner in decision-making at all levels and will be satisfied with the services they receive.

- Community-based service systems will be organized so families can use them easily.

- All youth with special health care needs will receive the services necessary to make transitions to all aspects of adult life, including adult health care, work, and independence."

Children with chronic illness and disability also need assurance that they can continue to have full access to educational services through the Individuals with Disabilities Education Act. It is through community-based educational endeavors that children and youth experience intellectual and social growth.

Within hospital and community settings, there is a growing appreciation that the 5% to 6% of children with the most serious conditions often have quite extraordinary needs. The care of these children can require the input of multiple specialists, and when these children become sick, they often require high-intensity care within the hospital setting. Planning of pediatric service delivery and training is changing in the face of these needs. The Medical Home Learning Collaborative developed by the National Initiative for Children's Healthcare Quality[95] is one step toward increasing the skills of practicing pediatricians. It would be reasonable to introduce more training about the care of the complex child into medical schools and residencies as all indications point to a continuing and potentially increasing need in this area.

As policymakers and clinicians study the shape of current childhood morbidity, it is becoming increasingly clear that while all children must have access to health insurance and basic services, a one-size-fits-all model does not address the serious and increasing concerns of the nation's children with special health care needs. An approach that uses case identification and a series of tiered levels by severity would greatly improve the delivery of care and would ensure a more effective approach to service delivery.[96]

<u>Addressing Inequities</u>

The recognition and documentation of inequities in health care outcomes are the first steps toward rectifying the inequities. The new data systems for amassing and depicting health data (such as is done in this volume) are a major step in a forward direction. Unfortunately, just documenting inequity is not enough. There needs to be a direct and concerted attack on the causes of unequal

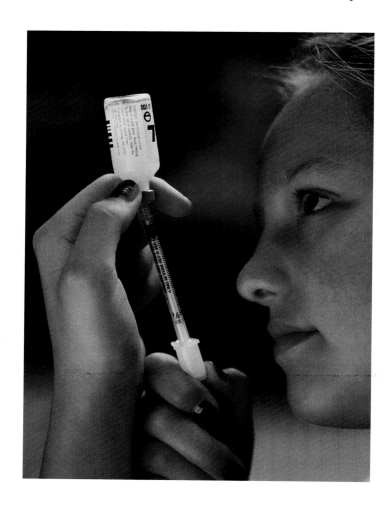

treatment and disparate outcomes. U.S. Surgeon General David Satcher sounded the clarion call with his campaign, Closing the Gap.[97] The elements of the attack are (a) assurance of equal access to health care for all people, (b) elimination of communication and cultural barriers, (c) outreach to groups at increased chance of particular disorders (poor families, teenage parents, immigrants, people who have experienced trauma, and families at known genetic risk), and (d) other targeted interventions to eliminate disparities. Recently, the American Academy of Pediatrics instituted special measures to ensure that Black children receive the pneumococcal vaccine. This intervention has resulted in the closing of a considerable disparity gap, demonstrating that such a targeted and explicit approach can be successful.[98]

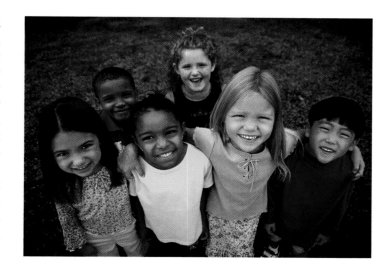

With the ever-increasing diversity of the U.S. population, inequality in health care access and outcomes is bound to be a perennial and vexing concern for some time to come. Future directions in health care delivery, therefore, need to include close monitoring of group (and subgroup) health care outcomes as well as those of individuals. Flexibility to increase surveillance and service levels will benefit children at the highest risks.

Conclusion

The health of children and youth depends on a large number of determinants: the community in which they live, the family that raises them, their own genetic makeup, as well as the particular secular trends of the chronological times they grow up in. Children and youth in the United States have grown through eras of great peril and distress as well as times of prosperity and promise. In this chapter,

The remarkable accomplishments in medical and surgical science of the 20th century have revolutionized the life chances for children with serious chronic illnesses and disabilities.

we have presented a brief cataloguing of the effects that living in these various eras has had on their health. Our own time will have its ups and downs, its forwards and backs. For the health of children and youth, it is essential that we capitalize on the forward movement while bolstering against the inevitable threats and ill consequences of setbacks.

The United States has the greatest biomedical research capacity in the world, the most highly trained health personnel, the most sophisticated health technology, as well as the greatest economic resources. The challenge for the future is to harness these resources in concert to ensure the health of our children and to work with our neighbors around the globe to promote the health of all children and youth.

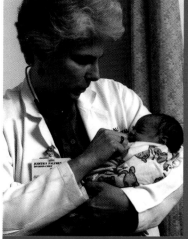

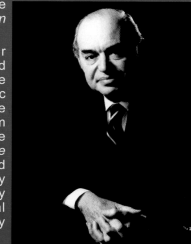

Judith S. Palfrey and Julius B. Richmond

Judith S. Palfrey, MD, is chief of the Division of General Pediatrics at Children's Hospital, Boston, and the T. Berry Brazelton Professor of Pediatrics at Harvard Medical School. Dr. Palfrey is the director of the National Program Office for the Dyson Foundation's Community Pediatrics Training Initiative. Among her many professional activities, she has served as the pediatric coordinator of the Brookline Early Education Project in Brookline, MA, and she developed and directed Project School Care to facilitate transitions from hospital to school for medical technology-dependent children. She is the author of *Community Child Health: An Action Plan for Today* and many articles and book chapters.

Julius B. Richmond, MD, is the John D. MacArthur Professor of Health Policy Emeritus at Harvard University. Dr. Richmond was a pioneer in the introduction of psychosocial development into pediatric education, research, and services and served as the first director of the national Head Start program. From 1977 to 1981, he was Surgeon General and Assistant Secretary for Health of the U.S. Department of Health and Human Services. His report, *Healthy People: The Surgeon General's Report on Health Promotion and Disease Prevention* established quantitative health goals for the nation—a process that has been institutionalized by the U.S. Public Health Service. His current interests are health policies, particularly those on health promotion and disease prevention, and the developmental antecedents of habituation from conceptual, methodological, and public policy approaches.

References

Introduction Andrews & Greenberg

1. Shonkoff JP, Phillips DA, eds. *From Neurons to Neighborhoods: The Science of Early Childhood Development*. Washington, DC: National Academy Press; 2000.

2. World Health Organization. Constitution of the World Health Organization as adopted by the International Health Conference, New York, 1946.

3. Bronfenbrenner U. *The Ecology of Human Development*. Cambridge, MA: Harvard University Press; 1979.

4. Bronfenbrenner U. Environments in development perspective: theoretical and operational models. In: Friedman SL, Wachs TD, eds. *Measuring Environment Across the Life Span: Emerging methods and concepts*. Washington, DC: American Psychological Association Press; 1999:3-28.

5. Andrews AB. Securing adequate living conditions for each child's development. In: Andrews AB, Kaufman NH, eds. *Implementing the U.N. Convention on the Rights of the Child. A Standard of Living Adequate for Development*. Westport, CT: Praeger; 1999:3.

6. Qvortrup J, Bardy M, Sgritta GB, Wintersberger H, eds. *Childhood Matters: Social Theory, Practice, and Politics*. Vienna: Avebury; 1994.

7. The United Nations. Convention on the rights of the child. [UNICEF Web site]. 1989. Available at: http://www.unicef.org/crc/crc.htm. Accessed May 26, 2004.

8. Gruskin S, Taranta D. Health and Human Rights. In: Detels R, Beaglehole R, eds. *Oxford Textbook on Public Health*. Oxford: Oxford University Press; 2001:311-335.

Chapter 1 De Graaf/Childhood "Affluenza"

1. Cowley G, Begley S. Fat for life. *Newsweek*; July 3, 2000.

2. de Graaf J. Affluenza TV Program. The Public Broadcasting Service, 1997.

3. de Graaf J, Wann D, Naylor TH. *Affluenza*. San Francisco: Berrett-Koehler Publishers, Inc.; 2001.

4. de Graaf J. *Take Back Your Time*. San Francisco: Berrett-Koehler Publishers; 2003.

5. de Graaf J. Affluenza Commercial Alert. Available at: http://www.commercialalert.org. Accessed May 24, 2004.

6. Doherty W. *Take Back Your Kids*. Notre Dame, Indiana: Sorin Books; 2000.

7. Korten D. *The Post Corporate World*. San Francisco: Berrett-Koehler; 1999.

8. Molnar A. *Giving Kids the Business*. New York: Westview; 1996.

9. Pipher M. *In the Shelter of Each Other: Rebuilding Our Families*. New York: Ballantine Books; 1996.

10. Walsh D. *Selling Out America's Children*. Minneapolis: Fairview Press; 1995.

11. Walsh D. *Designer Kids*. Minneapolis: Deaconess Press; 1990.

Chapter 2 Molnar/Advertising in Schools

1. Brown L, ed. *The New Shorter Oxford English Dictionary*. Oxford: Clarendon Press; 1993.

2. Twitchell JB. *Lead Us Into Temptation*. New York: Columbia University Press; 1999.

3. McNeal JU. *Kids As Customers: A Handbook of Marketing to Children*. New York: Lexington Books; 1992.

4. Moran C. *Education or Indoctrination? Motives Questioned for Some Lessons Kids Taught on Environment*: Copley News Service; 2002.

5. Molnar A. *No Child Left Unsold: The Sixth Annual Report on Schoolhouse Commercialism Trends, Year 2002-2003*. Tempe, AZ: Education Policy Studies Laboratory, Arizona State University; 2003.

6. Molnar A. *Sponsored Schools and Commercialized Classrooms: Tracking Schoolhouse Commercializing Trends*. Milwaukee: Center for the Analysis of Commercialism in Education, University of Wisconsin-Milwaukee; 1998.

7. Molnar A. *Cashing in on Kids: Second annual report on trends in schoolhouse commercialism*. Milwaukee: Center for the Analysis of Commercialism in Education, University of Wisconsin-Milwaukee; 1999.

8. Molnar A, Morales J. *Commercialism@School.com. Third annual report on trends in schoolhouse commercialism*. Milwaukee: Center for the Analysis of Commercialism in Education, University of Wisconsin-Milwaukee; 2000.

9. Molnar A, Reaves JA. *Buy Me! Buy Me! Fourth Annual Report on Trends in Schoolhouse Commercialism*. Tempe, AZ: Education Policy Studies Laboratory, Arizona State University; 2001.

10. Molnar A. *What's in a Name? The Corporate Branding of America's Schools*. Tempe, AZ: Education Policy Studies Laboratory, Arizona State University; 2002.

11. National Center for Health Statistics. Prevalence of overweight among children and adolescents: United States, 1999-2000. [Centers for Disease Control and Prevention Web site]. October 24, 2002. Available at: http://www.cdc.gov/nchs/products/pubs/pubd/hestats/overwght99.htm. Accessed February 26, 2004.

12. Kaufman M. Pop culture: Health advocates sound alarm as schools strike deals with Coke and Pepsi [The Washington Post Web site]. 1999. Available at: http://www.washingtonpost.com/wp-srv/national/colawars032399.htm. Accessed February 26, 2004.

13. Jacobson MF. Liquid candy. How soft drinks are harming Americans' health [Center for Science in the Public Interest Web site]. 1998. Available at: http://www.cspinet.org/sodapop/liquid_candy.htm. Accessed February 26, 2004.

14. Nagourney E. Cola is no boon for bones, study says. *The New York Times*. June 20, 2000:D8.

15. Wyshak G. Teenaged girls, carbonated beverage consumption, and bone fractures. *Arch Pediatr Adolesc Med*. 2000;154(6):610-613.

16. Jensen JJ. Olchefske given a 'D' on removing school ads. *The Seattle Times*. December 13, 2002:B5.

17. DiMassa CM, Hayasaki E. LA schools set to can soda sales. *Los Angeles Times*. August 25, 2002;1.

18. DiMassa CM. Sale of junk food at school banned. *Los Angeles Times*. October 29, 2003;B1.

19. Snyder S. Views vary on school soda sales. *The Philadelphia Inquirer*. August. 27, 2003.

20. Reuters. School vending machines losing favor [CNN Web site]. July 14, 2003. Available at: http://www.cnn.com/2003/EDUCATION/07/14/food.vending.reut/. Accessed February 26, 2004.

21. Spake A, Marcus MB. A fat nation. *U.S. News & World Rep.* 2002;33(7):40.

22. Ishibashi L, Woldow D, Grannan C. K-12 At a crossroads: one school's uncanny success with junk-food ban. [Arizona State University Web site]. April 2003. Available at: http://www.asu.edu/educ/epsl/CERU/Articles/CERU-0304-50-OWI.doc. Accessed February 26, 2004.

23. Molnar A.Commercialism in Education Research Unit, Education Policy Studies Laboratory. What's in a name? The corporate branding of America's schools: the fifth annual report on trends in schoolhouse commercialism, year 2001-2002 [Arizona State University Web site]. September 2002. Available at: http://www.asu.edu/educ/epsl/CERU/Annual%20reports/EPSL-0209-103-CERU.rtf. Accessed February 26, 2004.

24. National Association of State Boards of Education. Sample policies to encourage healthy eating [Web site]. Available at: http://www.nasbe.org/HealthySchools/healthy_eating.html. Accessed February 26, 2004.

25. Reid L, Gedissman A. Required TV program in schools encourages poor lifestyle choices [The American Academy of Pediatrics Web site]. 2000. Available at: http://www.aap.org/advocacy/reid1100.htm. Accessed February 26, 2004.

26. US General Accounting Office. Public education: commercial activities in schools [Web site]. 2000. Available at: http://www.gao.gov/new.items/he00156.pdf. Accessed February 26, 2004.

27. American School Food Service Association. Gov. Davis signs California Childhood Obesity Prevention Act [Web site]. 2003. Available at: http://www.asfsa.org/newsroom/sfsnews/casb677.asp. Accessed February 26, 2004.

28. Molnar A. *School Commercialism, Student Health, and the Pressure To Do More With Less.* Tempe, AZ: Education Policy Studies Laboratory, Arizona State University; 2003.

29. American Quality Beverages. Suit claims school soda contracts are illegal [Empire Information Services web site]. 2003. Available at: https://www.eisinc.com/eis-cgi-bin/displaystory.cgi?story=DFINYS.010&btdate=Wednesday+February+19. Accessed February 26, 2004.

30. Circuit Court for the State of Oregon. Complaint for injunctive and declaratory relief [Commercial Alert Web site]. 2003. Available at: http://www.commercialalert.org/orcomplaint.pdf. Accessed February 26, 2004.

Molnar Data References

1. Centers for Disease Control and Prevention. Fact sheet: foods and beverages sold outside of the school meal programs. [Arizona State University Web site]. 2001. Available at: http://www.asu/Educ/epsl/CERU/Articles/CERU-0302-29-OWI.pdf. Accessed March 22, 2004.

2. Molnar A. No student left unsold. The sixth annual report on schoolhouse commercialism trends [Arizona State University Web site]. 2003. Available at: http://www.asu.edu/educ/epsl/CERU/Annual%20reports/EPSL-0309-107-CERU.doc. Accessed April 14, 2004.

3. Sawicky M, Molnar A. The hidden costs of Channel One: estimates for the fifty states [Arizona State University Web site]. 1998. Available at: http://www.asu.edu/educ/epsl/CERU/documents/cace-98-02/cace-98-02.htm. Accessed March 22, 2004.

Chapter 3 Calvert/Interactive Media and Well-being

1. Rideout V, Vandewater E, Wartella E. Zero to six: electronic media in the lives of infants, toddlers, and preschoolers [Kaiser Family Foundation Web site]. 2003. Available at: http://www.kff.org/entmedia/loader.cfm?url=/commonspot/security/getfile.cfm&PageID=22754. Accessed February 5, 2004.

2. Azzarone S. *Tweens, Teens, and Technology: What's Important Now.* Paper presented at: Exploring the Digital Generation, White House Conference Center, 2003; Washington, DC.

3. Bumatay M, Heineman M. Nielsen report [Netratings Web site]. 2003. Available at: http://www.netratings.com/pr/pr_030618_us.pdf. Accessed November 6, 2003.

4. Greenspan R. African-Americans create online identity [Cyberatlas Web site]. 2003. Available at: http://cyberatlas.internet.com/big_picture/demographics/article/0,,5901_3084241,00.html. Accessed November 6, 2003.

5. Bruner JS, Olver RR, Greenfield PM. *Studies in Cognitive Growth.* New York: Wiley; 1968.

6. Calvert SL. *Children's Journeys through the Information Age.* Boston: McGraw Hill; 1999.

7. Malone T. Toward a theory of intrinsically motivating instruction. *Cognitive Sci.* 1981;4:333-369.

8. Gross EF, Juvonen J, Gable SE. Online communication and well being in early adolescence: the social function of instant messages. *J Soc Issues.* 2002;58:75-90.

9. Turkle S. Construction and reconstructions of self in virtual reality: playing in MUDs. In: Kiesler S, ed. *Culture of the Internet.* Mahwah, NJ: Erlbaum; 1997.

10. Calvert SL, Mahler BA, Zehnder SM, Jenkins A, Lee M. Gender differences in preadolescent children's online interactions: symbolic modes of self-presentation and self-expression. *J Appl Del Psychol.* 2003;24:627-644.

11. Montgomery K. Digital kids: the new on-line children's consumer culture. In: Singer D, Singer J, eds. *Handbook of Children and the Media.* Thousand Oaks, CA: Sage; 2001.

12. Anderson C, Bushman B. Effects of violent video games on aggressive behavior, aggressive affect, physiological arousal, and prosocial behavior: a meta-analytic review of the scientific literature. *Psychol Sci.* 2001;12:353-359.

13. Borzekowski D, Rickert V. Adolescents, the Internet, and health: issues of access and content. In: Calvert SL, Jordan AB, Cocking RR, eds. *Children In the Digital Age: Influences of Electronic Media on Development.* Westport, CT: Praeger; 2002.

Calvert Data References

1. Rideout VJ, Vandewater EA, Wartella EA. Zero to six: electronic media in the lives of infants, toddlers, and preschoolers [The Henry J. Kaiser Family Foundation Web site]. 2003. Available at: http://www.kff.org/content/2003/3378/0to6Report.pdf. Accessed January 14, 2004.

2. US Department of Commerce, Telecommunications and Information Administration. *Falling Through the Net: Toward Digital Inclusion.* Washington, DC. 2000. Available at: http://www.ntia.doc.gov/ntiahome/ftn00/Falling.htm. Accessed February 10, 2004.

3. US Department of Commerce, Telecommunications and Information Administration. *A Nation Online: How Americans Are Expanding Their Use of the Internet.* Washington, DC. 2002. Available at: http://www.ntia.doc.gov/ntiahome/dn/anationonline2.pdf. Accessed February 10, 2004.

Chapter 4 Robinson & Sargent/Children and Media

1. Roberts DF, Foehr UG, Rideout VJ, Brodie M. *Kids & Media @ the New Millennium: A Comprehensive National Analysis of Children's Media Use.* Menlo Park, CA: The Henry J. Kaiser Family Foundation; 1999.

2. Robinson TN. Television viewing and childhood obesity. *Pediatr Clin N Am.* 2001;48:1017-1025.

3. Sargent JD, Dalton MA, Beach ML. Viewing tobacco use in movies: does it shape attitudes that mediate adolescent smoking? *Am J Prev Med.* 2002;22(3):137-145.

4. Huston AC, Donnerstein D, Fairchild H. *Big World, Small Screen: The Role of Television in American Society.* Lincoln, NE: University of Nebraska Press; 1992.

5. Pearl D, Bouthilet L, Lazar J, eds. *Television and Behavior: Ten Years of Scientific Progress and Implications for the Eighties.* Rockville, MD: National Institute of Mental Health, U.S. Dept of Health and Human Services; 1982. DHHS Publication No. (ADM) 82-1196.

6. Robinson TN, Wilde ML, Navracruz LC, Haydel KF, Varady A. Effects of reducing children's television and video game use on aggressive behavior: a randomized controlled trial. *Arch Pediatr Adolesc Med.* 2001;155:17-23.

7. Robinson TN. Reducing children's television viewing to prevent obesity: a randomized controlled trial. *JAMA.* 1999;282:1561-1567.

8. Robinson TN, Chen HL, Killen JD. Television and music video exposure and risk of adolescent alcohol use. *Pediatr.* 1998;102(5):e54.

9. Sargent JD, Dalton MA, Heatherton T, Beach ML. Modifying exposure to movie smoking: a novel approach to preventing adolescent smoking. *Arch Pediatr Adolesc Med.* 2003;157:643-648.

10. Sargent JD, Beach ML, Dalton MA, Tickle J, Ahrens B, Heatherton T. Effect of seeing tobacco use in films on trying smoking among adolescents: cross sectional study. *BMJ.* 2001;323:1394-1397.

11. Dalton M, Sargent JD, Beach M, Ahrens B, Tickle J, Heatherton T. Relation between parental restrictions on movies and adolescent use of tobacco and alcohol. *Eff Clin Pract.* 2002;5(1):1-10.

12. Smoke Free Movies [Web site]. Avaiable at: http://www.smokefreemovies.ucsf.edu. Accessed March 15, 2004.

13. Comstock G, Paik H. *Television and the American Child.* San Diego, CA: Academic Press; 1991.

14. Williams P, Haertel G, Wahlberg H. The impact of leisure time television on school learning: a research synthesis. *Am Educ Res J.* 1982;19:19-50.

15. Kunkel D, Roberts D. Young minds and marketplace values: issues in children's television advertising. *J Social Issues.* 1991;47:57-72.

16. Atkin CK. Effects of media alcohol messages on adolescent audiences. *Adolesc Med.* October 1993;4(3):527-542.

17. Robinson TN, Saphir MN, Kraemer HC, Varady A, Haydel KF. Effects of reducing television viewing on children's requests for toys: a randomized controlled trial. *J Dev Behav Pediatr.* 2001;22:179-184.

Robinson & Sargent Data References

1. Roberts DF, Foehr UG, Rideout VJ, Brodie M. *Kids & Media at the New Millennium: A Comprehensive National Analysis of Children's Media Use.* Menlo Park, CA: The Henry J. Kaiser Family Foundation; 1999.

2. Robinson TN, Stanford University School of Medicine. Unpublished Author Calculations. Stanford, CA;1999.

3. Robinson TN, Wilde, Navracruz, et al. Unpublished Author Calculations; 2001.

4. Robinson TN, Chen HL, Killen JD. Television and music video exposure and risk of adolescent alcohol use. *Pediatr.* 1998;102(5):e54.

5. Sargent JD, Beach ML, Dalton MA, et al. Effect of seeing tobacco use in films on trying smoking among adolescents: cross sectional study. *BMJ.* 2001;323:1394-1397. Unabridged Version Available at: http://bmj.com/cgi/reprint/323/7326/1394.pdf. Accessed on April 7, 2004.

6. US Department of Commerce, Telecommunications and Information Administration. *A Nation Online: How Americans Are Expanding Their Use of the Internet.* Washington, DC. 2002. Available at: http://www.ntia.doc.gov/ntiahome/dn/anationonline2.pdf. Accessed February 10, 2004.

Chapter 5 Groves/Violence in the Lives of Children

1. Cohen R, Smolan L. *A Day In the Life of America.* New York: Collins Publishers; 1986.

2. Children's Defense Fund [Web site]. Protect children instead of guns. 2001. Available at: http://www.childrendefense.org/. Accessed December 12, 2003.

3. Bernard-Bonnin AC, Gilbert S, Rousseau E, Masson P, Maheux B. Television and the three-to-ten year old child. *Pediatrics.* 1991;88(1):48-54.

4. Brown BV, Bzostek S. Violence in the lives of children [Child Trends Databank Web site]. 2003. Available at: http://www.childtrendsdatabank.org/PDF/Violence.pdf. Accessed February 16, 2004.

5. Meyrowitz J. *No Sense of Place: The Impact of Electronic Media on Social Behavior.* New York: Oxford University Press; 1985.

6. Comstock G, Strasburger V. Deceptive appearances: television violence and aggressive behavior. *J Adolesc Health Care.* 1990;11(1):31-44.

7. Sege R, Dietz W. Television viewing and violence in children: the pediatrician as agent for change. *Pediatrics.* 1994;94(4):600-606.

8. Drabman RS, Thomas MH. Does media violence increase children's tolerance for real-life aggression? *Dev Psychol.* 1974;10:418-421.

9. Huesman LR, Moise-Titus J, Podolski CL, Eron LD. Longitudinal relations between children's exposure to TV violence and their aggressive and violent behavior in young adulthood:1977-1992. *J Dev Psychol.* 2003;39(2):201-221.

10. Taylor L, Zuckerman B, Harik V, Groves B. Exposure to violence among inner city parents and young children. *Dev Behav Pediatrics.* 1994;15(1):20-123.

11. Ahren J, Galea S, Resnick H, Kilpatrick D, Bucuvalas M, Gold J. Television images and psychological symptoms after September 11 terrorist attacks. *Psychiatr.* 2002;65(4):289-300.

12. Pfefferbaum B, Doughty DE, Reddy C, et al. Exposure and posttraumatic response as predictors of posttraumatic stress in children following the 1995 Oklahoma City bombing. *J Urban Health.* 2002;79(3):354-363.

13. Pfefferbaum B, Nixon S, Tivis RD, et al. Television exposure in children after a terrorist incident. *Psychiatr.* 2001;64(3):202-211.

14. Collins, KS. *Health Concerns Across a Woman's Life Span: 1998 Survey of Women's Health.* New York: The Commonwealth Fund; 1999.

15. Edelson J. Children's witnessing of adult domestic violence. *J Interpersonal Violence.* 1999;13(8):839-870.

16. Groves B. *Children Who See Too Much: Lessons From the Child Witness To Violence Project.* Boston: Beacon Press; 2002.

17. Felitti VJ, Anda RF, Nordenberg D, et al. Relationship of childhood abuse and household dysfunction to many of the leading causes of death in adults. *Am J Prev Med.* 1998;14(4):254-258.

18. American Psychological Association. *Report of the American Psychological Association on Violence and Youth (Vol. 1).* Washington, DC: American Psychological Association Press; 1993.

19. Scheeringa MS, Zeanah CH. Symptom expression and trauma variables in children under 48 months of age. *Infant Ment Health J.* 1995;16(4):259-269.

20. Scheeringa MS, Zeanah CH. A relational perspective on PTSD in early childhood. *J Trauma Stress.* 2001;14(4):799-815.

Groves Data References

1. US Bureau of Justice Statistics [Web site]. The number of arrests for violent crimes of juveniles (under age 18) and adults (age 18 or older), 1970-99, 10/00 spreadsheet. February 6, 2004. Available at: http://www.ojp.usdoj.gov/bjs/dtdata.htm. Accessed February 17, 2004.

2. US Bureau of Justice Statistics [Web site]. State level homicide trends and characteristics. January 16, 2003. Available at: http://bjsdata.ojp.usdoj.gov/dataonline/Search/Homicide/State/StateHomicide.cfm. Accessed February 19, 2004.

3. Centers for Disease Control and Prevention (CDC). Compressed mortality file: underlying cause-of-death mortality for 1979-1998 with ICD 9 codes [CDC Wonder database online]. November 03, 2003. Available at: http://wonder.cdc.gov/mortSQL.html. Accessed February 17, 2004.

4. Centers for Disease Control and Prevention [Web site]. Youth risk behavior survey. May 27, 2003. Available at: http://apps.nccd.cdc.gov/YRBSS/ChangeRptBySiteV.asp?X=1&Site=XX&Year1=2001&Year2=1991. Accessed February 17, 2004.

5. Centers for Disease Control and Prevention (CDC). Compressed mortality file: underlying cause-of-death mortality for 1979-1998 with ICD 9 codes [CDC Wonder database online]. November 03, 2003. Available at: http://wonder.cdc.gov/mortSQL.html. Accessed February 17, 2004.

6. Office of Juvenile Justice and Delinquency Prevention [Web site]. Statistical briefing book. September 30, 1999. Available at: http://ojjdp.ncjrs.org/ojstatbb/html/qa117.html. Accessed February 20, 2004.

7. Office of Juvenile Justice and Delinquency Prevention [Web site]. Statistical briefing book. September 30, 1999. Available at: http://ojjdp.ncjrs.org/ojstatbb/html/qa125.html. Accessed February 18, 2004.

Chapter 6 Redlener/Children in a Post-9/11 World

1. Schuster MA, Stein BD, Jaycox LH, et al. A national survey of stress reactions after the September 11, 2001, terrorist attacks. *NEJM.* 2001;345:1507-1512.

2. Centers for Disease Control and Prevention. Psychological and emotional effects of the September 11 attacks on the World Trade Center - Connecticut, New Jersey, and New York, 2001. *MMWR Morb Mortal Wkly Rep.* 2002.

3. Galea S, Ahern J, Resnick H, et al. Psychological sequelae of the September 11 terrorist attacks in New York City. *NEJM*.346:982-987.

4. Centers for Disease Control and Prevention, Morbidity and Mortality Weekly Review. September 11, 2002. Community needs assessment of lower Manhattan residents following the World Trade Center attacks - Manhattan, New York, 2001. *JAMA*. 2002;288:1227-1228.

5. New York City Department of City Planning. Manhattan Community District One profile, New York City Department of City Planning. [The Official New York City Web site]. 2004. Available at: http://www.nyc.gov/html/dcp/pdf/lucds/mnlprofile. Accessed May 19, 2004.

6. New York City Department of Education. New York City Education Department data for Manhattan Community School District Two 2001-2002 [Web site]. Available at www.nycenet.edu/OurSchools /default.htm. Accessed May 19 2004.

7. Ahern J, Galea S, Resnick H, et al. Television images and psychological symptoms after the September 11 terrorist attacks. *Psychiatry*. 2002;65(289-300).

8. Putnam FW. Televised trauma and viewer PTSD: implications for prevention. Commentary on "Television images and psychological symptoms after the September 11 terrorist attacks." *Psychiatry*. 2002;65:310-312.

9. Applied Research and Consulting, LLC, Columbia University Mailman School of Public Health and New York State Psychiatric Institute. Effects of the World Trade Center attack on NYC public school students: initial report to the New York City Board of Education [New York Department of Education Web site]. 2002. Available at: http://www.nycenet.edu/offices/spss/wtc_needs/ firstrep.pdf. Accessed May 19, 2004.

10. Cieslak TJ, Henretig FM. Ring-a-ring-a-roses: bioterrorism and its peculiar relevance to pediatrics. *Curr Opinion Pediatr*. 2002;15:107-111.

11. American Academy of Pediatrics, Committee on Environmental Health and Committee on Infectious Diseases. Chemical-biological terrorism and its impact on children: a subject review. *Pediatr*. 2000;105:662-669.

12. Redlener I, Grant R. The 9/11 terror attacks: emotional consequences persist for children and their families. *Contemp Pediatr*. 2002;19:43-59.

Redlener Data References

1. The nation's children still feeling the effects of terrorist attacks, according to Children's Health Fund/Marist Poll [press release]. New York: The Children's Health Fund; August 2002. Available at: http://www.childrenshealthfund.org/marist4.htm. Accessed May 24, 2004.

2. Two years after 9/11, Americans lack confidence in the U.S. healthcare system's capacity to respond effectively to at terror or biological attack [press release]. New York: National Center for Disaster Preparedness/The Children's Health Fund; September 8, 2003. Available at: http://www.childrenshealthfund.org/ NCDPMaristsurvey.htm. Accessed May 24, 2004.

3. US Bureau of the Census [Web site]. Summary file 3. 2000. Available at: http://www.census.gov/main/www/cen2000.html. Accessed May 5, 2004.

Chapter 7 Vachio/Children of Incarcerated Parents

1. Adalist-Estrin A. Children of incarcerated parents: at risk and forgotten [Family and Corrections Network Web site]. 2003. Available at: http://www.fcnetwork.org. Accessed February 6, 2004.

2. Adalist-Estrin A. Children of Prisoners Library. Tips for caregivers—from caregivers [Family and Corrections Network Web site]. 2003. Available at: http://www.fcnetwork.org/cpl/CPL204-TipsFromCaregivers.html. Accessed February 6, 2004.

3. Bosley B, Donner C, McLean C, Toomey-Hale E. Parenting from prison: a resource guide for parents incarcerated in Colorado [Colorado Dept of Human Services Web site]. 2002. Available at: http://www.cdhs.state.co.us/cyf/cwelfare/CW%20Web%20pages/Pa renting%20From%20Prison%201.3.pdf. Accessed February 6, 2004.

4. Brown S, Winchester-Silbaugh J, Vachio A. *Improving the Lives of Children of Prisoners*. Final Report to the National Institute of Corrections, 2003; Washington, DC.

5. Bush-Baskette S. *The Evaluation of Demonstration Sites Working with Children of Incarcerated Parents: One-Year Progress Report*. Oakland, CA: National Council on Crime and Delinquency; 2002.

6. Butterfield F. Parents in prison: As inmate population grows, so does focus on children. [New York Times Company Web site]. April 1999. Available at: http://psych.colorado.edu/~blechman/Th4-3.html. Accessed February 3, 2004.

7. Child Welfare League of America. Parents in prison: children in crisis [Web site]. 2003. Available at: http://www.cwla.org/ programs/incarcerated/issuebrief.htm. Accessed February 3, 2004.

8. DeAngelis T. Punishment of the innocents: children of parents behind bars. *Monitor Psychol*. 2002;32(5):56-59.

9. Family Corrections Network. African American families and communities. Proceedings from the National Summit on the Impact of Incarceration on African American Families and Communities, 2002; Washington, DC.

10. Johnson D. Developmental issues in practice of children of criminal offenders. Proceedings from the National Summit on the Impact of Incarceration on African American Families and Communities, 2003; Washington, DC.

11. Johnston D. *Children of Offenders*. Pasadena, CA: Pacific Oaks Center for Children of Incarcerated Parents; 1992.

12. Johnston D. Research on children of incarcerated parents [Family and Corrections Network Web site]. 1998. Available at: http://www.fcnetwork.org/5thconf/5fullagenda.html. Accessed February 6, 2004.

13. Locy T. Like mother, like daughter. *U.S. News and World Report*. Vol 10.4; 1999:18-21.

14. Mumola M. Incarcerated parents and their children [Bureau of Justice Statistics Web site]. September 22, 2000. Available at: http://www.ojp.usdoj.gov/bjs/abstract/iptc.htm. Accessed February 3, 2004.

15. Mauer M. *Race to Incarcerate*. New York: New York Press; 1999.

16. US Department of Justice, National Institute of Corrections. Children of prisoners: children of promise. National Institutes of Corrections Videoconference, 2003; Proceedings from National Satellite and Internet Broadcast.

17. Nolan C. Children of arrested parents: strategies to improve their safety and well-being [California Research Bureau Web site]. July 2003. Available at: http://www.library.ca.gov/crb/03/11/03-011.pdf. Accessed February 5, 2004.

18. Simmons C. Children of incarcerated parents [California Research Bureau Web site]. March 2000. Available at: http://www.library. ca.gov/crb/00/notes/v7n2.pdf. Accessed February 5, 2004.

19. Slavin P. Children with parents behind bars: they serve a sentence of their own. *Children's Voice*. Child Welfare League of America. 2000;9(5).

20. Travis J, Waul M, Solomon A. *The Impact of Incarceration and Reentry on Children, Families, and Communities*. Background paper for the US Dept of Health and Human Services "From Prison to Home" Conference; 2002.

21. Wright L, Seymour C. *Working With Children and Families Separated by Incarceration*. Washington, DC: CWLA Press; 2000.

Vachio Data References

1. Bonczar, TP. *Bureau of Justice Statistics Bulletin, Prevalence of Imprisonment in the U.S. Population, 1974-2001*. Washington, DC: U.S. Department of Justice; August 2003. Available at: http://www.ojp.usdoj.gov/bjs/pub/pdf/piusp01.pdf. Accessed February 8, 2004.

2. Greenfeld L, Snell, T. Women offenders [U.S. Department of Justice Web site]. 1999. Available at: http://www.ojp.usdoj.gov/ bjs/pub/pdf/wo.pdf. Accessed January 25, 2004.

3. Harrison PM, Beck AJ. *Bureau of Justice Statistics Bulletin, Prisoners in 2002*. Washington, DC: U.S. Department of Justice; July 2003. Available at: http://www.ojp.usdoj.gov/bjs/ pub/pdf/p02.pdf. Accessed February 8, 2004.

4. Mumola, C. Incarcerated parents and their children [U.S. Department of Justice Web site]. 2000. Available at: http://www.ojp.usdoj.gov/bjs/pub/pdf/iptc.pdf. Accessed January 25, 2004.

Chapter 8 Cisneros/Urban Housing

1. Beaumont CE, Pianca EG. *Why Johnny Can't Walk to School: Historic Neighborhood Schools in the Age of Sprawl.* 2nd ed. Washington, DC: National Trust for Historic Preservation; 2002.

2. US Department of Housing and Urban Development. Hope IV, Public and Indian housing [Web site]. Updated March 25, 2004. Available at: http://www.hud.gov/offices/pih/programs/ph/hope6/index.cfm. Accessed May 18, 2004.

3. Kotlowitz A. *There Are No Children Here: The Story of Two Boys Growing Up in the Other America.* Garden City, NY: Anchor Books; 1992.

4. US Bureau of the Census. The housing survey. [Web site] updated March 5, 2004. Available at: http://www.census.gov/hhes/www/ahs.html. Accessed May 18, 2004.

5. US Department of Housing and Urban Development Data. [Web site]. Updated January 19, 2004. Available at: http://www.hud.gov. Accessed May 18, 2004.

Cisneros Data References

1. National Low Income Housing Coalition [Web site]. Out of reach 2003: America's housing wage climbs. 2003. Available at: http://www.nlihc.org/oor2003/. Accessed January 27, 2004.

2. US Bureau of the Census [Web site]. Summary file 3. 2000. Available at: http://www.census.gov/main/www/cen2000.html. Accessed January 27, 2004.

3. US Bureau of the Census Bureau [Web site]. Historical census of housing tables: homeownership. August 22, 2002. Available at: http://www.census.gov/hhes/www/housing/census/historic/hograph.html. Accessed January 27, 2004.

Chapter 9 Redlener/Homelessness and Its Consequences

1. U.S. Department of Human Resources, Department of Homeless Services. New York City Data. Washington, DC: U.S. Department of Human Resources; 2003.

2. Urban Institute [Web site]. What will it take to end homelessness? 2001. Available at: http://www.urban.org/UploadedPDF/end_homelessness.pdf. Accessed March 2, 2004.

3. The United States Conference of Mayors [Web site]. Hunger and homelessness survey: a status report on hunger and homelessness in America's cities. Available at: http://www.usmayors.org/uscm/hungersurvey/2003/onlinereport/HungerAndHomelessnessReport2003.pdf. Accessed May 19, 2004.

4. New York City Department of Housing Preservation and Development. Housing New York City 1996: summary report [The Official New York City Web site]. 1999. Available at: http://www.ci.nyc.ny.us/html/hpd/pdf/hvs-summary-1996.pdf. Accessed May 19, 2004.

5. US Department of Health and Human Services, Administration for Children, Youth, and Families. Fact sheet: runaway and homeless youth program [Administration for Children, Youth, and Families Web site]. 2000. Available at: http://www.acf.hhs.gov/news/facts/youth.htm. Accessed May 19, 2004.

6. Parker RM, Rescola LA, Finkelstein JA, Barnes N, Holmes JH, Stolley PD. A survey of the health of homeless children in Philadelphia shelters. *Am J Dis Child.* 1991;145:520-526.

7. Grant R. The special needs of homeless children: early intervention at a welfare hotel. *Top Early Child Special Educ.* 1991;10(4):76-91.

8. Zima BT, Wells KB, Freeman HE. Emotional and behavioral problems and severe academic delays among sheltered homeless children in Los Angeles County. *Am J Public Health.* 1994;84:260-264.

9. Zima BT, Wells KB, Benjamin B, Duan N. Mental health problems among homeless mothers: relationship to service use and child mental health problems. *Arch Gen Psychiatry.* 1996;53:332-338.

10. Zima BT, Bussing R, Forness SR, Benjamin B. Sheltered homeless children: their eligibility and unmet need for special education evaluations. *Am J Public Health.* 1997;87:236-240.

11. McLean DE, Bowen S, Drezner K, et al. Asthma among the homeless: undercounting and undertreating the underserved. *Arch Pediatr Adolesc Med.* 2004;158:244-249.

Redlener Data References

1. Interagency Council on the Homeless. *Homelessness: Programs and the People They Serve: Findings of the National Survey of Homeless Assistance Providers and Clients, Summary.* Washington, DC: Interagency Council on the Homeless; 1999.

2. The United States Conference of Mayors. A status report on hunger and homelessness in America's cities [Various years] [The United States Conference of Mayors Web site]. 1998-2002. Available at: http://usmayors.org. Accessed February 2, 2004.

Chapter 10 Weitzman & Kavanaugh/Tobacco and Health

1. Cameron P, Kostin J, Zaks JM. The health of nonsmokers' children. *J Allergy.* 1969;43:336-341.

2. Cameron P. The presence of pets and smoking as correlates of perceived disease. *J Allergy.* 1967;4:12-15.

3. Simpson WJ. A preliminary report on cigarette smoking and the incidence of prematurity. *Am J Obstet Gynecol.* 1957;73:808-815.

4. US Department of Health, Education, and Welfare. *Smoking and Health: Report of the Advisory Committee to the Surgeon General of the Public Health Service.* Washington, DC: US Dept of Health, Education, and Welfare; 1964. Public Health Service Publication No. 1103.

5. US Department of Health and Human Services. *Healthy People 2010.* McLean, VA: International Medical Publishing; 2001.

6. Anderson HR. Passive smoking and sudden infant death syndrome: review of the epidemiological evidence. *Thorax.* 1997;52(11):1003-1009.

7. National Cancer Institute. *Health Effects of Exposure to Environmental Tobacco Smoke: The Report of the California Environmental Protection Agency.* Bethesda, MD: US Dept of Health and Human Services, National Institutes of Health, National Cancer Institute; 1999. NIH Pub. No. 99-4645.

8. Mitchell E. Commentary: cot death - the story so far. *Br Med J.* 1999;319(7723):1461-1462.

9. Cook DG, Strachan DP. Summary of effects of parental smoking on respiratory health of children and implications for research. *Thorax.* 1999;54(4):357-365.

10. Aligne CA, Moss ME, Auinger P, Weitzman M. Association of pediatric dental caries with passive smoking. *JAMA.* 2003;289(10):1258-1264.

11. Weitzman M, Gortmaker S, Walker DK. Maternal smoking and childhood asthma. *Pediatrics.* 1990;85(4):505-511.

12. Mannino DM, Homa DM, Akinbami LJ, Moorman JE, Gwynn C, Redd SC. Surveillance for asthma—United States, 1980-1999. *MMWR.* 2002;51(SS01):1-13.

13. Finkelstein JA, Davis RL, Dowell SF, et al. Reducing antibiotic use in children: a randomized trail in 12 practices. *Pediatrics.* 2001;108(1):U113-U119.

14. Finkelstein JA, Metlay JP, Davis RL, Rifas-Shiman SL, Dowell SF, Platt R. Antimicrobial use in defined populations of infants and young children. *Arch Pediatr Adolesc Med.* 2000;154(4):395-400.

15. Weitzman M, Byrd RS, Aligne CA, Moss ME. The effects of tobacco exposure on children's behavioral and cognitive functioning: implications for clinical and public health policy and future research. *Neurotoxicol Teratol.* 2002;24(3):397-406.

16. Gilliland FD, Berhane K, Islam T, et al. Environmental tobacco smoke and absenteeism related to respiratory illness in schoolchildren. *Am J Epidemiol.* 2003;157(10):861-869.

17. Aligne CA, Stoddard JJ. Tobacco and children: an economic evaluation of the medical effects of parental smoking. *Arch Pediatr Adolesc Med.* 1997;151(10):648-653.

18. Cook J, Owen P, Bender B, et al. State-specific prevalence of cigarette smoking among adults, and children's and adolescents' exposure to environmental tobacco smoke - United States, 1996. *MMWR.* 1997;46(44):1038-1043.

19. Woollery T, Trosclair A, Husten CG, Caraballo RC, Kahende J. Cigarette smoking among adults—United States, 2001. *MMWR.* 2003;52(40):953-980.

20. Pirkle JL, Flegal KM, Bernert JT, Brody DJ, Etzel RA, Maurer KR. Exposure to the US population to environmental tobacco smoke - The Third National Health and Nutrition Examination Survey, 1988 to 1991. *JAMA.* 1996;275(6):1233-1240.

21. Public Health Service. *Healthy People 2000: National Health Promotion and Disease Prevention Objectives.* Washington, DC: Dept of Health and Human Services, Public Health Service; 1991. DHHS publication no. (PHS) 91-50212.

22. Matthews TJ. Smoking during pregnancy in the 1990s. *Natl Vital Stat Rep.* 2001;49(7):1-14.

23. DiFranza J, Aligne CA, Weitzman M. Prenatal and environmental tobacco smoke exposure and children's health. *Pediatrics.* 2004;113:1007-1015.

24. Conrad KM, Flay BR, Hill D. Why children start smoking cigarettes: predictors of onset. *Br J Addict.* 1992;87(12):1711-1724.

25. Grunbaum JA, Kann L, Kinchen SA, et al. Youth risk behavior surveillance—United States, 2001. *MMWR.* 2002;51(4):1-62.

26. Office on Smoking and Health and Div of Adolescent and School Health, National Center for Chronic Disease Prevention and Health Promotion, Centers for Disease Control and Prevention. Trends in cigarette smoking among high school students—United States, 1991-2001. *MMWR.* 2002;51(19):409-412.

27. Office on Smoking and Health, National Center for Chronic Disease Prevention and Health Promotion, American Legacy Foundation, CDC Foundation, Macro International, State Youth Tobacco Survey Coordinators. Youth tobacco surveillance - United States, 2000. *MMWR CDC Surveillance Summaries.* 2001;50(4):1-84.

28. Gilpin EA, Choi WS, Berry C, Peirce JP. How many adolescents start smoking each day in the United States? *J Adolesc Health.* 1999;25(4):248-255.

29. Healton C, Messeri P, Reynolds J, et al. Tobacco use among middle and high school students — United States, 1999. *MMWR.* 2000;49(3):49-53.

30. US Department of Health and Human Services. *Youth and Tobacco: Preventing Tobacco Use Among Young People: A Report of the Surgeon General.* Atlanta, GA: US Dept of Health and Human Services, Centers for Disease Control and Prevention, National Center for Chronic Disease Prevention and Health Promotion, Office on Smoking and Health; 1995.

31. Glantz SA. Smoking in movies: a major problem and a real solution. *Lancet.* 2003;362(9380):258-259.

32. Tobacco-Free Kids. Campaign for Tobacco-free Kids (R): Tobacco company marketing to kids [Web site]. 2003. Available at: http://www.tobaccofreekids.org/research/factsheet/pdf/0008.pdf. Accessed February 2, 2003.

33. Biener L, Siegel M. Tobacco marketing and adolescent smoking: more support for a casual inference. *Am J Public Health.* 2000;90(3):407-411.

34. Smoke-Free Movies. Fact sheet [Web site]. 2003. Available at: http://www.smokefreemovies.ucsf.edu. Accessed February 2, 2003.

35. Choi WS, Pierce JP, Gilpin EA, Farkas AJ, Berry C. Which adolescent experimenters progress to establish smoking in the United States. *Am J Prev Med.* 1997(5):385-391.

36. US Department of Health and Human Services. *Preventing Tobacco Use Among Young People. A Report of the Surgeon General.* Atlanta, GA: US Dept of Health and Human Services, Public Health Service, Centers for Disease Control and Prevention, National Center for Chronic Disease Prevention and Health Promotion, Office on Smoking and Health; 1994.

37. Stolerman IP, Jarvis MJ. The scientific case that nicotine is addictive. *Psychopharmacol.* 1995;117(1):2-10.

38. DiFranza J, Savageau JA, Rigotti NA, et al. Development of symptoms of tobacco dependence in youth: 30 month follow up data from the DANDY study. *Tobacco Control.* 2002;11(3):228-235.

39. Moss AJ, Allen KF, Giovino GA, Mills SL. *Recent Trends in Adolescent Smoking, Smoking-uptake Correlates, and Expectations about the Future.* Hyattsville, MD: National Center for Health Statistics. Advance Data from Vital and Health Statistics; 1992. No 221,1-28.

40. US Department of Health and Human Services. Reducing tobacco use. A report of the Surgeon General. Executive Summary. *MMWR Recommendations and Reports.* 2000;49(RR-16):1-27.

41. Evans CA, Fielding JE, Brownson RC, et al. Recommendations regarding interventions to reduce tobacco use and exposure to environmental tobacco smoke. *Am J Prev Med.* 2001;20(2):10-15.

42. American Lung Association. State legislated actions on tobacco issues [Web site]. 2002. Available at: http://slati.lungusa.org/StateLegislateAction.asp. Accessed February 2, 2003.

43. American Lung Association. State legislative actions on tobacco issues midterm [Web site]. May 2003. Available at: http://slati.lungusa.org/reports/midtermupdate.pdf. Accessed February 2, 2003.

44. Fiore MC, Bailey WC, Cohen SJ, et al. *Treating Tobacco Use and Dependence: A Clinical Practice Guideline.* Rockville, MD: US Dept of Health and Human Services, Public Health Services; 2000.

45. Etzel RA, Balk SJ, Bearer CF, Miller MD, Shea KM, Simon PR. Environmental tobacco smoke: a hazard to children. *Pediatrics.* 1997;99(4):639-642.

46. Newacheck PW, Stoddard JJ, Hughes DC, Pearl M. Health insurance and access to primary care for children. *N Engl J Med.* 1998;338(8):513-519.

47. Tanski SE, Klein JD, Winickoff JP, Auinger P, Weitzman M. Tobacco counseling at well-child and tobacco-influenced illness visits: opportunities for improvement. *Pediatrics.* 2003;111(2):e162-e167.

48. Zapka JC, Fletcher K, Pbert L, Druker SK, Ockene JK, Chen L. The perceptions and practices of pediatricians: tobacco intervention. *Pediatrics.* 1999;103(5):e65.

49. National Center for Tobacco-Free Kids. Estimated New Revenues, Cost Savings, and Benefits from Federal Cigarette Tax Increases [Tobacco-Free Kids Web site]. 2003. Available at: http://www.tobaccofreekids.org/research/factsheets/pdf/0149.pdf. Accessed February 2, 2003.

50. Substance Abuse and Mental Health Services Administration, US Dept of Health and Human Services. Implementing the synar requirements of the substance abuse prevention and treatment block grant: fact sheet [Substance Abuse and Mental Health Services Administration Web site]. 1998. Available at: http://www.samhsa.gov/centers/csap/SYNAR/fctsheet.htm. Accessed February 2, 2003.

Weitzman & Kavanaugh Data References

1. American Lung Association [Web site]. State legislative actions on tobacco issues: midterm update, May 2003. Available at: http://slati.lungusa.org/reports/midtermupdate.pdf. Accessed January 24, 2004.

2. Centers for Disease Control and Prevention [Web site]. Trends in cigarette smoking among high school students—United States, 1991–2001 *MMWR Morb Mortal Wkly Rep.* 2002;51:409-412. Available at: http://www.cdc.gov/mmwr/preview/mmwrhtml/mm5119a1.htm. Accessed May 24, 2004.

3. Centers for Disease Control and Prevention [Web site]. State-specific prevalence of cigarette smoking among adults, and children's and adolescents' exposure to environmental tobacco smoke—United States, 1996. *MMWR Morb Mortal Wkly Rep.* 1997;46:1038-1043. Available at: http://www.cdc.gov/mmwr/preview/mmwrhtml/00049780.htm#00002762.htm. Accessed January 24, 2004.

4. Federal Trade Commission [Web site]. Cigarette Report for 2001. 2003. Available at: http://www.ftc.gov/os/2003/06/2001cigreport.pdf. Accessed January 24, 2004.

5. Johnston LD, O'Malley PM, Bachman JG. *Monitoring the Future National Survey Results on Drug Use, 1975-2002. Volume I: Secondary school students* [NIH Publication No. 03-5375]. Bethesda, MD: National Institute on Drug Abuse; 2003. Available at: http://monitoringthefuture.org/pubs/monographs/vol1_2002.pdf. Accessed May 28, 2004.

6. Mathews TJ. National Center for Health Statistics. *National Vital Statistics Report.* Smoking during pregnancy in the 1990s. Washington, DC: Centers for Disease Control and Prevention. 2001;49:1-15. Available at: http://www.cdc.gov/nchs/data/nvsr/nvsr49/nvsr49_07.pdf. Accessed January 24, 2004.

Chapter 11 Leshner/Substance Abuse

1. Johnston LD, O'Malley PM, Bachman JG. Monitoring the future national results on adolescent drug use: overview of key findings (NIH Publication No. 02-5105) [National Institute on Drug Abuse Web site]. 2001. Available at: http://www.nida.nih.gov/PDF/overview2001.pdf. Accessed June 15, 2003.

2. Glantz MD, Pickens RW. Vulnerability to drug abuse: introduction and overview. In: Glantz MD, Pickens RW, eds. *Vulnerability to Drug Abuse.* Washington, DC: American Psychological Press; 1992.

3. Glantz MD, Hartel CR. *Drug Abuse: Origins and Interventions.* Washington, DC: American Psychological Press; 1999.

4. National Institute on Alcoholism and Alcohol Abuse. Drinking and your pregnancy (NIH Publication No. 96-4101) [National Institutes of Health Web site]. 1996. Available at: http://www.niaaa.nih.gov/ publications/brochures.htm. Accessed June 15, 2003.

5. Chavkin W, Wise PH, Elman D. Where do we go from here and how do we get there? Round Table 6. *Ann N Y Acad Sci.*. 1998;846:348-354.

6. Lester BM, Das A, LaGasse LL, Seifer R, Bauer CR, Shankaran S. Prenatal Cocaine Exposure and 7-year Outcome: IQ and Special Education.: Paper presented at: Meeting of the Society for Pediatric Research; May, 2003; Seattle, WA.

7. Giedd JN, Blumenthal J, Jefferies NO, Castellanos FX, Lui H, Zijdenbos A. Brain development during childhood and adolescence: a longitudinal MRI study. *Nat Neurosci.* 1999;2:861-863.

8. National Institute on Drug Abuse. Preventing drug abuse among children and adolescents: a research-based guide [National Institutes of Health Web site]. 1997. Available at: http://www.nida.nih.gov. Accessed June 15, 2003.

Leshner Data References

1. Johnston LD, O'Malley PM, Bachman JG. Demographic subgroup trends for various licit and illicit drugs, 1975-2002. Monitoring the Future occasional paper No. 59 [Monitoring the Future Web site]. 2003. Available at: http://monitoringthefuture.org/pubs.html#papers. Accessed January 22, 2004.

2. National Institute on Drug Abuse [Web site]. High school and youth trends. Data reported from Monitoring the Future Study. Updated June 25, 2003. Available at: http://www.drugabuse.gov/Infofax/ HSYouthtrends.html. Accessed January 22, 2004.

3. Substance Abuse and Mental Health Services Administration [Web site]. Pregnancy and illicit drug use. July 13, 2001. Available at: http://www.samhsa.gov/oas/2k2/pregDU/pregDU.htm. Accessed January 22, 2004.

4. Wright, D. State estimates of substance use from the 2000 National Household Survey on Drug Abuse: Volume I. findings. DHHS Publication No. SMA 02-3731, NHSDA Series H-15 [Substance Abuse and Mental Health Service Administration Web site]. 2002. Available at: http://www.samhsa.gov/oas/2kState/PDF/Vol1/ 2kSAEv1W.pdf. Accessed January 22, 2004.

Chapter 12 Moore & Vandivere/Turbulence: The Effects of Change

1. Starfield B. The importance of primary care to health [The Medical Reporter Web site]. June 1999. Available at: http://medicalreporter. health.org/tmr0699/importance_of_primary_care_to_he.htm. Accessed February 12, 2004.

2. Scanlon E, Devine K. Residential mobility and youth well-being: research, policy, and practical issues. *J Sociol Soc Welfare.* 2001;28(1):119-138.

3. Lippman L, Burns S, McArthur E. *Urban Schools: The Challenge of Location and Poverty.* Washington, DC: U.S. Department of Education, Office of Educational Research and Improvement; 1996.

4. Hayes CD, Palmer JL, Zaslow MJ, eds. *Who Cares for America's Children?* Washington, DC: National Academy Press; 1990.

5. Carollee H, Hamilton CE. The changing experience of child care: Changes in teachers and in teacher-child relationships and children's social competence with peers. *Early Child Res Q.* 1993;8(1):15-32.

6. Seltzer JA. Consequences of marital dissolution for children. *Ann Rev Sociol.* 1994;20:235-266.

7. Amato PR. The consequences of divorce for adults and children. *J Marriage Fam.* 2000;62(4):1269-1287.

8. Cherlin AJ, Frustenburg FF, Jr. Stepfamilies in the United States: a reconsideration. *Ann Rev Sociol.* 1994;20:359-381.

9. Teachmean J. Childhood living arrangements and the formation of co-residential unions. *J Marriage Fam.* 2003;65(3):507-524.

10. Seltzer JA. Families formed outside of marriage. *J Marriage Fam.* 2000;62(4):1247-1268.

11. Moore KA, Ehrle J, Vandivere S. Turbulence and child well-being [The Urban Institute Web site]. 2000. Available at: http://www.urban.org/Uploadedpdf/anf_b16.pdf. Accessed February 12, 2004.

12. Moore KA, Vandivere S, Reed Z. *Cumulative Measures of Stress, Risk, Turbulence and Social Disconnectedness: Item Choice, Reliability and Validity. (Assessing the New Federalism).* Washington, DC: The Urban Institute; Forthcoming.

13. Quint JC, Bos JM, Polit DF. *New Chance: Final Report on a Comprehensive Program for Young Mothers in Poverty and Their Children.* New York: Manpower Demonstration Research Corporation; 1997.

Moore & Vandivere Data References

1. Moore K, Vandivere S. Turbulence and child well-being [The Urban Institute Web site]. 2000. Available at: http://www.urban.org/ UploadedPDF/anf_b16.pdf. Accessed February 2, 2004.

2. US Bureau of the Census [Web site]. Geographical mobility/migration. 2003. Available at: http://www.census.gov/ population/www/socdemo/migrate.html. Accessed February 2, 2004.

3. US Bureau of the Census [Web site]. Summary file 3. 2000. Available at: http://www.census.gov/main/www/cen2000.html. Accessed February 15, 2004.

Chapter 13 Wertsch/Children of the Fortress: America's Most Invisible Culture

1. US Department of Defense. 2001 Demographics Report [Military Family Resource Research Center Web site]. Updated August 12, 2001. Available at: http://www.mfrc-dodqol.org/stat.cfm. Accessed October 7, 2003.

2. Collins JJ, Dorn E, Graves HD, Jacobs TO, Ulmer WJ. *American Military Culture in the Twenty-First Century: A Report of the CSIS International Security Program.* Washington, DC: Center for Strategic and International Studies; 2000.

3. Congressional Record, Air Force Retention Issue. Remarks of Rep. Duncan Hunter [U.S. House of Representatives Web site]. May 12, 1998. Available at: http://www.house.gov/hunter/stm3-af.htm. Accessed October, 27, 2003.

4. Kozaryn LD. Department of Defense plans minor 1999-2000 child care fee hike [US Department of Defense Web site]. January 14, 2003. Available at: http://www.defenselink.mil/news/Jul1999/ n07061999_9907061.html. Accessed October 27, 2003.

5. Research Triangle Institute. *1998 Department of Defense Survey of Health Related Behaviors among Military Personnel.* Research Triangle Park, North Carolina: Research Triangle Institute; March 1999. Report No. RTI/7034/006-FR.

6. Kozaryn LD. Military child care: the best is yet to come [US Department of Defense Web site]. May 18, 2000. Available at: http://www.defenselink.mil/news/May2000/n05182000_20005185.ht ml. Accessed October 27, 2003.

7. Association of the US Army [Web site]. HASC will work to close military pay gap. January 10, 2003. Available at: http://www.ausa.org/www/news.nsf/0/55dc82472b61c34d85256caa 005aa3cd?OpenDocument&AutoFramed. Accessed October 27, 2003.

8. Chittum R, Starkman D. Victory on the home front in military housing [*Wall Street Journal* Online]. April 23, 2003. Available at: http://www.joneslanglasalle.com/news/2003/06JUN/WSJ_ victory.pdf. Accessed October 27, 2003.

Wertsch Data References

1. Bureau of Transportation Statistics [Web site]. Military base boundaries. 2002 National transportation atlas data. 2002. Available at: http://www.bts.gov/gis/download_sites/ntad02/ newusdownloadform.html. Accessed January 30, 2004.

2. Military Family Resource Center [Web site]. Active duty families. Profile of the military community: 2001. 2002. Available at: http://www.mfrc-dodqol.org/WordFiles/ III_Active_Duty_Families.doc. Accessed January 30, 2004.

3. Military Family Resource Center [Web site]. Department of Defense: supporting military youth. 1999. Available at: http://www.mfrc-dodqol.org/pdffiles/Military_youth_fs.pdf. Accessed January 30, 2004.

4. US Bureau of the Census. *Statistical Abstract of the United States, 2001.* United States Military and Civilian Personnel in Installations: 1999. Table No. 501. Washington, DC: Bureau of the Census. 2001;10:330. Available at: http://www.census.gov/prod/ 2003pubs/02statab/defense.pdf. Accessed on February 5, 2004.

5. US Department of Defense [Web site]. Base structure report, fiscal year 2003 baseline. 2003. Available at: http://www.defenselink.mil/news/Jun2003/basestructure2003.pdf. Accessed January 30, 2004.

6. US Department of Defense [Web site]. Active duty military personnel and their dependents. 1998. Available at: http://www.defenselink.mil/pubs/almanac/. Accessed January 30, 2004.

Chapter 14 Wallerstein/The Consequences of Divorce

1. Amato PR. The consequences of divorce for adults and children. *J Marriage Fam.* 2000;62(4):1269-1287.

2. Amato PR, Booth A. *A Generation At Risk: Growing Up In An Era of Family Upheaval.* Cambridge, MA and London: Harvard University Press; 1997.

3. Amato PR, DeBoer DD. The transition of marital stability across generations: relationship skills or commitment to marriage. *J Marriage Fam.* 2001;63(4):1038-1051.

4. Buchanan CM, Maccoby EE, Dirnbusch SM. *Adolescents After Divorce.* Cambridge, MA and London: Harvard University Press; 1996.

5. Cherlin AJ, Chase-Lansdale PL, McRae C. Effects of parental divorce on mental health throughout the life course. *Am Sociol Rev.* 1998;63:239-249.

6. Cherlin AJ, Kiernan KE, Chase-Lansdale PL. Parental divorce in childhood and demographic outcomes in young adulthood. *Demogr.* 1995;32:299-318.

7. Hetherington EM, Kelly J. *For Better Or Worse. Divorce Reconsidered.* New York and London: W.W. Norton; 2002.

8. Johnston JM. Research update: Children's adjustment in sole custody families and principles for custody decision-making. *Fam Conciliation Court Rev.* 1995;33:420-421.

9. Maccoby EE, Mnookin RH. *Dividing the Child: Social and Legal Dilemmas of Custody.* Cambridge, MA and London: Harvard University Press; 1992.

10. McLanahan S, Sandefur G. *Growing Up With a Single Parent: What Hurts, What Helps.* Cambridge, MA and London: Harvard University Press; 1994.

11. US Bureau of the Census. Estimates of figures for adults ages 18-44. National Survey of Families and Households and Statistical Abstract of the US Census Bureau [Web site]. 2003. Available at: http://www.census.gov/population/www/socdemo/age.html. Accessed February 13, 2004.

12. Resnick MD. Protecting adolescents from harm: Findings from the national longitudinal study on adolescent health. *JAMA.* 1997;278(10):823-832.

13. Wallerstein JS, Blakeslee S. *Second Chances: Men, Women, and Children a Decade After Divorce.* Boston: Houghton Mifflin; 1989.

14. Wallerstein JS, Blakeslee S. *What About the Kids: Raising Your Children Before, During, and After Divorce.* New York: Hyperion; 2003.

15. Wallerstein JS, Blakeslee S. *Surviving the Breakup: How Parents and Children Cope with Divorce.* New York: Basic Books; 1980.

16. Wallerstein JS, Lewis JM, Blakeslee S. *The Unexpected Legacy of Divorce. A 25-year Landmark Study.* New York: Hyperion; 2002.

Wallerstein Data References

1. Alexander, P. National Center for Health Statistics. 100 years of marriage and divorce statistics, United States, 1867-1967. Series 21, No. 24 [Centers for Disease Control and Prevention Web site]. 1973. Available at: http://www.cdc.gov/nchs/data/series/sr_21/sr21_024.pdf. Accessed February 17, 2004.

2. Centers for Disease Control and Prevention [Web site]. Families and living arrangements. 2003. Available at: http://www.census.gov/ population/www/socdemo/hh-fam.html. Accessed February 10, 2004.

3. National Center for Health Statistics. Supplements to the monthly vital statistics report. Series 24, No. 1. 1989. Available at: http://www.cdc.gov. Accessed February 2, 2004.

4. US Bureau of the Census [Web site]. Statistical abstract of the United States. 2000. Available at: http://www.censu.gov/prod/2001pubs/statab/sec02.pdf. Accessed February 2, 2004.

5. US Bureau of the Census [Web site]. Families, by presence of own children under 18: 1950 to present. 2003. Available at: http://www.census.gov/population/socdemo/hh-fam/tabFM-1.pdf. Accessed February 10, 2004.

6. US Bureau of the Census [Web site]. Summary file 3. 2000. Available at: http://www.census.gov/main/www/cen2000.html. Accessed May 14, 2004.

Chapter 15 Butts & Peterson/Grandparents Raising Grandchildren

1. Bryson KR, Casper LM. *Current Population Reports.* Co-resident Grandparents and Their Grandchildren. Washington, DC: US Bureau of the Census, 1999. Special Studies, P23-198.

2. Fields J. *Children's Health Insurance Coverage by Presence of Parents, Gender, Race, and Hispanic Origin for Selected Characteristics.* Washington, DC: US Bureau of the Census; 2002.

3. Fuller-Thomson E, Minkler M, Driver D. A profile of grandparents raising grandchildren in the United States. *The Gerontologist.* 1997;37(3):406-411.

4. Fuller-Thomson E, Minkler M. Housing issues and realities facing grandparent caregivers who are renters. *The Gerontologist.* 2003;43:92-98.

5. Butts D. Generations United. *Grandparents and Other Relatives Raising Children: An Intergenerational Action Agenda.* Washington, DC: 1998.

6. Butts D. Generations United. *Grandparents and Other Relatives Raising Children: Support in the Workplace.* Washington, DC: 2002.

7. Lee S, Colditz G, Berkman L, Kawachi I. Caregiving to children and grandchildren and risk of coronary heart disease in women. *Am J Public Health.* 2003;93(11):1939-1944.

8. Simmons T, Dye JL. *Grandparents living with grandchildren: 200).* Washington, DC: US Bureau of the Census; 2003. Census 2000 Brief, C2KBR-31

9. US Bureau of the Census. *March 1997 Current Population Survey.* Washington, DC: US Bureau of the Census; 1997.

10. US Bureau of the Census. *Relationship by Household Type for Population Under 18 Years* (Census 2000 Summary File 1, Table P28). Washington, DC: US Bureau of the Census; 2000.

11. US Bureau of the Census. *Children in Kinship Care for the Population Under 18 Years* (Census 2000 Summary File 2, table PCT20). Washington, DC: US Bureau of the Census; 2000.

12. US Bureau of the Census. *Grandparents Responsible for Own Grandchildren Under 18 Years by Marital Status of Grandparents in Households* (Data Set: 2002 American Community Survey Summary Table PCT017). Washington, DC: US Bureau of the Census; 2002.

13. US Bureau of the Census. *Grandparents Responsible for Own Grandchildren Under 18 Years by Employment Status of Grandparents in Households* (Data Set: 2002 American Community Survey Summary Table PCT018). Washington, DC: US Bureau of the Census; 2002.

14. US Department of Health and Human Services. *AFCARS - Adoption and Foster Care Analysis and Reporting System March 2003 Estimates.* Washington, DC: US Dept of Health and Human Services; 2003.

15. White House Conference on Aging. *The Road to Aging Policy for the 21st Century: Executive Summary.* Washington, DC: White House Conference on Aging; 1996.

Butts & Peterson Data References

1. Simmons T, Dye J. Grandparents living with grandchildren: 2000 [US Bureau of the Census Web site]. 2003. Available at: http://www.census.gov/prod/2003pubs/c2kbr-31.pdf. Accessed March 18, 2004.

Chapter 16 M. Szilagyi/Foster Care

1. American Academy of Pediatrics. Committee on Early Childhood Adoption and Dependent Care. Policy statement: health care of children in foster care. *Pediatr.* 1994;93:335-338.

2. American Academy of Pediatrics, Committee on Early Childhood Adoption and Dependent Care. Developmental issues for young children in foster care. *Pediatr.* 2000;106:1145-1150.

3. Blatt S, Saletsky RD, Meguid V, et al. A comprehensive, multidisciplinary approach to providing health care for children in out-of-home care. *Child Welfare.* 1997;76(2):331-347.

4. Child Welfare League of America. *Standards for Health Care Services for Children in Out-of-Home Care.* Washington, DC: Child Welfare League of America, Inc; 1988.

5. Dubowitz H, Feigelman S, Zuravin S, Tepper V, Davidson N, Lichenstein R. The physical health of children in kinship care. *Am J Dis Child.* 1992;146(5):603-610.

6. Halfon N, Berkowitz G, Klee L. Children in foster care in California: an examination of Medicaid reimbursed health services utilization. *Pediatr.* 1992;89(6 Pt 2):1230-1237.

7. Halfon N, Berkowitz G, Klee L. Mental health service utilization by children in foster care in California. *Pediatr.* 1992;89(6,Pt.2):1238-1244.

8. Harman JS, Childs GE, Kelleher KJ. Mental health care utilization and expenditures by children in foster care. *Arch Pediatr Adolesc Med.* 2000;154:1114-1117.

9. Horwitz SM, Owens P, Simms MD. Specialized assessments for children in foster care. *Pediatr.* 2000;106(1,Pt.1):59-66.

10. Leslie LK, Gordon JG, Ganger W, Gist K. Developmental delay in young children in child welfare by initial placement type. *Infant Ment Health J.* 2002;23(5):496–516.

11. Leslie LK, Hurlburt MS, Landsverk J, Rolls JA, Wood PA, Kelleher KJ. Comprehensive assessments for children entering foster care: a national perspective. *Pediatr.* 2003;112(1):134-142.

12. Leslie LK, Kelleher KJ, Burns B, Landsverk J, Rolls JA. Medicaid managed care: issues for children in foster care. *Child Welfare.* 2003;82(3):367-392.

13. Leslie LK, Landsverk J, Ezzet-Lofstrom R, Tschann JM, Slymen DJ, Garland AF. Children in foster care: factors influencing outpatient mental health service use. *Child Abuse Negl.* 2000;24(4):465-476.

14. Silver J, Haecker T, Forkey H. Health care for young children in foster care. In: Silver J, Amster B, Haecker T, eds. *Young Children and Foster Care.* Baltimore, MD: Paul H. Brookes Publishing Co.; 1999:161-193.

15. Stein BD, Zima BT, Elliot MN, et al. Violence exposure among school-age children in foster care: relationship to distress symptoms. *J Am Acad Child Adol Psychiatr.* 2001;40(5):588-594.

16. Szilagyi M. The pediatrician and the child in foster care. *Pediatr Rev.* 1998;19(2):39-50.

17. Simms MD, Dubowitz H, Szilagyi M. Health care needs of children in the foster care system. *Pediatr.* 2000;16(4 Suppl):909-918.

18. Takayama JI, Wolfe E, Coulter KP. Relationship between reason for placement and medical findings among children in foster care. *Pediatr.* 1998;101(2):201-207.

19. Takayama JI, Bergman AB, Connell FA. Children in foster care in the state of Washington: health care utilization and expenditures. *JAMA.* 1994;271(23):1850-1855.

20. US Department of Health and Human Services, Administration for Children and Families, Administration on Children, Youth and Families, Children's Bureau [Administration for Children and Families Web site]. The AFCARS Report. May 22, 2001. Available at: http://www.acf.dhhs.gov/programs/cb/publications/afcars/june2001.htm. Accessed September 30, 2003.

21. US General Accounting Office. *Foster Care: Health Needs of Many Young Children are Unknown and Unmet.* Washington, DC: US Government Printing Office; 1995.

M. Szilagyi Data References

1. US Department of Health and Human Services, Administration for Children and Families, Administration on Children, Youth and Families, Children's Bureau. National adoption and foster care statistics. [Administration for Children and Families Web site]. 2003. Available at: http://www.acf.hhs.gov/programs/cb/dis/afcars/publications/afcars.htm. Accessed May 28, 2004.

2. US Department of Health and Human Services, Administration for Children and Families, Administration on Children, Youth and Families, Children's Bureau. The AFCARS report. 1998 Estimates as of January 1999 [Administration for Children and Families Web site]. 2000. Available at: http://www.acf.hhs.gov/programs/cb/publications/afcars/rpt0199/ar0199.htm. Accessed February 5, 2004.

3. US Department of Health and Human Services, Administration for Children and Families, Administration on Children, Youth and Families, Children's Bureau. The AFCARS report. 2001 Estimates as of March 2003 [Administration for Children and Families Web site]. 2003. Available at: http://www.acf.hhs.gov/programs/cb/publications/afcars/report8.htm. Accessed February 5, 2004.

4. US Department of Health and Human Services, Administration for Children and Families, Administration on Children, Youth and Families, Children's Bureau. Adoptions of children with public child welfare agency involvement by state, FY 1995-FY 2002 [Administration for Children and Families Web site]. 2003. Available at: http://www.acf.dhhs.gov/programs/cb/dis/adoptchild03b.pdf. Accessed April 23, 2004.

5. US Department of Health and Human Services, Administration for Children and Families, Administration on Children, Youth and Families, Children's Bureau. National foster care and adoption information [Federal Foster Care Expenditures] [Administration for Children and Families Web site]. 2003. Available at: http://www.acf.dhhs.gov/programs/cb/dis/tables/sec11gb/national.htm#welfare. Accessed April 23, 2004.

Chapter 17 Camarota/Children of Immigrants

1. Camarota SA, Center for Immigration Studies. Unpublished Author Calculations Based on Public Use Decennial Census Data, 1970-2000. Washington, DC: US Bureau of the Census; 2003.

2. Camarota, SA, Center for Immigration Studies. Unpublished Author Calculations Based on US Bureau of the Census Current Population Reports, 2003. Washington, DC: US Bureau of the Census; 2003.

3. Schmidley DA, US Bureau of the Census, *Current Population Reports.* Profile of the Foreign-born Population in the United States: 2000. Washington, DC 2001. Series P23-206.

Camarota Data References

1. Camarota SA, Center for Immigration Studies. Author Calculations Based on Public Use Decennial Census Data, 1970-2000. Washington, DC: US Bureau of the Census; 2003.

2. Camarota, SA, Center for Immigration Studies. Author Calculations Based on U.S. Census Bureau Current Population Reports, 2003. Washington, DC: US Bureau of the Census; 2003.

3. Fields J. *Current Population Reports.* Children's Living Arrangements and Characteristics: March 2002. Washington, DC: US Bureau of the Census; 2003. Series P20-547. Available at: http://www.census.gov/prod/2003pubs/p20-547.pdf. Accessed February 10, 2004.

4. Inter-university Consortium for Political and Social Research [Web site]. Immigrants admitted to the United States, 1990-1998 [Immigration and Natralization Service Data]. Available at: http://www.icpsr.umich.edu/. Accessed May 2002.

5. US Bureau of the Census. Percent of state population that is foreign born, 2000. Summary file 3 [US Bureau of the Census Web site]. Available at: http://www.census.gov/main/www/cen2000.html. Accesses February 11, 2004.

Chapter 18 Belle & Phillips/Experiences in the After-school Hours

1. Heymann J. *The Widening Gap: Why America's Working Families Are in Jeopardy and What Can Be Done About It.* New York: Basic Books; 2000.

2. Furstenberg FF. History and current status of divorce in the United States. *Future of Child.* 1994;4(1):29-43.

3. Garey AI. Social domains and concepts of care: protection, instruction, and containment in after-school programs. *J Fam Issues.* 2002;23:768-788.

4. Mishel L, Bernstein J, Schmitt J. *The State of Working America: 1998-1999.* Economic Policy Institute Series, Ithaca, NY: Cornell University Press; 1999.

5. Halpern R. After-school programs for low-income children: promise and challenges. *Future of Child.* 1999;9(2):81-95.

6. Belle D. *The After-school Lives of Children: Alone and With Others While Parents Work.* Mahway, NJ: Lawrence Erlbaum Associates; 1999.

7. Stewart R. Adolescent self-care: reviewing the risks. *Families in Society: J Contemp Hum Serv.* 2001;82(2):119-126.

8. Flannery DJ, Williams LL, Vazsonyi AT. Who are they with and what are they doing? Delinquent behavior, substance use, and early adolescents' after-school time. *Am J Orthopsychiatry.* 1999;69(2):247-253.

9. Steinberg L. Latchkey children and susceptibility to peer pressure: an ecological analysis. *Dev Psychol.* 1986;22:433-439.

10. Galambos NL, Maggs JL. Out-of-school care of young adolescents and self-reported behavior. *Dev Psychol.* 1991;27:644-655.

11. Marshall N, Coll CG, Marx F, McCartney K, Keefe N, Ruh J. After-school time and children's behavioral adjustment. *Merrill-Palmer Q.* 1997;43:497-514.

12. Pettit GS, Laird RD, Bates JE, Dodge KA. Patterns of after-school care in middle childhood: risk factors and developmental outcomes. *Merrill-Palmer Q.* 1997;43:515-538.

13. Vandell DL, Shumow L. After-school child care programs. *Future of Child.* 1999;9(2):64-80.

14. McLaughlin M, Irby M, Langman J. *Urban Sanctuaries: Neighborhood Organizations in the Lives and Futures of Inner City Youth.* San Francisco: Jossey-Bass; 1994.

Belle & Phillips Data References

1. Mott Foundation. Afterschool alert, poll report: a report of findings from the 1999 Mott Foundation/JC Penny nationwide survey on afterschool programs [Afterschool Alliance Web site]. Page 3 Graph [Responsibility for setting up afterschool programs]. January 2000. Available at: http://www.afterschoolalliance. org/poll.pdf. Accessed January 30, 2004.

2. Smith, K. *Current Population Reports.* Who's Minding the Kids? Child Care Arrangements: Spring 1997. Washington, DC: US Bureau of the Census; 2002. Available at: http://www.census.gov/prod/2002pubs/p70-86.pdf. Accessed January 30, 2004.

3. Urban Institute. National survey of American families, 1999. Child Public Use Data File [Urban Institute Web site]. Available at: http://www.urban.org/Content/Research/NewFederalism/NSAF/Overview/NSAFOverview.htm. Accessed January 30, 2004.

4. US Department of Education. Providing quality afterschool learning, opportunities for America's families [US Dept of Education Web site]. 2000. Available at: http://www.ed.gov/pubs/Providing_Quality_Afterschool_Learning/report2000.pdf. Accessed January 30, 2004.

5. US Department of Education. The condition of education, 2003 [National Center for Education Statistics Web site]. NCES #2003067. Available at: http://nces.ed.gov/pubsearch/. Accessed February 5, 2004.

Chapter 19 Blank/Challenges of Child Care

1. Federal Interagency Forum on Child and Family Statistics [Web site]. America's children: key national indicators of well-being, 2002. Available at: http://www.nichd.nih.gov/publications/pubs/childstats/report2002.pdf. Accessed February 12, 2004.

2. Cubed M. The national economic impacts of the child care sector [National Child Care Association Web site]. Fall 2002. Available at: http://www.nccanet.org/NCCA%20IMPACT%20Study.pdf . Accessed February 12, 2004.

3. Denton K, West J. *Children's Reading and Mathematics Achievement in Kindergarten and First Grade.* Washington, DC: US Dept of Education, National Center for Educational Statistics; 2002.

4. Bowman B, Donovan MS, Burns MS, eds. *Eager to Learn: Educating our Preschoolers.* Washington, DC: National Research Council; 2000.

5. Peisner-Feinberg ES, Clifford RM, Culkin ML, et al. *The Children of Cost, Quality, and Outcomes Study Go to School.* Chapel Hill, NC: University of North Carolina; 1999.

6. Karoly LA, Greenwood PW, Everingham SS, Hoube J, Kilburn MR, Rydell M, Sanders M, Chiesa J. *Investing in Our Children: What We Know and Don't Know about the Costs and Benefits of Early Childhood Interventions.* Santa Monica, CA: Rand; 1998.

7. Children's Defense Fund. Calculations from U.S. Department of Health and Human Services FY Budget in Brief. Paper presented at: State Administrators meeting; August 13, 2001; Washington, DC.

8. Mitchell A, Stoney L, Dichter H. *Financing Child Care in the United States: An Illustrative Catalog of Current Strategies.* Philadelphia, PA: The Pew Charitable Trusts and The Ewing Marion Kauffman Foundation; 1979.

9. Schulman K. *The High Cost of Child Care Puts Quality Care Out of Reach for Many Families.* Washington, DC: Children's Defense Fund; 2000.

10. Children's Defense Fund. Presence of Related Children Under 18 Years Old-All Families, by Total Money Income in 2001, Type of Family Work Experience in 2001, Race and Hispanic Origin of Reference Person. Table FINC-03. [US Bureau of the Census Web site]. 2002. Available at: http://www.census.gov/. Accessed February 12, 2004.

11. Coltoff P, Torres J, Lifton N. *The Human Cost of Waiting for Child Care: A Study.* New York, NY: Children's Aid Society; December 1999.

12. Gulley J, Hilbig A. *Waiting List Survey: Gulf Coast Workforce Development Area.* Houston, TX: Neighborhoods Centers, Inc.; November 1999.

13. Schlik D, Daly M, Bradford L. *Faces on the Waiting List: Waiting for Child Care Assistance in Ramsey County.* Survey conducted by Minnesota Center for Survey research at the University of Minnesota. Ramsey County, MN: Ramsey County Human Services; 1999.

14. Lyons JD, Russell SD, Gilgor C, Staples AH. *Child Care Subsidy: The Costs of Waiting.* Chapel Hill, NC: Day Care Services Association; September 1998.

15. Coonerty C, Levy T. *Waiting for Child Care: How Do Parents Adjust to Scarce Options in Santa Clara County?* Berkeley, CA: Policy Analysis for California Education; 1998.

16. Philadelphia Citizens for Children and Youth, Greater Minneapolis Day Care Association. *Valuing Families: The High Cost of Waiting for Child Care Sliding Fee Assistance.* Minneapolis, MN; 1995.

17. Helburn S, Culkin ML, Howes C, et al. *Cost, Quality, and Child Outcomes in Child Care Centers, Executive Summary.* Denver, CO: University of Colorado; 1995.

18. US General Accounting Office. *Child Care: States Face Difficulties Enforcing Standards and Promoting Quality.* Washington, DC: US General Accounting Office; 1992. Publication GAO/HRD 93-13.

19. National Institute of Child Health and Human Development. *Preschoolers Who Experience Higher Quality Care Have Better Intellectual and Language Skills.* Washington, DC: National Institute of Child Health and Human Development; April 19, 2001.

20. Children's Defense Fund. Analysis of data compiled by the National Child Care Information Center from licensing regulations [The National Resource Center for Health and Safety in Child Care Web site]. November 2002. Available at: http://nrc.uchsc.edu. Accessed February 12, 2004.

21. Phillips DA, ed. *Quality in Child Care: What Does the Research Tell Us?* Washington, DC: National Association for the Education of Young Children; 1987.

22. Whitebrook M, Howes C, Phillips D. *National Child Care Staffing Study: Who Cares? Child Care Teachers and the Quality of Care in America.* Washington, DC: Center for Child Care Workforce; 1989.

23. Kagan SL, Cohen NE. *Not by Chance: Creating and Early Care and Education System for America's Children.* New Haven, CT: Bush Center in Child Development and Social Policy at Yale University; 1997.

24. Whitebook M, Howes C, Phillips D. *Worthy Work, Unlivable Wages: The National Child Care Study, 1988-1997.* Washington, DC: Center for Child Care Workforce; 1998.

25. Helburn S, Culkin C, Howes C, et al. *Cost, Quality, and Child Outcomes Study.* Denver, CO: University of Colorado; 1995.

26. Personal Communication. Norma Lee, Executive Director, Cosmetology Advancement Foundation. December 18, 2001.

Blank Data References

1. O'Neill G, O'Connell M. Establishment Types per 1,000 Children Under Five: 1987, 1992, and 1997. Washington, DC: U.S. Census Bureau; 2001. Working Paper Series No. 55. Available at: http://www.census.gov/population/www/documentation/twps0055.html. Accessed February 12, 2004.

2. Smith K. *Current Population Reports.* Who's Minding the Kids? Child Care Arrangements: Fall 1995. Table 1B. Washington, DC: US Bureau of the Census; 2000. Series P70-70PPL. Available at: http://www.census.gov/prod/2000pubs/p70-70.pdf . Accessed February 18, 2004.

3. US Bureau of the Census. Primary child care arrangements used by employed mothers of preschoolers: 1985 to 1999 [US Bureau of the Census Web site]. October 28, 2003. Available at: http://www.census.gov/population/socdemo/child/ppl-168/tabH-1.pdf. Accessed February 11, 2004.

5. US Bureau of the Census. Who's minding the kids? Child care arrangements: spring 1999 [US Bureau of the Census Web site]. January 24, 2003. Available at: http://www.census.gov/population/www/socdemo/child/ppl-168.html. Accessed May 28, 2004.

6. US Bureau of the Census. Primary child care arrangements used for preschoolers by families with employed mothers: selected years, 1977 to 1994 Table A. [U.S. Census Bureau Web site]. 2003. Available at: http://www.census.gov/population/socdemo/child/p70-62/tableA.txt. Accessed February 11, 2004.

Chapter 20 Galinsky/Gender Roles

1. Barnett R, Rivers C. *Same Difference: How the Myth of Gender Differences Are Hurting Our Relationships, Our Children, and Our Jobs*. New York: Basic Books; 2004.

2. Pipher M. *Reviving Ophelia: Saving the Selves of Adolescent Girls*. New York: Ballantine Books; 1995.

3. Pollock WS. *Real boys: Rescuing our Sons from the Myths of Boyhood*. New York: Henry Holt & Company, Inc; 1999.

4. Kindlon D, Thompson M, Barker T. *Raising Cain. Protecting the emotional life of boys*. New York: The Random House Publishing Group; 2000.

5. Galinsky E. *Ask the Children: The Breakthrough Study that Reveals How to Succeed at Work and Parenting*. New York: Quill; 2000.

6. Galinsky E, Kim SS, Bond JT, Salmond K. *Youth & Employment: Today's Students, Tomorrow's Workforce*. New York: Families and Work Institute; 2001.

7. Families and Work Institute. *Women: The New Providers (The Whirlpool Study, Part One)*. Benton Harbor, MI: The Whirlpool Foundation; 1995.

8. Bond JT, Thompson C, Galinsky E, Prottas D. *Highlights of the National Study of the Changing Workforce*. New York: Families and Work Institute; 2003.

Galinsky Data References

1. Galinsky E. *Ask the Children: The Breakthrough Study that Reveals How to Succeed at Work and Parenting*. New York: Quill; 2000.

2. US Bureau of the Census [Web site]. Summary file 3. 2000. Available at: http://www.census.gov/main/www/cen2000.html. Accessed May 13, 2004.

3. Galinsky E, Kim SS, Bond JT, Salmond K. *Youth & Employment: Today's Students, Tomorrow's Workforce*. New York: Families and Work Institute; 2001.

Chapter 21 Wertheimer/Poverty

1. US Bureau of the Census. CPS annual demographic survey, March supplement [Web site]. September 23, 2002. Available at: http://ferret.bls.census.gov/macro/032002/pov/toc.htm. Accessed February 12, 2004.

2. Korenman S, Miller JE. Effect of long-term poverty on physical health of children in the National Longitudinal Survey of Youth. In: Duncan GJ, Brooks-Gunn J, eds. *Consequences of Growing Up Poor*. New York: Russell Sage Foundation; 1997.

3. Wertheimer R. Poor families in 2001: parents working less and children continue to lag behind [Child Trends Web site]. 2003. Available at: https://secure.webfirst.com/childtrends.org/onlinecart/viewcategory.cfm. Accessed February 12, 2004.

4. Smith JR, Brooks-Gunn J, Klebanov PK. Consequences of living in poverty for young children's cognitive and verbal ability and early school achievement. In: Duncan GJ, Brooks-Gunn J, eds. *Consequences of Growing Up Poor*. New York: Russell Sage Foundation; 1997.

5. Haveman R, Wolfe B, Wilson K. Childhood poverty and adolescent schooling and fertility outcomes: reduced-form and structural estimates. In: Duncan GJ, Brooks-Gunn J, eds. *Consequences of Growing Up Poor*. New York: Russell Sage Foundation; 1997.

6. Rector RA, Hederman RS. The role of parental work in child poverty [The Heritage Foundation Web site]. January 29, 2003. Available at: http://www.heritage.org/Research/Family/cda-03-01.cfm. Accessed February 12, 2004.

7. Sawhill I, Thomas A. A hand up for the bottom third: toward a new agenda for low-income working families [The Brookings Institution Web site]. 2001. Available at: http://www.brook.edu/dybdocroot/views/papers/sawhill/20010522.pdf. Accessed February 12, 2004.

Wertheimer Data References

1. Federal Interagency Forum on Child and Family Statistics [Web site]. America's children: key national indicators of well-being, 2002. Available at: http://www.nichd.nih.gov/publications/pubs/childstats/report2002.pdf. Accessed February 12, 2004.

2. US Bureau of Labor Statistics, US Bureau of the Census. CPS annual demographic survey, March supplement. 2002. Available at: http://ferret.bls.census.gov/macro/032002/pov/new01_007.htm. Accessed May 24, 2004.

3. US Bureau of the Census [Web site]. Poverty status of people by age, race, and Hispanic origin, 1959-2002 [Historic poverty tables]. Table 3. 2003. Available at: http://www.census.gov/hhes/poverty/histpov/hstpov3.html. Accessed January 25, 2004.

4. US Bureau of the Census [Web site]. Poverty status of families, by type of family, presence of related children, race, and Hispanic origin, 1959-2002. Table 4. 2003. Available at: http://www.census.gov/hhes/poverty/histpov/hstpov4.html. Accessed January 25, 2004.

5. US Bureau of the Census [Web site]. Poverty in the United States. Current Population Reports, P60-222 [U.S. Census Web site]. 2003. Available at: http://www.census.gov/prod/2003pubs/p60-222.pdf. Accessed January 25, 2004.

6. US Bureau of the Census [Web site]. Poverty-poverty dynamics, 1996-99. Table 4. 2003. Available at: http://www.census.gov/hhes/www/sipp96/table04.html. Accessed on January 25, 2004.

7. US Bureau of the Census [Web site]. Small area income and poverty estimates, 2000 state and county FTP files and description. 2000. Available at: http://www.census.gov/housing/saipe/ estmod00/est00ALL.dat. Accessed on January 25, 2004.

Chapter 22 Casey/Food Insecurity

1. Bickel G, Nord M. Measuring food security in the United States: guide to measuring household food security [US Department of Agriculture, Food, and Nutrition Web site]. 2000. Available at: http://www.fns.usda.gov/fsec/FILES/FSGuide.pdf. Accessed February 19, 2004.

2. Keenan DP, Olson CM, Hersey JC, Parmer SM. Measures of food insecurity/security. *J Nutr Education*. 2001;33:S49-S58.

3. Nord M, Andrews M, Carson S. *Household Food Security in the United States* 2002 [US Dept of Agriculture, Economic Research Service Web site]. 2003. Available at: http://www.ers.usda.gov/publications/fanrr35/. Accessed May 24, 2004.

4. Briefel RR, Woteki CE. Development of the food insufficiency questions for the third National Health and Nutrition Examination Survey. *J Nutr Education*. 1992;24:S24-S28.

5. Nord M, Andrews M, Winick J. Frequency and duration of food insecurity and hunger in US households. *J Nutrit Educ Behav*. 2002;34:194-201.

6. Campbell CC. Food insecurity: a nutritional outcome or predictor variable? *J Nutr*. 1991;121:408-415.

7. Casey PH, Szeto K, Lensing MS, Bogle ML, Weber J. Children in food-insufficient, low income families: prevalence, health and nutrition status. *Arch Pediatr Adoles Med*. 2001;155(508-517).

8. Matheson DM, Varady J, Varady A, Killen JD. Household food security and nutritional status of Hispanic children in the fifth grade. *Am J Clin Nutr*. 2002;76:210-217.

9. Dixon LB, Wikleby MA, Radimer KL. Dietary intakes and serum nutrients differ between adults from food-insufficient and food-sufficient families. *J Nutr*. 2001;131:1232-1246.

10. Rose D, Oliveira V. Nutrient intakes of individuals from food-insufficient households in the United States. *Am J Public Health*. 1997;87:1956-1961.

11. Pheley AM, Holben DH, Graham AS, Simpson C. Food Security and perceptions of health status: a preliminary study in rural Appalachia. *J Rural Health*. 2002;18:447-454.

12. Vozaris NT, Tarasuk VS. Household food insufficiency is associated with poorer health. *J Nutr.* 2003;133:120-126.

13. Townsend MS, Peerson J, Love B, Achterberg C, Murphy SP. Food insecurity is positively related to overweight in women. *J Nutr.* 2001;131:1738-1745.

14. Alaimo K, Olson CM, Frongillo EA, Briefel RB. Food insufficiency, family income, and health in U.S. preschool and school aged children. *Am J Public Health.* 2001;91:781-786.

15. Alaimo K, Olson CM, Frongillo EA. Family food insufficiency, but not low family income, is positively associated with dysthmia and suicide symptoms in adolescents. *J Nutr.* 2002;132:719-725.

16. Alaimo K, Olson CM, Frongillo EA. Food insufficiency and American school-aged children's cognitive, academic, and psychosocial development. *Pediatrics.* 2001;108:44-53.

17. Kaiser LL, Melgar-Quinonez HR, Lamp CL. Food security and nutritional outcomes of pre-school aged Mexican-American children. *J Am Diet Assoc.* 2002;102:924-929.

18. Alaimo K, Olson CM, Frongillo EA. Low income and food insufficiency in relation to overweight in U.S. children. *Arch Pediatr Adoles Med.* 2001;155:1161-1167.

19. Willis E, Kliegman RM, Meurer JR, Perry JM. Welfare reform and food insecurity: influence on children. *Arch Pediatr Adoles Med.* 1997;151:871-875.

20. Cook JT, Frank DA, Berkowitz C, et al. Welfare reform and the health of young children. *Arch Pediatr Adoles Med.* 2002;156:678-684.

21. Rose D, Habicht JP, Devaney B. Household Participation in the food stamp and WIC programs increases the nutrient intakes of preschool children. *J Nutr.* 1998;128:548-555.

22. Jones SL, Jahns L, Laraia BA, Haughton B. Lower risk of overweight in school-aged food insecure girls who participate in food assistance. *Arch Pediatr Adoles Med.* 2003;157:780-784.

Casey Data References

1. Federal Interagency Forum on Child and Family Statistics. America's children: key national indicators of well-being, 2002 [National Institute of Child Health and Human Development Web site]. 2002. Available at: http://www.nichd.nih.gov/publications/pubs/childstats/report2002.pdf. Accessed February 12, 2004.

2. Nord M, Andrews M, Carlson S. Household food security in the United States, 2002. Report No. 35 [Economic Research Service Web site]. 2002. Available at: http://www.ers.usda.gov/publications/fanrr35/fanrr35.pdf. Accessed February 12, 2004.

Chapter 23 Guyer & Wigton/Child Health: An Evaluation of the Last Century

1. Benson V, Marano MA. *Vital Statistics of the United States, 1998.* Current estimates for the National Health Interview Survey,1995. Hyattsville, MD: National Center for Health Statistics. 1998;10(199):1-428.

2. Bloom B, Cohen RA, Vickerie JL, Wondimu EA. *Vital Statistics of the United States, 2003.* Summary health statistics for U.S. children: National Health Interview Survey, 2001. Hyattsville, MD: National Center for Health Statistics. 2003;10(216).

3. Centers for Disease Control and Prevention. Measuring childhood asthma prevalence before and after the 1997 redesign of the National Health Interview Survey—United States. *MMWR Morb Mortal Wkly Rep.* 2000;49:908-911.

4. Guyer B, Freedman MA, Strobino DM, Sondik EJ. Annual summary of vital statistics: trends in the health of Americans during the 20th century. *Pediatrics.* 2000;106(6):1307-1317.

5. Guyer B, Minkovitz CS, Strobino DM. Morbidity and mortality among the young. In: Hoekelman RA, Adam HM, Nelson NM, Weitzman ML, Wilson MH, eds. *Primary Pediatric Care.* 4th ed. St. Louis: Mosby Press; 2001.

6. Lesesne C, Abramowitz A, Perou R, Brann E. *Attention Deficit/Hyperactivity Disorder: A Public Health Research Agenda.* Washington, DC: Centers for Disease Control and Prevention; 2000.

7. MacDorman MF, Miniño AM, Guyer B. Annual summary of vital statistics-2001. *Pediatrics.* 2002;110(6):1037-1052.

8. Mannino DM, Homa DM, Akinbami LJ, Moorman JE, Gwynn C, Redd SC. Surveillance for asthma—United States, 1980-1999. *MMWR Morb Mortality Weekly Report (MMWR).* 2002;51(SS01):1-13.

9. Miniño AM, Arias E, Kochanek KD, Murphy SL, Smith BL. *National Vital Statistics Report.* Deaths: Final Data for 2000. Washington, DC: Centers for Disease Control and Prevention. 2002;50(15).

10. Murphy SL. *National Vital Statistics Report.* Deaths: Final Data for 1998. Washington, DC: Centers for Disease Control and Prevention. 2000;48(11).

11. National Center for Health Statistics. *Prevalence of overweight among children and adolescents: United States 1999-2000.* Hyattsville, MD: National Center for Health Statistics; 2001.

12. National Center for HIV, STD and TB Prevention, Division of HIV/AIDS Prevention. *Status of Prenatal HIV Prevention: US Declines Continue.* Washington, DC: Centers for Disease Control and Prevention; 1999.

13. National Center for HIV, STD and TB Prevention, Division of HIV/AIDS Prevention. *US HIV and AIDS Cases reported through December 2001. Year-end edition. HIV/AIDS Surveillance Report.* Washington, DC: Centers for Disease Control and Prevention; 2001.

14. National Center for HIV, STD and TB Prevention, Division of HIV/AIDS Prevention. *Young People at Risk: HIV/AIDS among America's Youth.* Washington, DC: Centers for Disease Control and Prevention; 2002.

15. National Institute of Neurological Disorders and Stroke. *NINDS Attention Deficit-Hyperactivity Disorder Information Page.* Bethesda, MD: National Institutes of Health; 2003.

16. Newacheck PW, Strickland B, Shondoff JP, et al. An epidemiological profile of children with special health care needs. *Pediatrics.* 1998;102:117-123.

17. Rowland AS, Lesesne CA, Abramowitz AJ. The epidemiology of attention-deficit/hyperactivity disorder (ADHD): a public health view. *Ment Retard Developmental Disabilities Res Rev.* 2002;8(3):162-170.

18. US Department of Health and Human Services, Office of the Surgeon General. *The Surgeon General's call to action to prevent and decrease overweight and obesity.* Washington, DC: US Dept of Health and Human Services; 2001.

Guyer & Wigton Data References

1. Centers for Disease Control and Prevention. Infant mortality and low birth weight among black and white infants—United States, 1980-2000. *MMWR Morb Mortal Wkly Rep.* 2002;51(27):589-592. Available at: http://www.cdc.gov/mmwr/preview/mmwrhtml/m m5127a1.htm. Accessed May 21, 2004.

2. Guyer B, Johns Hopkins Bloomberg School of Public Health. Unpublished tabulations, 1900 to 1998 [Childhood mortality rates by age]. Washington, DC: National Center for Health Statistics; 2003.

3. Guyer B, Johns Hopkins Bloomberg School of Public Health. Published and Unpublished Calculations from National Vital Statistics Data, 1900 to 1998. Washington, DC: National Center for Health Statistics; 2003.

4. Murphy SL. *Vital Statistics of the United States.* Deaths: Final Data for 1998. Hyattsville, MD: National Center for Health Statistics; 2000;48(11).

5. National Center for Health Statistics. *Vital Statistics of the United States, 1992, Volume II, Mortality, Part A.* Hyattsville, MD: National Center for Health Statistics; 1996.

6. Pastor PN, Makuc DM, Reuben C, Xia H. Chartbook on trends in the health of Americans. Health, United States, 2002 [Centers for Disease Control and Prevention Web site]. 2002. Available at: http://www.cdc.gov/nchs/data/hus/tables/2002/02hus071.pdf. Accessed April 8, 2004.

Chapter 24 Edelstein/Tooth Decay: The Best of Times, the Worst of Times

1. Edelstein BL. Dental care considerations for young children. *Spec Care Dentist.* 2002;22:11S-25S.

2. US Department of Health and Human Services. Healthy People 2010 [Web site]. 2000. Available at: http://www.healthypeople.gov/document/html/volume2/21Oral.htm. Accessed May 24 2004.

3. US Department of Health and Human Services. *Oral Health in America: A Report of the Surgeon General.* Rockville, MD: US Dept of Health and Human Services, National Institute of Dental and Craniofacial Research, National Institutes of Health; 2000.

4. Zavras T, Edelstein BL, Vamvakidis T. Health care savings from microbiologic caries risk screening of toddlers: a cost estimation model. *J Public Health Dent.* 2000;60:182-188.

Edelstein Data References

1. Apanian D, Malvitz D, Presson S. Populations receiving optimally fluoridated public drinking water—United States, 2000. *MMWR Morb Mortal Wkly Rep.* 2002;51(07): 144-147. Available at: http://www.cdc.gov/mmwr/preview/mmwrhtml/mm5107a2.htm. Accessed February 20, 2004.

2. Children's Dental Health Project (CDHP). Unpublished Calculations Based on Medical Expenditure Panel Survey Data Using Methodology Developed by CDHP with Urban Institute and the National MCHP Oral Health Policy Center. Rockville, MD: Medical Expenditure Panel Survey Data; 2003.

3. US Department of Health and Human Services. *Healthy People 2010: Understanding and Improving Health.* 2nd ed. Washington, DC: US Dept of Health and Human Services; 2000.

Chapter 25 Dietz/Overweight: An Epidemic

1. Ogden CL, Flegal KM, Carroll MD, Johnson CL. Prevalence and trends in overweight among US children and adolescents, 1999-2000. *JAMA.* 2002;288(14):1728-1732.

2. Whitaker RC, Wright JA, Pepe MS, Seidel KD, Dietz WH. Predicting obesity in young adulthood from childhood and parental obesity. *N Engl J Med.* 1997;337(13):869-873.

3. Whitaker RC, Dietz WH. Role of the prenatal environment in the development of obesity. *J Pediatr.* 1998;132(5):768-776.

4. Must A, Jacques PF, Dallal GE, Bajema CJ, Dietz WH. Long term morbidity and mortality of overweight adolescents: a follow-up of the Harvard Growth Study, 1922 to 1935. *N Engl J Med.* 1992;327(19):1379-1380.

5. Freedman DS, Khan LK, Dietz WH, Srinivasan SR, Berenson GS. Relationship of childhood obesity to coronary heart disease risk factors in adulthood: the Bogalusa Heart Study. *Pediatr.* 2001;108(3):712-718.

6. Flegal KM, Carroll MD, Ogden CL, Johnson CL. Prevalence and trends in obesity among US adults, 1999-2000. *JAMA.* 2002;288(14):1723-1727.

7. Freedman DS, Dietz WH, Srinivasan SR, Berenson GS. The relation of overweight to cardiovascular risk factors among children and adolescents: the Bogalusa Heart Study. *Pediatr.* 1999;103(6 Pt 1):1175-1182.

8. Cook S, Weitzman M, Auinger P, Nguyen M, Dietz WH. Prevalence of a metabolic syndrome phenotype in adolescents: findings from the third National Health and Nutrition Examination Survey. *Arch Pediatr Adolesc Med.* 2003;157(8):821-827.

9. Fagot-Campagna A, Pettit DJ, Engelgau MM, et al. Type 2 diabetes among North American children and adolescents; an epidemiologic review and a public health perspective. *Pediatr.* 2000;136(5):664-672.

10. Krakoff J, Lindsay RS, Looker HC, Nelson RG, Hanson RL, Knowler WC. Incidence of retinopathy and nephropathy in youth-onset compared with adult-onset type 2 diabetes. *Diabetes Care.* 2003;26(1):76-81.

11. Wang G, Dietz WH. Economic burden of obesity in youths aged 6 to 17 years: 1979-1999 [Pediatrics Web site]. 2002. Available at: www.Pediatrics.org/cgi/content/full/109/5/e81. Accessed March 30, 2004.

12. US Department of Health and Human Services. *Healthy People 2010, 2nd ed. with Understanding and Improving Health and Objectives for Improving Health (2 vols)*. Washington DC: U.S. Dept of Health and Human Services; 2000.

13. Kahn EB, Ramsey LT, Brownson RC, et al. The effectiveness of interventions to increase physical activity. a systematic review. *Am J Prev Med.* 2002;22(4 Suppl):73-107.

14. Dellinger AM. Barriers to children walking and biking to school - United States, 1999. *MMWR Morb Mortal Wkly Rep.* 2002;51(32):701-704.

15. Dietz WH, Gortmaker SL. Do we fatten our children at the television set? Obesity and television viewing in children and adolescents. *Pediatr.* 1985;75(5):807-812.

16. Andersen RE, Crespo CJ, Bartlett SJ, Cheskin LJ, Pratt M. Relationship of physical activity and television watching with body weight and level of fatness among children: results from the Third National Healthy and Nutrition Examination Survey. *JAMA.* 1998;279(12):938-942.

17. Berkey CS, Rockett HR, Gillman MW, Colditz GA. One-year changes in activity and inactivity among 10- to 15-year-old boys and girls: relationship to change in body mass index. *Pediatr.* 2003;111(4 Pt 1):836-843.

18. Robinson TN. Reducing children's television viewing to prevent obesity: a randomized controlled trial. *JAMA.* 1999;282(16):1561-1567.

19. Epstein LH, Valoski AM, Vara LS, et al. Effects of decreasing sedentary behavior and increasing activity on weight change in obese children. *Health Psychol.* 1995;14(2):109-115.

20. Gortmaker SL, Peterson K, Wiecha J. Reducing obesity via a school-based interdisciplinary intervention among youth: Planet Health. *Arch Pediatr Adolesc Med.* 1999;153(4):409-418.

21. Committee on Public Education, American Academy of Pediatrics. Children, adolescents and the media. *Pediatr.* 2001;107:423-426.

22. Dewey KG. Is breast feeding protective against child obesity? *J Hum Lact.* 2003;19(1):9-18.

23. Satter E. *How to Get Your Kid to Eat...but Not Too Much.* Palo Alto, CA: Bull Publishing Company; 1987.

24. Dietz WH, Stern L, eds. *Guide to Your Child's Nutrition.* New York: Villard Books; 1999.

25. Fisher JO, Birch LL. Restricting access to palatable foods affects children's behavioral response, food selection, and intake. *Am J Clin Nutr.* 1999;69(6):1264-1272.

26. Johnson SL, Birch LL. Parents' and children's adiposity and eating style. *Pediatr.* 1994;94(5):653-661.

Dietz Data References

1. Centers for Disease Control and Prevention [Web site]. Prevalence of overweight among children and adolescents: United States, 1999-2000. October 24, 2002. Available at: http://www.cdc.gov/nchs/products/pubs/pubd/hestats/overwght99.htm. Accessed February 3, 2004.

2. Federal Interagency Forum on Child and Family Statistics [Web site]. America's children: key national indicators of well-being, 2003. 2003. Available at: http://www.childstats.gov/ac2003/pdf/ac2003.pdf. Accessed March 3, 2004.

3. Wang G, Dietz WH. Economic burden of obesity in youths aged 6 to 17 years: 1979-1999 [*Pediatrics* Web site]. 2002. Available at: www.Pediatrics.org/cgi/content/full/109/5/e81. Accessed March 3, 2004.

4. Centers for Disease Control and Prevention [Web site]. Youth risk behavior surveillance survey. 1991-2001. Available at: http://www.cdc.gov/nccdphp/dash/yrbs/. Accessed May 28, 2004.

Chapter 26 Kelly/Asthma

1. Centers for Disease Control and Prevention. Measuring childhood asthma prevalence before and after the 1997 redesign of the National Health Interview Survey—United States. *MMWR Morb Mortal Wkly Rep.* 2000;49:908-911.

2. Pew Environmental Health Commission. Attack asthma: why America needs a public health system to battle environmental threats [Web site]. Available at: http://www.pewenvirohealth.jhsph.edu. Accessed May, 2003.

3. Centers for Disease Control and Prevention. Asthma prevalence, health care use and mortality, 2000-2001 [Web site]. January 28, 2003. Available at: http://www.cdc.gov/nchs/products/pubs/pubd/hestats/asthma/asthma.htm. Accessed May, 2003.

4. Akinbami LJ, Schoendorf KC. Trends in childhood asthma: prevalence, health care utilization, and mortality. *Pediatrics.* 2002;110:315-322.

5. US Department of Health and Human Services. *National Asthma Education and Prevention Program Expert Panel Report 2: Guidelines for the Diagnosis and Management of Asthma.* NIH Publication No. 97-4051. Bethesda, MD: US Dept of Health and Human Services; 1997.

6. Newacheck PW, Halfon N. Prevalence, impact, and trends in childhood disability due to asthma. *Arch Pediatr Adolesc Med.* 2000;154:287-293.

7. Weiss KB, Sullivan SD, Lyttle CS. Trends in the cost of illness for asthma in the United States, 1985-1994. *J Allergy Clin Immunol.* 2000;106:493-499.

8. Murphy S, Kelly HW, eds. *Pediatric Asthma. Lung Biology in Health and Disease Series/126.* New York: Marcel Dekker, Inc.; 1999.

9. von Mutius E. The environmental predictors of allergic disease. *J Allergy Clin Immunol.* 2000;105:9-19.

10. Aligne CA, Auinger P, Byrd RS, Weitzman M. Risk factors for pediatric asthma: contributions of poverty, race, and urban residence. *Am J Respir Crit Care Med.* 2000;162:873-877.

11. Ledogar RJ, Penchaszadeh A, Garden CCI, Acosta LG. Asthma and Latino cultures: different prevalence reported among groups sharing the same environment. *Am J Public Health.* 2000;90:929-935.

12. Liu LL, Stout JW, Sullivan M, Solet D, Shay DK, Grossman DC. Asthma and bronchiolitis hospitalizations among American Indian children. *Arch Pediatr Adolesc Med.* 2000;154:991-996.

13. Bloomberg GR, Trinkaus KM, Fisher Jr. EB, Musick JR, Strunk RC. Hospital readmissions for childhood asthma: a 10-year metropolitan study. *Am J Respir Crit Care Med.* 2003;167:1068-1076.

14. Lieu TA, Lozano P, Finkelstein JA, et al. Racial/ethnic variation in asthma status and management practices among children in managed Medicaid. *Pediatrics.* 2002;109:857-865.

15. National Institutes of Health, National Heart, Lung, and Blood Institute. *Global Strategy for asthma management and prevention revised.* NIH Publication No. 02-3659. Bethesda, MD: National Heart, Lung, and Blood Institute/World Health Organization; 2002.

16. Lara M, Rosenbaum S, Rachelefsky G, Morton S, Vaiana ME, Genovese B. Improving childhood asthma outcomes in the United States: a blueprint for policy action. *Pediatrics.* 2002;109:919-930.

Kelly Data References

1. Blackwell DL, Tonthat L. Summary health statistics for US children: National Health Interview Survey, 1999. National Center for Health Statistics. Vital Statistics of the United States. 2003;10(210). Available at: http://www.cdc.gov/nchs/data/series/sr_10/sr10_210.pdf. Accessed January 22, 2004.

2. Centers for Disease Control and Prevention. Measuring childhood asthma prevalence before and after the 1997 redesign of the National Health Interview Survey—United States. *MMWR Morb Mortal Wkly Rep.* 2000;49:908-11. Available at: http://www.cdc.gov/mmwr/preview/mmwrhtml/mm4940a2.htm#fig1. Accessed January 23, 2004.

3. Centers for Disease Control and Prevention [Web site]. Asthma Prevalence, Health Care Use and Mortality, 2000-2001. Updated January, 2003. Available at: http://www.cdc.gov/nchs/products/pubs/pubd/hestats/asthma/asthma.htm. Accessed January 23, 2004.

4. Centers for Disease Control and Prevention [Web site]. Behavioral Risk Factor Surveillance System. 2002. Available at: http://ftp.cdc.gov/pub/Data/Brfss/cdbrfs2002asc.exe. Accessed January 23, 2004.

5. US Department of Health and Human Services, Centers for Disease Control and Prevention (CDC), National Center for Health Statistics, Office of Analysis, Epidemiology, and Health Promotion. Compressed mortality file (CMF) compiled from CMF 1968-88, Series 20, No. 2A 2000, CMF 1989-98, Series 20, No. 2E 2003 and CMF 1999-2000, Series 20, No. 2F 2003 [CDC Wonder database online]. November, 2003. Available at: http://wonder.cdc.gov/mortSql.html. Accessed February 8, 2004.

Chapter 27 Arango/Special Health Care Needs

1. Beers NS, Kemeny A, Sherrit L, Palfery JS. Variations in state-level definitions: children with special health care needs. *Public Health Rep.* 2003;118(5):434-447.

2. Bishop KK, Taylor MS, Arango P. *Partnerships at Work.* Burlington, VT: The University of Vermont; 1997.

3. Bishop KK, Woll J, Arango P. *Family/Professional Collaboration.* Burlington, VT: University of Vermont; 1993.

4. Children's Defense Fund. *A Report on Child Status from the National Child Advocacy Group.* Washington, DC: Children's Defense Fund; 2001.

5. Family Voices of California, Brandeis University. Your voice counts!! Family survey report to California participants [Family Voices Web site]. 2000. Available at: http://www.familyvoicesofca.org/ PDFs/YourVoiceCountsFull.pdf. Accessed May 13, 2004.

6. National Center for Health Statistics. The national survey of children with special health care needs [Centers for Disease Control and Prevention Web site]. 2004. Available at: http://www.cdc.gov/nchs/about/major/slaits/cshcn.htm http. Accessed April 6, 2004.

7. Newacheck PW, Halfon N. Prevalence and impact of disabling chronic condition in childhood. *Am J Public Health.* 1998;98(4):610-617.

8. Newacheck PW, Strickland B, Shonkoff JP, et al. An epidemiologic profile of children with special health care needs. *Pediatrics.* 1998;102(1):117-121.

9. Perrin JM. Health services research for children with disabilities. *Milbank Q.* 2002;80(2):303-324.

10. Shenkman E, Vogel B, Brooks R, Wegener DH, Naff R. Race and ethnicity and the identification of special needs children. *Health Care Financing Rev.* 2001;23(2):35-51.

11. Stein REK, Shenkman E, Wegener DH, Silver EJ. Health of children in Title XXI: Should we worry? [*Pediatrics* Web site]. 2003. Available at: http://pediatrics.aappublications.org/cgi/content/abstract/112/2/e112?maxtoshow=&HITS=10&hits=10&RESULTFORMAT=&author1=Stein%2C+Ruth+&andorexactfulltext=and&searchid=1081278918435_14355&stored_search=&FIRSTINDEX=0&sortspec=relevance&resourcetype=1&journalcode=pediatrics. Accessed April 6, 2004.

12. The Research Consortium on Chronic Conditions in Childhood. *Chart book on Children with Chronic Conditions.* Boston, MA: The Research Consortium on Chronic Conditions in Childhood; 2002.

Arango Data References

1. National Center for Health Statistics. National survey of children with special health care needs, 2001 [Web site]. Available at: http://www.sscnet.ucla.edu/issr/da/index/techinfo/H90051.HTM. Accessed February 13, 2004.

2. van Dyck, Peter C. 2003. Presentation for DataSpeak—May, 2003 [Health Resources and Services Administration, Maternal and Child Health Information Resource Center Web site]. 2003. Available at: http://www.mchirc.net/dataspeak/Archive/events/feb_2003/ppt/vanDyck.ppt. Accessed April 19, 2004.

Chapter 28 Rivara/Impact of Injuries

1. Centers for Disease Control and Prevention [Web site]. Web-based Injury Statistics Query and Reporting System. January 13, 2004. Available at: http://www.cdc.gov/ncipc/wisqars. Accessed May 1, 2003.

2. Fingerhut LA, Cox CS, Warner M. *International Comparative Analysis of Injury Mortality: Findings from the ICE on Injury Statistics. Advance Data from Vital and Health Statistics, No. 303.* Hyattsville, MD: National Center for Health Statistics; 1998.

3. Maricin JP, Schembri MS, He J, Romano JS. A population-based analysis of socioeconomic status and insurance status and their relationship with pediatric trauma hospitalization and mortality rates. *Am J Public Health.* 2003;93:461-466.

4. McLoughlin E, Clarke N, Stahl K, Crawford JD. One pediatric burn unit's experience with sleepwear related injuries. 1977. *Inj Prev.* 1998;4(4):313-316.

5. Peden M, McGee K, Krug E, eds. *Injury: A Leading Cause of the Global Burden of Disease, 2000.* Geneva: World Health Organization; 2002.

6. Rivara FP, Cummings P, Koespell TD, Grossman DC, Maier RV, eds. *Injury Control: A Guide to Research and Program Evaluation.* New York: Cambridge University Press; 2001.

7. Rivara FP, Thompson DC, Beahler C, MacKenzie, EJ. Systematic reviews of strategies to prevent motor vehicle injuries. *Am J Prev Med.* 1999;16(1 suppl):1-5.

8. Rodgers GB. The effectiveness of child-resistant packaging for aspirin. *Arch Pediatr Adolesc Med.* 2002;156:929-933.

9. Schieber RA, Gilchrist J, Sleet DA. Legislative and regulatory strategies to reduce childhood unintentional injuries. *Future Child.* 2000;10(1):111-136.

10. Thompson DC, Rivara FP, Thompson RS. Effectiveness of bicycle safety helmets in preventing head injuries. A case-control study. *JAMA*. 1996;276(24):1968-1973.

11. Thompson RS, Rivara FP, Thompson DC. A case-control study of the effectiveness of bicycle safety helmets. *New Engl J Med*. 1989;320:1361-1367.

Rivara Data References

1. Centers for Disease Control and Prevention [Web site]. Web-based injury statistics query and reporting system. 2002. Available at: http://www.cdc.gov/ncipc/wisqars. Accessed January 25, 2004.

2. US Department of Transportation. Fatality Analysis Reporting System (FARS) Web Based Encyclopedia. 2002. Available at: http://www-fars.nhtsa.dot.gov/. Accessed February 5, 2004.

Chapter 29 Block & Reece/Maltreatment

1. American Academy of Pediatrics, Committee on Child Abuse and Neglect. When inflicted skin injuries constitute child abuse. *Pediatrics*. 2002;110(3):644-645.

2. American Academy of Pediatrics, Committee on Child Abuse and Neglect. Distinguishing sudden infant death syndrome from child abuse fatalities. *Pediatrics*. 2001;107(2):437-441.

3. American Academy of Pediatrics, Committee on Child Abuse and Neglect. Distinguishing sudden infant death syndrome from child abuse fatalities addendum. *Pediatrics*. 2001;108(3):812.

4. American Academy of Pediatrics, Committee on Child Abuse and Neglect, Committee on Children with Disabilities. Assessment of maltreatment of children with disabilities. *Pediatr*. 2001;108(2):508-512.

5. American Academy of Pediatrics, Committee on Child Abuse and Neglect. Shaken baby syndrome: rotational cranial injuries-technical report. *Pediatrics*. 2001;108(1):206-210.

6. American Academy of Pediatrics, Committee on Child Abuse and Neglect, Committee on Bioethics. Forgoing life-sustaining medical treatment in abused children. *Pediatrics*. 2000;106(5):1151-1153.

7. American Academy of Pediatrics, Committee on Child Abuse and Neglect, Committee on Community Health Services. Investigation and review of unexpected infant and child deaths. *Pediatrics*. 1999;104(5):1158-1160.

8. American Academy of Pediatrics, Committee on Child Abuse and Ad Hoc Work Group on Child Abuse and Neglect. Oral and dental aspects of child abuse and neglect. *Pediatrics*. 1999;104(2):348-350.

9. American Academy of Pediatrics, Committee on Child Abuse and Neglect. Guidelines for the evaluation of sexual abuse of children: subject review. *Pediatrics*. 1999;103(1):186-191.

10. American Academy of Pediatrics, Committee on Child Abuse and Neglect. The role of the pediatrician in recognizing and intervening on behalf of abused women. *Pediatrics*. 1998;101(6):1091-1092.

11. American Academy of Pediatrics, Committee on Hospital Care, Committee on Child Abuse and Neglect. Medical necessity for the hospitalization of the abused and neglected child. *Pediatrics*. 1998;101(4):715-716.

12. American Academy of Pediatrics, Committee on Child Abuse and Neglect. Gonorrhea in prepubertal children. *Pediatrics*. 1998;101(1):134-135.

13. Dubowitz H, ed. *Neglected Children: Research, Practice and Policy*. Thousand Oaks, CA: Sage Publications; 1999.

14. Giardino AP, Finkel MA, Giardino ER, Seidl T, Ludwig S, eds. *A Practical Guide to the Evaluation of Sexual Abuse in the Prepubertal Child*. Thousand Oaks, CA: Sage Publications; 1992.

15. Giardino AP, Christian CW, Giardino ER, eds. *A Practical Guide to the Evaluation of Child Physical Abuse and Neglect*. Thousand Oaks, CA: Sage Publications; 1997.

16. Helfer ME, Kempe RS, Krugman RD, eds. *The Battered Child*. 5th ed. Chicago: The University of Chicago Press; 1997.

17. Kairys SW, Johnson CF, Committee on Child Abuse and Neglect. The psychological maltreatment of children. *Pediatrics*. 2002;109(4).

18. Myers JEB, Berliner L, Briere J, Hendrix CT, Jenny C, Reid T, eds. *The APSAC Handbook on Child Maltreatment*. 2nd ed. Thousand Oaks, CA: Sage Publications; 2002.

19. National Research Council. *Understanding Child Abuse and Neglect*. Washington, DC: National Academy Press; 1993.

20. Reece RM, ed. *Quarterly Child Abuse Medical Update*. Boston, MA: The Massachusetts Society for the Prevention of Cruelty to Children.

21. Reece RM, ed. *Treatment of Child Abuse: Common Ground for Mental Health, Medical, and Legal Practitioners*. Baltimore, MD: The Johns Hopkins University Press; 2000.

22. Reece RM, Ludwig S, eds. *Child Abuse: Medical Diagnosis and Treatment*. 2nd ed. Philadelphia: Lipincott Williams & Wilkins; 2001.

23. US Department of Health and Human Services, Administration on Children, Youth and Families, National Child Abuse and Neglect Data System. Child Maltreatment in 2001 [Administration for Children and Families Web site]. March 10, 2003. Available at: http://www.acf.hhs.gov/programs/cb/publications/cm01/. Accessed February 17, 2004.

24. US Department of Health and Human Services, US Advisory Board on Child Abuse and Neglect. *Child Abuse and Neglect: Critical First Steps in Response to a National Emergency*. Washington, DC: US Dept of Health and Human Services; 1990.

25. US Department of Health and Human Services, US Advisory Board on Child Abuse and Neglect. *Creating Caring Communities: Blueprint for an Effective Federal Policy on Child Abuse and Neglect*. Washington, DC: US Dept of Health and Human Services; 1991.

Block & Reece Data References

1. US Department of Health and Human Services. Child maltreatment 2001. Figure 3-2:22, 28 [Administration for Children and Families Web site]. 2003. Available at: http://www.acf.dhhs.gov/programs/cb/publications/cm01/outcover.htm. Accessed February 17, 2004.

Chapter 30 Darden/Immunization Delivery

1. World Health Organization. Immunization, vaccines and biologicals. The history of vaccination [Web site]. 2004. Available at: http://www.who.int/vaccines-diseases/history/history.shtml. Accessed May 18, 2004.

2. Centers for Disease Control and Prevention. Ten great public health achievements—United States, 1900-1999. *MMWR Morb Mortal Wkly Rep*. 1999;48(12):241-243.

3. Centers for Disease Control and Prevention. Summary of notifiable diseases—United States, 2000. MMWR Morb Mortal Wkly Rep. 2002;49(53):i-100.

4. Henderson DA. Smallpox eradication. *Public Health Rep*. 1980;954(5):22-426.

5. World Health Organization, Polio Eradication Iniative. *Global Polio Eradication Initiative Strategic Plan, 2004-2008*. Geneva, Switzerland: World Health Organization; 2003.

6. Centers for Disease Control and Prevention. Global polio eradication initiative strategic plan, 2004. *MMWR Morb Mortal Wkly Rep*. 2004;53(5):107-108.

7. Barker LE, Luman E, Zhao Z, Smith P, Linkins R, Santoli J. National, state, and urban area vaccination coverage levels among children aged 19-35 months—United States, 2001. *MMWR Morb Mortal Wkly Rep*. 2002;51(30):664-666.

8. Centers for Disease Control and Prevention. Vaccination coverage of 2 year-old children—United States, 1991-1992. *MMWR Morb Mortal Wkly Rep*. 1994;42(51&52):985-988.

9. Barker LE, Luman ET. Changes in vaccination coverage estimates among children aged 19-35 months in the United States, 1996-1999. *Am J Prev Med*. 2001;20(4 Suppl):28-31.

10. US Department of Health and Human Services, Public Health Service. *Healthy people 2000; national health promotion and disease prevention objectives*. Washington, DC: US Dept of Health and Human Services, Public Health Service; 1990.

11. US Department of Health and Human Services. *Healthy People 2010* (Conference Edition, in Two Volumes). Washington, DC: US Dept of Health and Human Services; 2000.

12. Gangarosa EJ, Galazka AM, Wolfe CR. Impact of anti-vaccine movements on pertussis control: the untold story. *Lancet*. 1998;351(9099):356-361.

13. Jansen VA, Stollenwerk N, Jensen HJ, Ramsay ME, Edmunds WJ, Rhodes CJ. Measles outbreaks in a population with declining vaccine uptake. *Sci*. 2003; 301(5634):804.

14. Centers for Disease Control and Prevention. General recommendations on immunization. *MMWR Morb Mortal Wkly Rep.* 1983;32(1):1-7.

15. Centers for Disease Control and Prevention. FDA licensure of diphtheria and tetanus toxoids and acellular pertussis adsorbed, hepatitis B (recombinant), and poliovirus vaccine combined, (PEDIARIX) for use in infants. *MMWR Morb Mortal Wkly Rep.* 2003;52(10):203-204.

16. American Academy of Pediatrics, Committee on Infectious Diseases. Recommended childhood and adolescent immunization schedule—United States, January-June 2004. *Pediatr.* 2004;113(1 Pt.1):142-143.

17. Centers for Disease Control and Prevention. Recommended childhood immunization schedule—United States, January 1995. Advisory Committee on Immunization Practices. American Academy of Pediatrics. American Academy of Family Physicians. National Immunization Program, Centers for DC. *MMWR Morb Mortal Wkly Rep.* 1995;43(51-52):959-960.

18. Centers for Disease Control and Prevention. Recommended childhood and adolescent immunization schedule—United States, January-June 2004. *MMWR Morb Mortal Wkly Rep.* 2004;53(1):Q1-Q4.

19. Centers for Disease Control and Prevention. New recommended schedule for active immunization of normal infants and children. *MMWR Morb Mortal Wkly Rep.* 1986;35(37):577-579.

20. Taylor JA, Darden PM, Brooks DA, Hendricks JW, Wasserman RC, Bocian AB. Association between parents' preferences and perceptions of barriers to vaccination and the immunization status of their children: a study from Pediatric Research in Office Settings and the National Medical Association. *Pediatr.* 2002;110(6):1110-1116.

21. Taylor JA, Darden PM, Brooks DA, Hendricks JW, Baker AE, Wasserman RC. Practitioner policies and beliefs and practice immunization rates: a study from Pediatric Research in Office Settings and the National Medical Association. *Pediatr.* 2002;109(2):294-300.

22. Centers for Disease Control and Prevention. Combination vaccines for childhood immunization. Recommendations of the Advisory Committee on Immunization Practices, the American Academy of Pediatrics, and the American Academy of Family Physicians. *MMWR Morb Mortal Wkly Rep.* 1999;48(RR-5):1-14.

23. Postema AS, Myers MG, Breiman RF. Challenges in the development, licensure, and use of combination vaccines. *Clin Infect Dis.* 2001;33(Suppl 4):S261-S266.

24. LeBaron CW, Lyons B, Massoudi M, Stevenson J. Childhood vaccination providers in the United States. *Am J Public Health.* 2002;92(2):266-270.

25. Centers for Disease Control and Prevention. Estimated percentage of children 19-35 months with selected socio-demographic characteristics by state and immunization action plan area—US, National Immunization Survey, Q1/2002-Q4/2002 [Web site]. 2004. Available at: http://www2a.cdc.gov/nip/coverage/nis/nis_iap.asp?fmt=d&rpt=tab43_dem_iap&qtr=Q1/2002-Q4/2002. Accessed May 18, 2004.

26. American Academy of Pediatrics Committee on Infectious Diseases. Recommendations for the use of live attenuated varicella vaccine. American Academy of Pediatrics Committee on Infectious Diseases. *Pediatr.* 1995;95(5):791-796.

27. Centers for Disease Control and Prevention, Prevention of varicella. Recommendations of the advisory committee on immunization practices. *MMWR Morb Mortal Wkly Rep.* 1996;45(RR-11).

28. Centers for Disease Control and Prevention. National, state, and urban area vaccination levels among children aged 19-35 months—United States, 2002. *MMWR Morb Mortal Wkly Rep.* 2003;52(31):728-732.

29. Herrera GA, Smith P, Daniels D, Klevens RM, Coronado V, McCauley M. National, state, and urban area vaccination coverage levels among children aged 19-35 months—United States, 1998. *MMWR Morb Mortal Wkly Rep.* 2000;49(9):1-26.

30. Centers for Disease Control and Prevention, National Immunization Program. *Measles. Epidemiology and prevention of vaccine-preventable diseases.* Atlanta, GA: Centers for Disease Control and Prevention; 2004.

31. National Vaccine Advisory Committee. The measles epidemic. The problems, barriers, and recommendations. *JAMA.* 1991;266:1547-1552.

32. Centers for Disease Control and Prevention. Retrospective assessment of vaccination coverage among school-aged children—selected US cities, 1991. *MMWR Morb Mortal Wkly Rep.* 1992(43):103-107.

33. Centers for Disease Control and Prevention. Summary of notifiable diseases, United States, 1998. *MMWR Morb Mortal Wkly Rep.* 1999;47(53):ii-92.

34. Centers for Disease Control and Prevention, National Immunization Program. *Poliomyelitis. Epidemiology and prevention of vaccine-preventable diseases.* Atlanta, GA: Centers for Disease Control and Prevention; 2004.

35. Centers for Disease Control and Prevention. Update: polio eradication—the Americas, 1993. *MMWR Morb Mortal Wkly Rep.* 1993;42(35):685-686.

36. Rodewald LE, Santoli JM. The challenge of vaccinating vulnerable children. *J Pediatr.* 2001;139(5):613-615.

37. Klevens RM, Luman ET. US children living in and near poverty: risk of vaccine-preventable diseases. *Am J Prev Med.* 2001;20(4 Suppl):41-46.

38. Rodewald LE. Closing the gap: strategies for increasing immunization levels among at- risk populations. *Ethn Dis.* 2002;12(1):S2-S3.

39. Centers for Disease Control and Prevention. Vaccination coverage by race/ethnicity and poverty level among children aged 19-35 months—United States, 1996. *MMWR Morb Mortal Wkly Rep.* 1997;46(41):963-969.

40. Centers for Disease Control and Prevention. Vaccination coverage by race/ethnicity and poverty level among children aged 19-35 months—United States, 1997. *MMWR Morb Mortal Wkly Rep.* 1998;47(44):956-959.

41. Ortega AN, Stewart DC, Dowshen SA, Katz SH. The impact of a pediatric medical home on immunization coverage. *Clin Pediatr (Phila).* 2000;39(2):89-96.

42. Luman ET, Barker LE, Simpson DM, Rodewald L, Szilagyi PG, Zhao Z. National, state, and urban area vaccination coverage levels among children aged 19-35 months—United States, 1999. *Am J Prev Med.* 2001;20(4 Suppl):88-153.

43. Feikin DR, Lezotte DC, Hamman R, Salmon DA, Chen RT, Hoffman RE. Individual and community risks of measles and pertussis associated with personal exemptions to immunization. *JAMA.* 2000;284(24):3145-3150.

44. Edwards KM. State mandates and childhood immunization. *JAMA.* 2000;284(24):3171-3173.

45. Briss PA, Rodewald LE, Hinman AR. Reviews of evidence regarding interventions to improve vaccination coverage in children, adolescents, and adults. The Task Force on Community Preventive Services. *Am J Prev Med.* 2000;18(1 Suppl):97-140.

46. Task Force on Community Preventive Services. Recommendations regarding interventions to improve vaccination coverage in children, adolescents, and adults. *Am J Prev Med.* 2000;18(1 Suppl):92-96.

47. National Vaccine Advisory Committee. Standards for child and adolescent immunization practices. *Pediatr.* 2003;112(4):958-963.

48. Bordley WC, Margolis PA, Stuart J, Lannon C, Keyes L. Improving preventive service delivery through office systems. *Pediatr.* 2001;108(3):E41.

49. Goodwin MA, Zyzanski SJ, Zronek S. A clinical trial of tailored office systems for preventive service delivery. The study to enhance prevention by understanding practice (STEP-UP). *Am J Prev Med.* 2001;21(1):20-28.

50. Margolis PA, Lannon CM, Stuart JM, Fried BJ, Keyes-Elstein L, Moore DE, Jr. Practice based education to improve delivery systems for prevention in primary care: randomised trial. *BMJ.* 2004;328(7436):388.

51. Loeser H, Zvagulis I, Hercz L, Pless IB. The organization and evaluation of a computer-assisted, centralized immunization registry. *Am J Public Health.* 1983;73(11):1298-1301.

52. Ortega AN, Andrews SF, Katz SH. Comparing a computer-based childhood vaccination registry with parental vaccination cards: a population-based study of Delaware children. *Clin Pediatr (Phila).* 1997;36(4):217-221.

53. Cutts FT, Zell ER, Mason D, Bernier RH, Dini EF, Orenstein WA. Monitoring progress toward US preschool immunization goals. [Review]. *JAMA.* 1992;267(14):1952-1955.

54. Soljak MA, Handford S. Early results from the Northland immunisation register. *N Z Med J*. 1987;100(822):244-246.

55. Slifkin RT, Freeman VA, Biddle AK. Costs of developing childhood immunization registries: case studies from four All Kids Count projects. *J Public Health Manag Pract*. 1999;5(5):67-81.

56. Freeman VA, DeFriese GH. The challenge and potential of childhood immunization registries. *Annu Rev Public Health*. 2003;24:227-246.

57. Faherty KM, Waller CJ, DeFriese GH. Prospects for childhood immunization registries in public health assessment and assurance: initial observations from the All Kids Count initiative projects. *J Public Health Manag Pract*. 1996;2(1):1-11.

Darden Data References

1. Centers for Disease Control and Prevention. Ten great public health achievements—United States, 1900-1999. *MMWR Morb Mortal Wkly Rep*. 1999;48(12):241-243. Available at: http://www.cdc.gov/epo/mmwr/preview/mmwrhtml/00056796.htm. Accessed May 21, 2004.

2. Centers for Disease Control and Prevention. Summary of notifiable diseases—United States, 2000. *MMWR Morb Mortal Wkly Rep*. 2002;49(53):i-100. Available at: http://www.cdc.gov/mmwr/preview/mmwrhtml/mm4953a1.htm. Accessed May 21, 2004.

3. Centers for Disease Control and Prevention. Recommended childhood immunization schedule—United States, January 1995. *MMWR Morb Mortal Wkly Rep*. 1995;43(51-52):959-960. Available at: http://www.cdc.gov/mmwr/preview/mmwrhtml/00038256.htm. Accessed May 21, 2004.

4. Centers for Disease Control and Prevention. Recommended childhood and adolescent immunization schedule—United States, January-June 2004. *MMWR Morb Mortal Wkly Rep*. 2004;53(1):Q1-Q4. Available at: http://www.cdc.gov/mmwr/preview/mmwrhtml/mm5301-Immunizationa1.htm. Accessed May 21, 2004.

5. Centers for Disease Control and Prevention. New recommended schedule for active immunization of normal infants and children. *MMWR Morb Mortal Wkly Rep*. 1986;35(37):577-579. Available at: http://www.cdc.gov/mmwr/preview/mmwrhtml/00000805.htm. Accessed May 21, 2004.

6. Centers for Disease Control and Prevention. Summary of notifiable diseases—United States, 1998. *MMWR Morb Mortal Wkly Rep*. 1999;47(53):1-93. Available at: http://www.cdc.gov/mmwr/preview/mmwrhtml/mm4753a1.htm. Accessed May 21, 2004.

7. Jansen VA, Stollenwerk N, Jensen HJ, Ramsay ME, Edmunds WJ, Rhodes CJ, . Measles outbreaks in a population with declining vaccine uptake. *Sci*. 2003;301(5634):804. Available at: http://www.cdc.gov/mmwr/. Accessed May 21, 2004.

8. National Immunization Program. *Measles. Epidemiology and prevention of vaccine-preventable diseases*. Atlanta, GA: Dept of Health and Human Services, Centers for Disease Control and Prevention; 2004.

9. World Health Organization [Web site]. Vaccines, immunizations, and biologicals. Available at: http://www.who.int/vaccines-surveillance/StatsAndGraphs.htm. Accessed March 19, 2004.

Chapter 31 P. Szilagyi/Health Insurance

1. Children and Managed Health Care. *Future of Child*. 1998;8(Spring). No. 2.

2. Children and Managed Health Care. *Future of Child*. 1998;8(Summer/Fall). No. 2.

3. Dubay L, Haley JM, Kenney GM. *Children's Eligibility for Medicaid and SCHIP: A View from 2000*. Washington, DC: Urban Institute, March 2002. Assessing the New Federalism Policy Brief No. b-41. Available at: http://www.urban.org/template.cfm?NavMenuID=24&Template=/TaggedContent/ViewByPubID.cfm&PubID=310435. Accessed May 24, 2004.

4. Dubay L, Kenney GM. Health care access and use among low-income children: who fares best? *Health Aff*. 2001;20(January/February):112-21.

5. Health Insurance for Children. *Future of Child*. 2003:13(Spring).

6. Holl JL, Szilagyi PG, Rodewald LE, Byrd R, Weitzman M. Profile of uninsured children in the United States. *Arch Pediatr Adolesc Med*. 1995;149:398-406.

7. Institute of Medicine. *Health Insurance is a Family Matter*. Washington, DC: National Academies Press, 2002.

8. Szilagyi PG, Zwanziger J, Rodewald LE, et al. Evaluation of a state health insurance program for low-income children: implications for State Child Health Insurance Programs (SCHIP). *Pediatrics*. 2000;105:363-371.

9. Szilagyi PG. Managed care for children: effect on access to care and utilization of services. *Future of Child*. 1998;Summer/Fall:39-59.

P. Szilagyi Data References

1. Bhandari S, Gifford E. *Current Population Reports*. Children with Health Insurance. Washington, DC: Bureau of the Census; 2003. Series P60-224. Available at: http://www.census.gov/prod/2003pubs/p60-224.pdf. Accessed February 11, 2003.

2. Cohen RA, Ni H, Hao C. Trends in health insurance coverage by poverty status among persons under 65 years of age [Centers for Disease Control Web site]. March 19, 2003. Available at: http://www.cdc.gov/nchs/products/pubs/pubd/hestats/insurance.htm#table1. Accessed February 11, 2003.

3. Dubay L, Kenney G. Health care access and use among low-income children: who fares best. *Health Aff*. 2001;20(January/February):112-121.

Chapter 32 Kelleher/Mental Health

1. Kelleher KJ, McInerny TK, Gardner WP, Childs GE, Wasserman RC. Increasing identification of psychosocial problems. 1979-1996. *Pediatr*. 2000;105(6):1313-1321.

2. Brandenburg NA, Friedman RM, Siber SE. Epidemiology of childhood psychiatric disorders: prevalence findings from recent studies. *J Am Acad Child Adolesc Psychiatry*. 1990;29(1):76-83.

3. National Institute of Mental Health. Brief notes on the mental health of children and adolescents [Web site]. 2003. Available at: http://www.nimh.nih.gov/publicat/childnotes.cfm. Accessed April 16, 2004.

4. Offord DR. Child psychiatric epidemiology: current status and future prospects. *Can J Psychiatry*. 1995;40(6):284-288.

5. Costello EJ, Costello AJ, Edelbroek C, et al. Psychiatric disorders in pediatric primary care. Prevalence and risk factors. *Arch Gen Psychiatry*. 1988;45(12):1107-1116.

6. Leslie LK, Hurlburt MS, Landsverk J, Rolls JA, Wood PA, Kelleher KJ. Comprehensive assessments for children entering foster care: a national perspective. *Pediatr*. 2003;112(1 Pt 1):134-142.

7. Teplin LA, Abram KM, McClelland GM, Duncan MK, Mericle AA. Psychiatric disorders in youth in juvenile detention. *Arch Gen Psychiatry*. 2002;59:1133-1143.

8. Burns BJ, Costello DJ, Angold A, et al. Children's mental health service use across sectors. *Health Aff*. 1995;14(3):147-159.

9. Garland AF, Hough RL, McCabe KM, Yeh M, Wood PA, Aarons GA. Prevalence of psychiatric disorders in youths across five sectors of care. *J Am Acad Child Adolesc Psychiatry*. 2001;40:409-418.

10. Regier DA, Narrow WE, Rae DS, Mandersheid RW, Locke BZ, Goodwin FK. The de facto US mental and addictive disorders service system. Epidemiologic catchment area prospective 1-year prevalence rates of disorders and services. *Arch Gen Psychiatry*. 1993;50:85-94.

11. Kelleher KJ, Childs GE, Harman JS. Health care costs for children with attention-deficit/hyperactivity disorder. *Economics Neurosci*. 2001;3(4):60-63.

12. Ringel JS, Sturn R. National estimates of mental health utilization and expenditures for children in 1998. *J Behav Health Services Res*. 2001;28(3):319-333.

13. Fergusson DM, Horwood LJ, Lynskey MT. The effects of conduct disorder and attention deficit in middle childhood on offending and scholastic ability at age 13. *J Child Psychol Psychiatry*. 1993;34(6):899-916.

14. Fischer M, Barkley RA, Fletcher KE, Smallish L. The adolescent outcome of hyperactive children: predictors of psychiatric, academic, social, and emotional adjustment. *J Am Acad Child Adolesc Psychiatry*. 1994;33(1):144-145.

15. Weller EB, Weller RA. Depression in adolescents: growing pains or true morbidity? *J Affect Disord*. 2000;61(Suppl 1):9-13.

16. Knapp M, McCrone P, Fombonne E, Beecham J, Wostear G. The Maudsley long-term follow-up of child and adolescent depression: impact of comorbid conduct disorder on service use and costs in adulthood. *Br J Psychiatry*. 2002;180:19-23.

17. Federation of Families for Children's Mental Health and Keys for Networking. *Blamed and Ashamed: The Treatment Experiences of Youth With Co-occurring Substance Abuse and Mental Health Disorders and Their Families.* Alexandria, VA: Federation of Families for Children's Mental Health; 2000.

18. Ormel J, Vorkoff M, Ustun TB, Pini S, Korten A, Oldehinkel T. Common mental disorders and disability across cultures. *JAMA.* 1994;272(22):1741-1748.

19. Sanderson K, Andrews G. Prevalence and severity of mental health-related disability and relationship to diagnosis. *Psychiatr Services.* 2002;53(1):80-86.

20. World Health Organization. *The World Health Report 2001 - Mental Health: New Understanding, New Hope.* Geneva: World Health Organization; 2001.

21. Halfon N, Newacheck PW. Prevalence and impact of parent-reported disabling mental health conditions among US children. *J Am Acad Child Adolesc Psychiatry.* 1999;38(5):600-609; discussion 610-3.

22. Peele PB, Lave JR, Kelleher KJ. Exclusions and limitations in children's behavioral health care coverage. *Psychiatr Services.* 2002;53(5):591-594.

23. Cheer SM, Figgitt DP. Spotlight on fluvoxamine in anxiety disorders in children and adolescents. *CNS Drugs.* 2002;16(2):139-144.

24. Pincus HA, Tanielian TL, Marcus SC, et al. Prescribing trends in psychotropic medications: primary care, psychiatry, and other medical specialties. *JAMA.* 1998;279(7):526-531.

25. Pine DS. Treating children and adolescents with selective serotonin reuptake inhibitors: how long is appropriate? *J Child Adolesc Psycholpharmacol.* 2002;12(3):189-203.

26. Wolraich ML. Annotation: The use of psychotropic medications in children: an American view. *J Child Psychol Psychiatry.* 2003;44(2):159-168.

27. Zito JM, Safer DJ, DosReis S, et al. Psychotropic practice patterns for youth: a 10-year perspective. *Arch Pediatr Adolesc Med.* 2003;157(1):17-25.

28. Strattera approved to treat ADHD. *FDA Consum.* 2003;37(2):4.

29. Weisz JR, Jensen PS. Efficacy and effectiveness of child and adolescent psychotherapy and pharmacotherapy. *Ment Health Serv Res.* 1999;1(3):125-157.

30. Santos AB, Henggeler SW, Burns BJ, Arana GW, Meisler N. Research on field-based services: models for reform in the delivery of mental health care to populations with complex clinical problems. *Am J Psychiatry.* 1995;152(8):1111-1123.

31. Safer DJ. Changing patterns of psychotropic medications prescribed by child psychiatrists in the 1990s. *J Child Adolesc Psycholpharmacol.* 1997;7(4):267-274.

32. Schweitzer JB, Holcomb HH. Drugs under investigation for attention-deficit hyperactivity disorder. *Curr Opin Investig Drugs.* 2002;3(8):1207-1211.

33. Olfson M, Gameroff MJ, Marcus SC, Jensen PS. National trends in the treatment of attention deficit hyperactivity disorder. *Am J Psychiatry.* 2003;160(6):1071-1077.

34. National Advisory Mental Health Council Workgroup on Child and Adolescent Mental Health Intervention and Deployment. *Blueprint for Change: Research on Child and Adolescent Mental Health.* Rockville, MD: National Institute of Mental Health; 2001.

35. US Department of Health and Human Services. *Report of the Surgeon General's Conference on Children's Mental Health.* Washington, DC; 2000.

36. Drake RE, Goldman HH, Leff HS, et al. Implementing evidence-based practices in routine mental health service settings. *Psychiatr Services.* 2001;52:179-182.

37. Hoge MA, Morris JA. Special double issue: behavioral health workforce education and training. *Adm Policy Ment Health.* 2002;29:295-439.

38. Weisz JR, Jensen AL. Child and adolescent psychotherapy in research and practice contexts: review of the evidence and suggestions for improving the field. *Eur Child Adolesc Psychiatry.* 2001;10(Suppl 1):112-118.

39. Duan N, Braslow JT, Weisz JR, Wells KB. Fidelity, adherence, and robustness of interventions. *Psychiatr Services.* 2001;52(4):413.

40. Horwitz SM, Kelleher KJ, Boyce T, et al. Barriers to health care for children and youth with psychosocial problems. *JAMA.* 2002;288(12):1508-1512.

41. Katon W, Von Korff M, Lin E, et al. Stepped collaborative care for primary care patients with persistent symptoms of depression: a randomized trial. *Arch Gen Psychiatry.* 1999;56:1109-1115.

42. Simon GE, VonKorff M. Recognition, management, and outcomes of depression in primary care. *Arch Fam Med.* 1995;4:99-105.

Kelleher Data References

1. Centers for Disease Control and Prevention [Web site]. School health policies and programs study, state-level summaries: mental health and social services. 2002. Available at: http://www.cdc.gov/nccdphp/dash/shpps/summaries/mental_health/index.htm. Accessed March 10, 2004.

2. The National Advisory Mental Health Council Workgroup on Child and Adolescent Mental Health Development and Deployment. Blueprint for change: research on child and adolescent mental health [The National Institute of Mental Health Web site]. 2001. Available at: http://www.nimh.nih.gov/child/blueprin.pdf. Accessed March 10, 2004.

Chapter 33 Olson/Maternal Depression

1. Murray L, Cooper PJ, eds. *Post Partum Depression and Child Development.* New York, NY: Guilford Press; 1997.

2. Beardslee WR, Versage EM, Gladstone TR. Children of affectively ill parents: a review of the past 10 years. *J Am Acad Child Adolesc Psychiatry.* 1998;37(11):1134-1141.

3. Halfon N, McLearn KT, Schuster MA, eds. *Child Rearing in America: Challenges facing parents with young children.* New York, NY: Cambridge University Press; 2002.

4. Kelley SA, Jennings KD. Putting the pieces together: Maternal depression, maternal behavior, and toddler helplessness. *Infant Ment Health J.* 2003;24(1):74-90.

5. Heneghan AM, Silver EJ, Bauman LJ, Stein RE. Do pediatricians recognize mothers with depressive symptoms? *Pediatr.* 2000;106(6):1367-1373.

6. Myers JK, Weissman MM, Tischler GL. Six-month prevalence of psychiatric disorders in three communities 1980 to 1982. *Arch Gen Psychiatry.* 1984;41:959-967.

7. Olson AL, DiBrigida LA. Depressive symptoms and work role satisfaction in mothers of toddlers. *Pediatr.* 1994;94(3):363-367.

8. Naerde A, Tambs K, Mathiesen KS, Dalgard OS, Samuelsen SO. Symptoms of anxiety and depression among mothers of pre-school children: effect of chronic strain related to children and child care-taking. *J Affect Disord.* 2000;58(3):181-199.

9. Pianta RC, Egeland B. Relation between depressive symptoms and stressful life events in a sample of disadvantaged mothers. *J Consult Clin Psychol.* 1994;62(6):1229-1234.

10. Prodromidis M, Abrams S, Field T, Scafidi F, Rahdert E. Psychosocial stressors among depressed adolescent mothers. *Adolescence.* 1994;29(114):331-343.

11. Reading R, Reynolds S. Debt, social disadvantage and maternal depression. *Soc Sci Med.* 2001;53(4):441-453.

12. Casey P, Goolsby S, Berkowitz C, et al. Maternal Depresion, Changing Public Assistance, Food Security, and Child Health Status. *Pediatr.* 2004;113(2):298-304.

13. O'Hara MW. *Postpartum Depression: Causes and consequences.* New York: Springer-Verlag; 1994.

14. Philipps LH, O'Hara MW. Prospective study of postpartum depression: 4 1/2-year follow-up of women and children. *J Abnorm Psychol.* 1991;100(2):151-155.

15. Beck D, Koenig H. Minor Depression: A review of the literature. *Int J Psychiatry Med.* 1996;26(2):179-211.

16. McLennan JD, Kotelchuck M. Parental prevention practices for young children in the context of maternal depression. *Pediatr.* 2000;105(5):1090-1095.

17. Grupp-Phelan J, Whitaker RC, Naish AB. Depression in mothers of children presenting for emergency and primary care; Impact on mothers' perception of caring for their children. *Ambul Pediatr.* 2003;3(3):142-146.

18. Beck CT. The effects of postpartum depression on child development: a meta-analysis. *Arch Psychiatr Nurs.* 1998;12(1):12-20.

19. Beck CT. Maternal depression and child behaviour problems: a meta-analysis. *J Adv Nurs.* 1999;29(3):623-629.

20. Civic D, Holt VL. Maternal depressive symptoms and child behavior problems in a nationally representative normal birthweight sample. *Matern Child Health J.* 2000;4(4):215-221.

21. Cairney J, Thorpe C, Rietschlin J, Avison WR. 12-month prevalence of depression among single and married mothers in the 1994 National Population Health Survey. *Can J Public Health.* 1999;90(5):320-324.

22. McLennan JD, Kotelchuck M, Cho H. Prevalence, persistence, and correlates of depressive symptoms in a national sample of mothers of toddlers. *J Am Acad Child Adolesc Psychiatry.* 2001;40(11):1316-1323.

23. Lyons-Ruth K. Parent Depression and Child Attachment:Hostile and helpless profiles of parent and child behavior among families at risk. In: Goodwin S, Gottlieb I, eds. *Childen of Depressed Parents: Mechanisms of Risk and Implications for Treatment.* Washington DC: American Psychological Association; 2002:97-104.

24. Lyons-Ruth K, Wolfe R. Depressive symptoms in parents of children under age three: Sociodemographic predictors, current correlates, and associated parenting behaviors. In: Halfon N, McLearn KT, Schuster MA, eds. *Child Rearing in America: Challenges facing parents with young children.* Cambridge: Cambridge University Press; 2003.

25. Sharp D, Hay DF, Pawlby S, Schmucker G, Allen H, Kumar R. The impact of postnatal depression on boys' intellectual development. *J Child Psychol Psychiatry.* 1995;36(8):1315-1336.

26. Hay DF, Pawlby S, Sharp D, Asten P, Mills A, Kumar R. Intellectual problems shown by 11-year-old children whose mothers had postnatal depression. *J Child Psychol Psychiatry.* 2001;42(7):871-889.

27. Miller L, Warner V, Wickramaratne P, Weissman MM. Self-esteem and depression: ten year follow-up of mothers and offspring. *J Affect Disord.* 1999;52(1-3):41-49.

28. Compas BE, Langrock AM. Children coping with parental depression: Processes of adaptation to family stress. In: Goodman SH, Gottlieb I, eds. *Children of Depressed Parents: Mechanisms of Risk and Implications for Treatment.* Washington, DC: American Psychological Association; 2001:227-254.

29. Lieb R, Isensee B, Hofler M, Pfister H, Wittchen HU. Parental Major Depression and the risk of depression and other mental disorders in offspring: a prospective-longitudinal community study. *Arch Gen Psychiatry.* 2002;59:365-374.

30. Olson AL, Kelleher KJ, Kemper KJ, Zuckerman BS, Hammond CS, Dietrich AJ. Primary care pediatricians' roles and perceived responsibilities in the identification and management of depression in children and adolescents. *Pediatr.* 2001;1(2):91-98.

31. Kahn RS, Wise PH, Finkelstein JA, Bernstein HH, Lowe JA, Homer CJ. The scope of unmet maternal health needs in pediatric settings. *Pediatr.* 1999;103(3):576-581.

32. Heneghan AM, Morton S. Do pediatricians and mothers share similar attitudes about discussing maternal depressive symptoms during a pediatric visit? *Pediatric Res.* 2003;53(2):73A.

33. Pignone MP, Gaynes BN, Rushton JL, et al. Screening for depression in adults: a summary of the evidence for the US Preventive Services Task Force. *Ann of Intern Med.* 2002;136:764-765.

34. Kroenke K, Spitzer RL, Williams JB. The Patient Health Questionnaire-2: Validity of a Two-Item Screener. *Med Care.* 2003;411(11):284-1292.

35. Minkovitz C, Hugart N. A practice-based intervention to enhance the quality of care in the first 3 years of life: The Healthy Steps for Young Children Program. *JAMA.* 2003;290(23):3081-3091.

Olson Data References

1. McMillen R., Southward L, Pascoe J. *Social Climate of Early Child Health and Well-being: A National Survey.* Mississippi State University, MS: Social Science Research Center & Wright State University; 2002.

Chapter 34 Doucette/Youth Suicide

1. Kienhorst CWM, De Wilde EJ, Diekstra RF, Wolter WHG. The adolescents' image of their suicide attempt. *J Am Acad Child Adolesc Psychiatry.* 1995; 34(5):623-628.

2. Blumenthal SJ. Youth suicide: risk factors, assessment, and treatment of adolescent and young adult suicidal patients. *Psychiatric Clin North Am.* 1990;13(3):511-556.

3. Miller KE, King CA, Shain BN, Naylor MW. Suicidal adolescents'

perceptions of their family environments. *Suicide and Life Threat Behav.* 1992;22(226-239).

4. Marttunnen MJ, Henriksson MM, Lonnqvist JK. Psychosocial stressors more common in adolescent suicides with alcohol abuse compared with depressive adolescent suicides. *J Am Acad Child Adolesc Psychiatry.* 1994;33(4):490-497.

5. Rutter M. Psychosical resilience and protective mechanisms. *Am J Orthopsychiatry.* 1987;57(316-331).

6. Tabachnick N. The interlocking psychologies of suicide and adolescence. *Adolesc Psychiatry.* 1981;10:399-410.

7. Orbach I, Rosenheim E, Hary E. Some aspects of cognitive functioning in suicidal children. *J Am Acad Child Adolesc Psychiatry.* 1987;26(2):181-185.

8. Hart EE, Williams CL, Davidson JA. Suicidal behavior, social networks, and psychiatric diagnosis. *Soc Psychiatr Epidemiol.* 1988;23:222-228.

9. Kahn AU. Heterogeneity of suicidal adolescents. *J Am Acad Child Adolesc Psychiatry.* 1987;1:92-96.

10. Withers LE, Kaplan DW. Adolescents who attempt suicide: a retrospective clinical chart review of hospitalized patients. *Professional Psychol: Res and Pract.* 1987;18:391-393.

11. Rotheram-Borus M, Trautman P. Hopelessness, depression, and suicidal intent among adolescent suicide attempters. *J Am Acad Child Adolesc Psychiatry.* 1988;27(6):700-704.

12. Hamburg D. Preparing for life: the critical transition of adolescence. In: Diekstra RFW, ed. *Preventive Interventions in Adolescence.* Toronto: Hogrefe & Huber; 1989.

13. Anderson RN, Smith BL. *National Vital Statistics Report.* Deaths: Leading Causes for 2001. Washington, DC: Centers for Disease Control and Prevention; 2003.

14. Vaillant GE, Blumenthal SJ. *Suicide Over the Life Cycle: Risk Factors and Life Span Development.* Washington, DC: American Psychiatric Press; 1990.

15. American Association of Suicidology [Web site]. 2004. Available at: www.suicidology.org. Accessed May 19, 2004.

16. Centers for Disease Control and Prevention. *The Youth Risk and Behavior Surveillance Survey, 2001.* Washington, DC: Centers for Disease Control and Prevention; 2001.

17. Kellerman AL, Rivara FP, Reay DT, Francisco J, Fligher C, Hackman BB. Suicide in the home in relationship to gun ownership. *N Engl J Med.* 1992;327:467-472.

Doucette Data References

1. Centers for Disease Control and Prevention [Web site]. *Youth risk behavior surveillance survey*, 1991-2001. Available at: http://www.cdc.gov/nccdphp/dash/yrbs/. Accessed May 28, 2004.

2. Centers for Disease Control and Prevention (CDC). Compressed mortality data: underlying cause of death [CDC Wonder database online]. 2003. Available at: http://wonder.cdc.gov/mortSQL.html. Accessed on December 3003.

3. US Department of Health and Human Services, Centers for Disease Control and Prevention (CDC), National Center for Health Statistics, Office of Analysis, Epidemiology, and Health Promotion. Compressed Mortality File. [CDC Wonder database online]. January 22, 2004. Available at: http://www.cdc.gov/nchs/products/elec_prods/subject/mcompres.htm. Accessed March 3, 2004.

Chapter 35 Wolraich/Attention Deficit Hyperactivity Disorder

1. Hoffman H. *Der Struwwelpeter.* Germany: 1848. Reprint, Mineola, NY: Dover Publishers; 1995:11-15.

2. Still G. The Coulstonian lectures on some abnormal physical conditions in children. *Lancet.* 1902;1:1008-1012.

3. Hohman LB. Post-encephalitic behavior disorder in children. *Johns Hopkins Hosp Bull.* 1922;33:372-375.

4. Ebaugh F. Neuropsychiatric sequelae of acute epidemic encephalitis in children. *Am J Dis Child.* 1923;25:89-97.

5. Clements SD. *Minimal Brain Dysfunction in Children: Terminology and Identification, NINDB Monograph #3.* Washington, DC: US Dept of Health, Education and Welfare; 1966.

6. American Psychiatric Association. *Diagnostic and Statistical Manual for Mental Disorders.* 2nd ed. Washington, DC: American Psychiatric Association; 1967.

7. Douglas V. Differences between normal and hyperkinetic children.

Clinical use of stimulant drugs in children. In: Conners C, ed. *Excerpta Medica*. Amsterdam; 1974:12-23.

8. Douglas V, Peters KG. Toward a clearer definition of the attention deficit of hyperactive children. In: Hale G, Lewis M, Eds. *Attention and the Development of Cognitive Skills*. New York: Plenum Press; 1979.

9. American Psychiatric Association. *Diagnostic and Statistical Manual for Mental Disorders*. 3rd ed. Washington, DC: American Psychiatric Association; 1980.

10. American Psychiatric Association. *Diagnostic and Statistical Manual of Mental Disorders*. 3rd ed. rev. Washington, DC: American Psychiatric Association; 1987.

11. American Psychiatric Association. *Diagnostic and Statistical Manual of Mental Disorders*. 4th ed. Washington, DC: American Psychiatric Association; 1994.

12. Gjone H, Stevenson J, Sundet JM. Genetic influence on parent-reported attention-related problems in Norwegian general population twin samples. *J Am Acad Child Adolesc Psychiatry*. 1996;35:588-596.

13. Alberts-Corush J, Firestone P, Goodman JT. Attention and impulsivity characteristics of the biological and adoptive parents of hyperactive and normal children. *Am J Orthopsychiatry*. 1986;56(3):413-423.

14. Morrison JR, Stewart MA. The psychiatric status of the legal families of adopted hyperactive child syndrome. *Arch Gen Psychiatry*. 1973;28:888-891.

15. Biederman J, Farone SV, Keenan K, et al. Further evidence for family-genetic risk factors in attention-deficit hyperactivity disorder: Patterns of comorbidity in probands and relatives in psychiatrically and pediatrically referred samples. *Arch Gen Psychiatry*. 1992;49(9):728-738.

16. Cook EJ, Stein MA, Krasowski MD, et al. Association of attention deficit disorder and the dopamine transporter gene. *Am J of Hum Genetics*. 1995;56(4):993-998.

17. Gill M, Daly G, Heron S, et al. Confirmation of an association between attention deficit/hyperactivity disorder and a dopamine transporter polymorphism. *Mol Psychiatry*. 1997;2(4):311-313.

18. Swanson J, Sunohara GA, Kennedy JL, et al. Association of the dopamine receptor D4 (DRD4) gene with a refined phenotype of attention deficit-hyperactivity disorder (ADHD): a family-based approach. *Mol Psychiatry*. 1998;3(1):38-41.

19. Klebanov PK, Brooks-Gunn J, McCormick MC. Classroom behavior of very low birth weight elementary school children. *Pediatr*. 1991;94(5):700-708.

20. Aylward E, Reiss AL, Reader MJ, et al. Basal ganglia volumes in children with attention deficit-hyperactivity disorder with normal controls. *J Child Neurol*. 1996;11(2):112-115.

21. Castellanos F, Giedd JN, Marsh WL, et al. Quantitative brain magnetic resonance imaging in attention deficit-hyperactivity disorder. *Arch Gen Psychiatry*. 1996;53(7):607-616.

22. Bradley C. The behavior of children receiving Benzedrine. *Am J Psychiatry*. 1937;94:577-585.

23. Greenhill LL. Attention-deficit hyperactivity disorder: the stimulants. *Child Adolesc Psychiatry Clin North Am*. 1995; 4:123-168.

24. Safer DJ, Zito JM, Fine EM. Increased methylphenidate usage for attention deficit disorder in the 1990's. *Pediatr*. 1996;98:1084-1088.

25. Rappley MD, Gardiner JC, Jetton JR, Houang RT. The use of methylphenidate in Michigan. *Arch Pediatr Adolesc Med*. 1995;149(6):675-679.

26. Diller LH. *The Run on Ritalin: Attention Deficit Disorder and Stimulant Treatment in the 1990's*. Hastings Center Report; 1996;26:12-18.

27. Dockx P. Are school children getting unnecessary drugs? *Sun Chronicle*, 1988: 15.

28. Ruel JM, Hickey P. Are too many children being treated with methylphenidate? *Can J Psychiatry*. 1992;37(8):570-572.

29. Jensen P, Xenakis SN, Shervette RE, Bain MW, Davis H. Diagnosis and treatment of attention deficit disorder in two general hospital clinics. *Hosp Commun Psychiatry*. 1989;40:708-712.

30. Perrin JM, Stein MT, Amler RW, et al. Diagnosis and evaluation of the child with attention-deficit/hyperactivity disorder. *Pediatr*. 2000;105:1158-1170.

31. Perrin JM, Stein MT, Amler RW. Clinical practice guideline: treatment of the school-aged child with attention-deficit/hyperactivity disorder. *Pediatr*. 2001;108(4):1033-1044.

Wolraich Data References

1. Bloom B, Cohen RA, Vickerie JL, Wondimu EA. Summary health statistics for U.S. children: National Health Interview Survey, 2001 [Centers for Disease Control and Prevention Web site]. 2003. Available at: http://www.cdc.gov/nchs/data/series/sr_10/sr10_216.pdf. Accessed March 31, 2004.

2. Pastor P. Attention deficit disorder and learning disability: United States, 1997-98 [Centers for Disease Control and Prevention Web site]. 2002. Available at: http://www.cdc.gov/nchs/data/series/sr_10/sr10_206.pdf. Accessed March 31, 2004.

Chapter 36 Bartkowski/Religion Among American Teens: Contours and Consequences

1. Regnerus M, Smith C, Fritsch M. Religion in the Lives of American Adolescents: A Review of the Literature. University of North Carolina: National Study of Youth and Religion; 2003. No. 3. Available at: http://www.youthandreligion.org/publications/docs/litreview.pdf. Accessed February 10, 2004. See also: Smith C, Faris R, Denton ML, Regnerus M. Mapping American adolescent subjective religiosity and attitudes of alienation toward religion: a research report. Sociol Religion. 2003;64:111-133.

2. Smith C, Faris R. Religion and American Adolescent Delinquency, Risk Behaviors and Constructive Social Activities. University of North Carolina: National Study of Youth and Religion; 2002. No. 1. Available at: http://www.youthandreligion.org/publications/docs/RiskReport1.pdf. Accessed February 10, 2004. See also: Smith C, Faris R. Religion and the Life Attitudes and Self-Images of American Adolescents. University of North Carolina: National Study of Youth and Religion; 2002. No. 2. Available at: http://www.youthandreligion.org/publications/docs/Attitudes.pdf. Accessed February 10, 2004. See also: Regnerus M, Smith C, Fritsch M. Religion in the Lives of American Adolescents: A Review of the Literature. University of North Carolina: National Study of Youth and Religion; 2003. No. 3:14. Available at: http://www.youthandreligion.org/publications/docs/litreview.pdf. Accessed February 10, 2004.

3. Regnerus M, Smith C, Fritsch M. Religion in the Lives of American Adolescents: A Review of the Literature. University of North Carolina: National Study of Youth and Religion; 2003. No. 3:14. Available at: http://www.youthandreligion.org/publications/docs/litreview.pdf. Accessed February 10, 2004.

4. Darnell A, Sherkat DE. The impact of Protestant fundamentalism on educational attainment. Am Sociol Rev. 1997;63:306-315. See also: Sherkat DE, Darnell A. The effect of parents' fundamentalism on children's educational attainment: examining differences by gender and children's fundamentalism. J Sci Stud Religion. 1999;38:23-35. See also: Regnerus M, Smith C, Fritsch M. Religion in the Lives of American Adolescents: A Review of the Literature. University of North Carolina: National Study of Youth and Religion; 2003. No. 3:16-19. Available at: http://www.youthandreligion.org/publications/docs/litreview.pdf. Accessed February 10, 2004.

5. Regnerus M, Elder GH Jr. Staying on track in school: religious influences in high- and low-risk settings. J Sci Stud Religion. 2003;42:633-649.

6. Smith C. Religious participation and network closure among American adolescents. J Sci Stud Religion. 2003;42:259-267.

7. Smith C. Religious participation and network closure among American adolescents. J Sci Stud Religion. 2003;42:260.

Bartkowski Data References

1. Johnston LD, Bachman JG, O'Malley PM. Monitoring the future: a continuing study of American youth. Ann Arbor, MI: University of Michigan Survey Research Center; 1996.

2. Kosmin BA, Mayer E, Keysar A. American religious identification survey, 2001. Exhibit 15: state by state distribution of selected religious groups [City University of New York Web site]. Available at: http://www.gc.cuny.edu/studies/key_findings.htm. Accessed February 8, 2004.

3. Penn State University. Interactive Maps and Reports for Religious Congregations and Membership, 1990-2000 [The American Religion Data Archive Web site]. Available at: http://www.thearda.com/. Accessed February 8, 2004.

4. Smith C, Faris R. Religion and American adolescent delinquency, risk behaviors and constructive social activities [National Study of Youth and Religion Web site]. 2002. Available at: http://www.youthandreligion.org/publications/docs/RiskReport1.pdf. Accessed January 30, 2004.

Chapter 37 Duncan & Kallock/Adolescent Sexuality: Beyound the Numbers

1. Centers for Disease Control and Prevention. *U.S. Pregnancy Rate Down from Peak; Births and Abortions on the Decline.* Hyattsville, MD: US Dept of Health and Human Services; 2003.

2. Sexuality Information and Education Council of the United States [Web site]. The truth about adolescent sexuality. 2003. Available at: http://www.siecus.org/pubs/fact/fact0020.html. Accessed May 13, 2004.

3. Kirby D. *Emerging Answers: Research Findings on Programs to Reduce Teen Pregnancy.* Washington, DC: National Campaign to Prevent Teenage Pregnancy; 2001.

4. National Campaign to Prevent Teenage Pregnancy. *Parent Power: What Parents Need to Know and Do to Help Teen Pregnancy.* Washington, DC: National Campaign to Prevent Teenage Pregnancy; 2003.

5. Albert B, Brown S, Flanigan C, eds. *14 and Younger: The Sexual Behavior of Young Adolescents.* Washington, DC: National Campaign to Prevent Teenage Pregnancy; 2003.

6. The Alan Guttmacher Institute. *Teenagers' Sexual and Reproductive Health: Developed Countries.* Washington, DC: The Alan Guttmacher Institute; 2003.

7. Ryan S, Manlove J, Franzetta K. *The First Time: Characteristics of Teens' First Sexual Relationships.* Washington, DC: Child Trends; 2003.

8. Brendtro LK, Brokenleg M, Van Bockern S. *Reclaiming Youth at Risk: Our Hope for the Future.* Bloomington, IN: National Education Service; 1992.

9. Simpson AR. *Raising Teens: A Synthesis of Research and a Foundation for Action.* Boston, MA: Center for Health Communication, Harvard School of Public Health; 2001.

10. National Campaign to Prevent Teenage Pregnancy. *Talking Back: What Teens Want Adults to Know About Teen Pregnancy.* Washington, DC: National Campaign to Prevent Teenage Pregnancy; 2003.

11. Moore KA, Zaff JF. *Building a Better Teenager: A Summary of "What Works" in Adolescent Development.* Washington, DC: Child Trends; 2002.

12. Miller KS, Kotchick BA, Dorsey S, Forehand R, Ham AY. Family communication about sex: what are parents saying and are their adolescents listening? *Fam Plann Perspective.* 1998;30(5):218-222.

13. Hoff T, Greene L, Davis J. National Survey of Adolescents and Young Adults: Sexual Health Knowledge, Attitudes and Experiences. Menlo Park, California: Kaiser Family Foundation; 2003.

14. Benson PL. All Kids Are Our Kids. San Francisco, CA: Jossey Bass; 1997.

15. Manlove J, Terry-Humen E, Papillo AR, et al. Preventing Teenage Pregnancy, Childbearing, and Sexually Transmitted Diseases: What the Research Shows. Washington, DC: Child Trends; 2003.

16. Lonczak H, Abbott R, Hawkins JD, et al. Effects of the Seattle Social Development Project on sexual behavior, pregnancy, birth, and sexually transmitted disease outcomes by age 21 years. Arch Pediatr Adolesc Med. 2002;156:438-447.

17. The National Campaign to Prevent Teen Pregnancy [Web site]. Ten Tips for Parents to Help Their Children Avoid Teen Pregnancy. June 21, 2004. Available at: http://www.teenpregnancy.org/resources/reading/tips/tips.asp. Accessed June 21, 2004.

18. Ryan C, Futterman D. Caring for gay and lesbian teens. Contemp Pediatr. 1998;15:107-130.

19. Earls, M. GLBTQ Youth: At Risk and Underserved. Washington, DC: Advocates for Youth; 2003.

Duncan & Kallock Data References

1. Centers for Disease Control and Prevention [Web site]. Youth Risk Behavior Surveillance Survey. May 4, 2004. Available at: http://www.cdc.gov/nccdphp/dash/yrbs/. Accessed April 7, 2004.

2. Centers for Disease Control and Prevention (CDC). Natality and census data. [CDC Wonder database online]. 2004. Available at: http://wonder.cdc.gov/nataJ.html and http://wonder.cdc.gov/census.html. Accessed April 7, 2004.

3. Maternal and Child Health Bureau [Web site]. Child health USA 2002. 2002. Available at: http://www.mchb.hrsa.gov/chusa02/main_pages/page_36.htm. Accessed April 7, 2004.

4. Ventura S, Joyce A, William M, Stanley H. Revised Pregnancy Rates, 1990-97, and New Rates for 1998-99: United States. National Vital Statistics Reports. Vital Statistics of the United States; 2003. Available at: http://www.cdc.gov/nchs/data/nvsr/nvsr52/nvsr52_07.pdf. Accessed April 7, 2004.

Chapter 38 Hein & Flasch/Youth as a Resource

1. United Nations Population Fund [Web site]. Fast Facts on Adolescents and Youth. 2001. Available at: http://www.unfpa.org/adolescents/facts.htm. Accessed May 15, 2003.

2. US Bureau of the Census [Web site]. Demographic Trends in the 20th Century. 2002. Available at: http://www.census.gov/prod/2002pubs/censr-4.pdf. Accessed February 16, 2004.

3. The Carnegie Corporation of New York. *The Civic Mission of School.* New York: The Carnegie Corporation of New York; 2003.

4. Woodard EH, Gridina N. *Media in the Home 2000.* Philadelphia: The Annenberg Public Policy Center; 2000.

5. Levin D, Arafeh S. *The Digital Disconnect: The Widening Gap Between Internet-Savvy Students and their School.* Washington, DC: Pew Internet and American Life Project; 2002: ii.

6. Levin D, Arafeh S. *The Digital Disconnect: The Widening Gap Between Internet-Savvy Students and their School.* Washington, DC: Pew Internet and American Life Project; 2002:7-8.

7. Gibson C. *From Inspiration to Participation.* New York: The Carnegie Corporation; 2001.

8. The Carnegie Corporation of New York. *The Civic Mission of Schools.* New York: The Carnegie Corporation; 2003:19.

9. The Carnegie Corporation of New York. *The Civic Mission of Schools.* New York: The Carnegie Corporation; 2003:17.

10. America's Promise [Web site]. Youth Partnership Team. 2003. Available at: http://www.americaspromise.org/about/youthPartnershipTeam.cfm. Accessed November 13, 2003.

11. Braken A. Need a grant? Ask a kid [Youth Today—Youth Tomorrow Web site]. 2000. Available at: http://www.ytyt.org/infobank/document.cfm/parent/185. Accessed February 16, 2004.

12. Massachusetts Department of Social Services [Web site]. DSS—Teens—Adolescent outreach. 2003. Available at: http://www.state.ma.us/dss/Teens/AS_Outreach.htm. Accessed November 13, 2003.

13. Yates R. Teen spending meets the 'stored-value card' [The Christian Science Monitor Web site]. 2001. Available at: http://csmweb2.emcweb.com/durable/2001/02/26/fp14s1-csm.shtml. Accessed June 4, 2003.

14. Eccles J, Gootman JA. *Community Programs to Promote Youth Development.* Washington, DC: National Academy Press; 2002:3.

15. Eccles J, Gootman JA. *Community Programs to Promote Youth Development.* Washington, DC: National Academy Press; 2002:8-10.

Hein & Flasch Data References

1. Federal Interagency Forum on Child and Family Statistics. America's children: key national indicators of well-being, 2002 [National Institute of Child Health and Human Development Web site]. 2002. Available at: http://www.nichd.nih.gov/publications/pubs/childstats/report2002.pdf. Accessed February 12, 2004.

2. Fields J. *Current Population Reports.* Children's Living Arrangements and Characteristics: March 2002. Washington, DC: US Bureau of the Census; 2003. Series P20-547. Available at: http://www.census.gov/prod/2003pubs/p20-547.pdf. Accessed April 16, 2004.

3. Kleiner B, Chapman C. Youth service-learning and community service among 6th- through 12th-grade students in the United States: 1996 and 1999 [National Center for Education Statistics Web site]. 1999. Available at: http://nces.ed.gov/pubs2000/2000028.pdf. Accessed April 16, 2004.

4. US Bureau of the Census. *Statistical Abstract of the United States*: 2004. Annual Expenditure Per Child by Husband-Wife Families, by Family Income and Category. Washington, DC: US Bureau of the Census; 2004.

5. US Department of Defense [Web site]. Population representation in the military services, various years. 2004. Available at: http://www.dod.mil/prhome/. Accessed February 23, 2004.

Chapter 39 Haycock & Yi/Access to Postsecondary Education

1. National Center for Education Statistics. Access to postsecondary education for the 1992 high school graduates [Web site]. 1997. Available at: http://nces.ed.gov/pubsearch/pubsinfo.asp?pubid=98105. Accessed April 14, 2004.

2. The National Center for Public Policy and Higher Education. *Measuring Up 2000: A state-by-state report card for higher education*. Washington, DC: The National Center for Public Policy and Higher Education; 2000.

3. US Department of Education. *The Digest of Education Statistics, 2002*. Washington, DC: US Dept of Education; 2003.

4. National Center for Education Statistics. *The Condition of Education, 2003*. Washington, DC: US Dept of Education; 2003.

5. Mortenson T. Postsecondary education opportunity. The Mortenson report on public policy analysis of opportunity for postsecondary education, 2003. *Post-Secondary Education Opportunity*. 2003;134:1.

6. The National Collegiate Athletic Association. NCAA college graduation rates reports [Web site]. 2003. Available at: http://www.ncaa.org/grad_rates/. Accessed April 14, 2004.

7. Mortenson T. Postsecondary education opportunity. The Mortenson report on public policy analysis of opportunity for postsecondary education, 2002. *Post-Secondary Education Opportunity*. 2002;117:1.

8. National Center for Education Statistics. *Coming of Age in the 1990s: The Eighth Grade Class of 1988, 12 Years Later*. Washington, DC: US Dept of Education; 2002.

9. National Center for Education Statistics. Remedial education at higher education institutions in fall 1995 [Web site]. 1999. Available at: http://nces.ed.gov/pubsearch/pubsinfo.asp?pubid=97584. Accessed April 14, 2004.

10. The College Board. Trends in student aid [Web site]. 2002. Available at: http://www.collegeboard.com/press/cost02/html/CBTrendsAid02.pdf. Accessed April 15, 2004.

11. Organisation for Economic Cooperation and Development. *Education at a Glance: OECD Indicators. 2002 Edition*. Paris, France: Centre for Educational Research and Innovation; 2002.

Haycock & Yi Data References

1. Choy S. Students whose parents did not go to college: postsecondary access, persistence, and attainment [National Center for Education Statistics Web site]. 2001. Available at: http://nces.ed.gov/pubs2001/2001126.pdf. Accessed February 26, 2004.

2. US Department of Education. Enrollment rates of 18- to 24-year-olds in degree-granting institutions, by sex and race/ethnicity: 1967 to 2001. Table 186 [National Center for Education Statistics Web site]. 2002. Available at: http://nces.ed.gov/programs/digest/. Accessed April 16, 2004.

3. US Department of Education. Enrollment rate charts [National Center for Education Statistics Web site]. 2002. Available at: http://nces.ed.gov/programs/digest/. Accessed March 2, 2004.

4. US Department of Education, National Center for Education Statistics. *The Condition of Education, 2002, NCES 2002-025*. Washington, DC: US Dept of Education; 2002.

Chapter 40 Bilchik/Children and the Law

1. Anderson JA. The need for interagency collaboration for children with emotional and behavioral disabilities and their families. *Families Soc*. 2000;81:484-494.

2. Braithwaite J. Restorative justice and a new criminal law on substance abuse. *Youth & Soc*. 2001;33:227-248.

3. Child Welfare League of America. *2000 Membership Trends and Issues Survey*. Washington, DC: Child Welfare League of America; 2001.

4. Child Welfare League of America. *Alcohol and Other Drug Survey of State Child Welfare Agencies*. Washington, DC: Child Welfare League of America; 1998.

5. Schwartz IM, Weiner NA, Enosh G. Myopic justice? The juvenile court and child welfare systems. *Ann Am Acad Political Soc Sci*. 1999;564:126-141.

Bilchik Data References

1. Child Welfare League of America [database online]. Available at http://cwla.org/. Accessed April 21, 2004.

2. National Center for Juvenile Justice. Easy access to FBI arrest statistics: 1994-2001 [Office of Juvenile Justice and Delinquency Prevention Web site]. Available at: http://www.ojjdp.ncjrs.org/ojstatbb/ezaucr/asp/ucr_display.asp?Select_State=0&Select_County=0&rdoData=3p&rdoYear=97. Accessed March 24, 2004.

Chapter 41 Lichter/Families: Diversity and Change

1. Federal Interagency Forum. America's children: Key national indicators of well-being, 2002 [National Institute of Child Health and Human Development Web site]. July, 2002. Available at: http://www.nichd.nih.gov/publications/pubs/childstats/Americas.htm. Accessed May 23, 2003.

2. US Bureau of the Census. *The Hispanic Population: Census 2000 Brief, C2KBR/01-3*. Washington, DC: Government Printing Office; 2001.

3. Annie E. Casey Foundation. Children at risk: state trends 1990-2000. A PRB/KIDS COUNT special report [Web site]. Updated 8/21/2002. Available at: http://www.aecf.org/kidscount/c2ss/index.htm.

4. US Bureau of the Census. Historical poverty tables. [Web site]. Updated October 6, 2003. Available at: http://www.census.gov/hhes/poverty/histpov/hstpov3.html. Accessed May 23, 2003.

5. Proctor BD, Dalaker J. Poverty in the United States. Current Population Reports. [US Bureau of the Census Web site] September, 2003. Available at: http://www.census.gov/prod/2003pubs/p60-2222.pdf. Accessed October 3, 2003.

6. Mather M, Rivers K. State profiles of child well-being: results from the 2000 census [Annie E. Casey Foundation Web site]. March, 2003. Available at: http://www.aecf.org/kidscount/census_2000_march_03.pdf. Accessed March, 2003.

7. Lichter DT, Crowley ML. Welfare reform and child poverty: effects of maternal employment, marriage, and cohabitation. *Soc Sci Res*. 2004;33(2): in press.

8. Forum on Children and Family Statistics. America's Children: Key National Indicators of Well-being 2002 (Highlights) [Childstats.gov Web site]. 2002. Available at: http://www.childstats.gov/ac2002/highlight.asp. Accessed May 13, 2003.

9. Ameristat. Traditional families account for only 7 percent of US households. Population Reference Bureau [Web site]. March, 2003. Available at: http://www.ameristat.org/Content/NavigationMenu/Ameristat/Topics1/MarriageandFamily/Traditional_Families_Account_for_Only_7_Percent_of_U_S__Households.htm. 2003.

10. Eggebeen DJ, Lichter DT. Race, family structure, and changing poverty among American children. *Am Sociol Rev*. 1991;56:801-807.

11. Dupree A, Primus W. *Declining Share of Children Lived with Single Mothers in the Late 1990s*. Center for Budget and Policy Priorities, Washington, DC; 2001.

12. Simmons T, O'Connell M. *Married-couple and Unmarried-partner Households: 2000, CENSR-5*. US Bureau of the Census, Washington, DC; 2003.

13. Manning WD, Lichter DT. Parental cohabitation and children's economic well-being. *J Marriage and the Fam*.1996;58:998-1010.

14. Manning WD, Brown SL. Children's conomic well-being in cohabiting parent families: an update and extension. Paper presented at: Annual meeting of the Population Association of America; 2003; Minneapolis, MN.

15. Graefe DR, Lichter DT. Life course transitions of American children: parental cohabitation, marriage, and single parenthood. *Demogr.* 1999;36:205-221.

16. Bumpass L, Lu HH. Trends in cohabitation and implications for children's family contexts. *Popul Stud.* 2000;54:29-41.

17. US Bureau of the Census. Household relationship and living arrangements of children under 18 years, by age, sex, race, Hispanic origin, and metropolitan residence. [Web site]. Available at: http://www.census.gov/population/socdemo/hh-fam/cps2002/tabC2-all.pdf. Accessed June 20, 2003.

18. US Bureau of the Census. Household relationship and living arrangements of children under 18 years, by age, sex, race, Hispanic origin, and metropolitan residence. [Web site]. Available at: http://www.census.gov/population/socdemo/hh-fam/cps2002/tabC2-black.pdf. Accessed June 20, 2003.

19. Grall T. Custodial mothers and fathers and their child support, 1999. Current Population Reports [US Bureau of the Census Web site]. October, 2002. Available at: http://www.census.gov/prod/2002pubs/p60-217.pdf.

20. Casper LM, Bryson KR. *Co-resident Grandparents and Their Grandchildren: Grandparent Maintained Families.* United States Bureau of Census, Washington, DC; 1998.

21. Pebley AR, Rudkin LL. Grandparents caring for grandchildren: what do we know? *J Fam Issues.* 1999;20(2):218-242.

Lichter Data References

1. Casper LM, Cohen PN. How does POSSLQ measure up? Historical estimates of cohabitation. Figure 3. *Demogr.* 2000;37:244.

2. Fields J. *Current Population Reports.* Children's Living Arrangements and Characteristics: March 2002. Washington, DC: US Bureau of the Census; 2003. Series P20-547. Available at: http://www.census.gov/prod/2003pubs/p20-547.pdf. Accessed January 22, 2004.

3. US Bureau of the Census [Web site]. Summary file 3. 2000. Available at: http://www.census.gov/main/www/cen2000.html. Accessed May 14, 2004.

4. Ventura SJ, Bachrach CA. Nonmarital childbearing in the United States,1940–99. Table 1. National Center for Health Statistics. Vital Statistics of the United States. 2000;48(16). Available at: http://www.cdc.gov/nchs/data/nvsr/nvsr48/nvs48_16.pdf. Accessed January 22, 2004.

Chapter 42 Murdock/Minority Child Population Growth

1. Cook PJ, Mizer KL. The Revised ERS County Typology: An Overview [National Agricultural Library Web site]. 1994. Available at: http://www.nal.usda.gov/ric/resources/backgrnd/counties/00typ.htm. Accessed February 6, 2004.

2. Hollmann FW, Mulder TJ, Kallan JE. *Population Projections of the United States: 1999-2100.* Washington, DC: US Bureau of the Census; 2000.

3. McGehee M. *Community Structure and Mortality: The Effect of Community Structure on the Health Status of Nonmetropolitan Minorities in Texas, 1990* [dissertation]. College Station, TX: Department of Sociology, Texas A&M University; 2001.

4. Murdock SH, Hoque N, Johnson K, McGehee MA. Net migration and natural increase by race and Hispanic origin for metropolitan and nonmetropolitan counties in the United States:1990-2000. Paper presented at: Annual Meeting of the Population Association of America; May 9-11, 2002; Atlanta.

5. Murdock SH, Hoque N, Johnson K. Racial/ethnic diversification and differentiation in metropolitan and nonmetropolitan population change in the United States: implications for health care provision in rural America. *J Rural Health.* 2003;.19(4),425-432.

6. Office of Management and Budget. *Revised Statistical Definitions for Metropolitan Areas.* Washington, DC: Office of Management and Budget; 1992. OMB Bulletin No. 93-05.

Murdock Data References

1. Murdock S. Unpublished Calculations Derived from the U.S. Census of Population and Housing for the Years Indicated. Washington, DC: U.S. Bureau of the Census; 2003.

2. US Bureau of the Census [Web site]. State estimates by demographic characteristics—single year of age, sex, race, and Hispanic origin. 2003. Available at: http://eire.census.gov/popest/data/states/files/STCH-6R.txt. Accessed February 9, 2004.

Chapter 43 O'Hare/Changes in the Well-being of Children

1. The Annie E. Casey Foundation. *2003 Kids Count Data Book.* Baltimore: The Annie E. Casey Foundation; 2003.

2. Proctor BD, Dalaker J. *Current Population Reports.* Poverty in the United States: 2002. Table A-2. Washington, DC: US Bureau of the Census; 2003. Series P60-222.

3. Land KC, Lamb VL, Mustillo SK. Child and youth well-being in the United States, 1975-1998: some findings from a new index. *Soc Indicators Res.* 2001;56:241-320.

4. Federal Interagency Forum on Child and Family Statistics [Web site]. America's children: key national indicators of well-being, 2002. Available at: http://www.nichd.nih.gov/publications/pubs/childstats/report2002.pdf. Accessed May 25, 2004.

5. Jamieson A, Curry A, Martinez G. *Current Population Reports.* School Enrollment in the United States—Social and Economic Characteristics of Students. Washington, DC: US Bureau of the Census; 2001. Series P20-533.

6. Fields J. *Current Population Reports.* Children's Living Arrangements and Characteristics: March 2002. Washington, DC: US Bureau of the Census; 2003. Series P20-547. Available at: http://www.census.gov/prod/2003pubs/p20-547.pdf. Accessed January 22, 2004.

7. US Department of Labor [Web site]. US Bureau of Labor Statistics. 2003. Available at: http://data.bls.gov/servlet/SurveyOutputServlet?data_tool=latest_numbers&series_id=LNS14000000. Accessed May, 2003.

8. DeNavas-Walt C, Cleveland RW, Webster BH, Jr. *Current Population Reports.* Money Income in the United States: 2002. Table A-1. Washington, DC: US Bureau of the Census; 2003. Series P60-221.

9. Jargowsky PA. *Stunning Progress, Hidden Problems: Dramatic Decline of Concentrated Poverty in the 1990s.* Washington, DC: Center on Urban and Metropolitan Policy, Brookings Institution; 2003.

10. O'Hare W, Mather M. *The Growing Number of Kids in Severely Distressed Neighborhoods: Evidence from the 2000 Census.* A KIDS COUNT/PRB Report. Washington, DC: Population Reference Bureau; 2003.

11. Harknett K, Garfinkel I, Bainbridge J, Smeeding T, Folbre N, McLanahan S. *Do Public Expenditures Improve Child Outcomes in the U.S.: A Comparison Across Fifty States.* Princeton, NJ; Princeton University; 2003.Working Paper No. 03-02.

12. Tax Policy Center [Web site]. EITC recipients 1975-2000. 2003. Available at: http://www.taxpolicycenter.org/TaxFacts/lowincome/eitc_recipients.cfm. Accessed May, 2003.

13. Duncan GJ, Yeung WJ, Brooks-Gunn J, Smith JR. How much does childhood poverty affect the life chances of children? *Am Sociol Rev.* 1998;63:406-423.

14. Mezey J. *Threatened Progress: U.S. in Danger of Losing Ground on Child Care for Low-Income Working Families.* Washington, DC: Childcare and Early Education Series; 2003. Brief No. 2.

15. The Kaiser Commission on Medicaid and the Uninsured. SCHIP program enrollment, June 2003 update [Kaiser Family Foundation Web site]. December, 2003. Available at: http://www.kff.org/medicaid/loader.cfm?url=/commonspot/security/getfile.cfm&pageID=28327. Accessed February 24, 2004.

16. The Urban Institute. *Protecting Vulnerable Children: Changes in State Financing of Child Welfare Services, 1998-2000.* Assessing the New Federalism. Washington, DC: The Urban Institute; 2003.

17. O'Hare W, Annie E. Casey Foundation. Author Calculations based on Kids Count data, 1990-2000. Baltimore, MD: Annie E. Casey Foundation; 2003.

18. Walsh MW. I.R.S. to ask working poor for proof on tax credits [*New York Times* Web site]. April 25, 2003. Available at: http://query.nytimes.com/gst/abstract.html?res=FB061EFB3C590C768EDDAD0894DB404482. Accessed February 12, 2004.

19. US General Accounting Office. *Child Care: Recent State Policy Changes Affecting the Availability of Assistance for Low-Income Families.* Washington, DC: US General Accounting Office; 2003:GAO-03-588.

20. Richer E, Rahmanou H, Greenberg M. Welfare caseloads increase in most states in fourth quarter [The Center for Law and Social Policy Web site]. April 29, 2003. Available at: http://www.clasp.org/DMS/Documents/1049386524.1/caseload_2002_Q4.pdf. Accessed May, 2003.

21. Lippman L, Guzman L, Moore KA, O'Hare W. Public Perceptions of Children's Well-being. Paper presented at: The Annual Meeting of the American Association of Public Opinion Research., 2003; Nashville, TN.

O'Hare Data References

1. Area Resource File Health Resources and Services Administration. *Area Resource File.* Washington, DC: Department of Health and Human Services; 2003.

2. Centers for Disease Control and Prevention. Infant mortality and low birth weight among black and white infants—United States, 1980-2000. *MMWR Morb Mortal Wkly Rep.* 2002;51(27):589-592. Available at: http://www.cdc.gov/mmwr/preview/mmwrhtml/mm5127a1.htm. Accessed May 21, 2004.

3. Centers for Disease Control and Prevention (CDC). Compressed mortality data: underlying cause of death. [CDC Wonder database online]. 2003. Available at: http://wonder.cdc.gov/mortSQL.html. Accessed December, 2003.

4. Population Reference Bureau [Web site]. U.S. fertility rates higher among minorities. 2001. Available at: http://www.prb.org/Content/NavigationMenu/Ameristat/Topics1/RaceandEthnicity/a-RACE_FertilityRates1.xls. Accessed February 17, 2004.

5. The Annie E. Casey Foundation [Web site}. Children at risk: state trends 1990-2000 [Annie E. Casey Foundation Web site]. 2002. Available at: http://www.aecf.org/kidscount/c2ss/. Accessed February 18, 2004.

6. The Kaiser Commission on Medicaid and the Uninsured. SCHIP program enrollment, June 2003 Update [Kaiser Family Foundation Web site]. December, 2003. Available at: http://www.kff.org/medicaid/loader.cfm?url=/commonspot/security/getfile.cfm&pageID=28327. Accessed February 24, 2004.

7. US Bureau of the Census [Web site]. Poverty status of people by age, race, and Hispanic origin, 1959-2002 [Historic poverty tables]. Table 3. 2003. Available at: http://www.census.gov/hhes/poverty/histpov/hstpov3.html. Accessed January 25, 2004.

8. US Bureau of the Census [Web site]. Summary file 3. 2000. Available at: http://www.census.gov/main/www/cen2000.html. Accessed February 18, 2004.

9. US Bureau of the Census [Web site]. Summary file 3. 1990. Available at: http://www.census.gov/main/www/cen1990.html. Accessed February 18, 2004.

10. Ventura SJ, Mathews TJ, Hamilton BE. Teenage Births in the United States: State Trends, 1991-2000. National Vital Statistics Reports. Vital Statistics of the United States. 2000;50(9). Available at: http://www.cdc.gov/nchs/data/nvsr/nvsr50/nvsr50_09.pdf. Accessed February 17, 2004.

11. Ventura SJ, Mathews TJ, Hamilton BE. Births to teenagers in the United States, 1940-2000. National Vital Statistics Reports. Vital Statistics of the United States. 2001;49(10). Available at: http://www.cdc.gov/nchs/data/nvsr/nvsr49/nvsr49_10.pdf. Accessed February 17, 2004.

Chapter 44 Wise/Medical Progress and Inequities in Child Health

1. Engels F. *The Condition of the Working-Class in England in 1844.* 1887. Reprint, Moscow: Progress; 1973.

2. Smedley BD, Stith AY, Nelson A, eds. *Unequal Treatment: Confronting Racial and Ethnic Disparities in Health Care.* Washington, DC: National Academy of Sciences Press; 2003.

3. Wise PH. The Anatomy of a Disparity in Infant Mortality. *Annu Rev Public Health.* 2003;24:114-136.

4. Lord W. *The Night Lives On.* New York: Morrow; 1986.

5. Hamvas A, Wise PH, Yang RK, Wampler NS, et al. The influence of the wider use of surfactant therapy on neonatal mortality among blacks and whites. *New Engl J Med.* 1996;334:1635-1640.

6. Nsiah-Jefferson L. 2001. Access to reproductive genetic services for low-income women and women of color. Fetal Diag Ther. 50(22):463-5.

7. Willinger M, Hoffman HJ, Wu KT, et al. Factors associated with the transition to nonprone sleep positions of infants in the United States: the National Infant Sleep Position Study. *JAMA.* 1998;280(4):329-335.

8. Flannery B, Schrag S, Bennett NM, et al. Impact of childhood vaccination on racial disparities in invasive Streptococcus pneumoniae infections. *JAMA.* 2004;291(18):2197-2203.

9. Rogers E.M. *The Diffusion of Innovations.* 2nd ed. New York: Free Press; 1983.

10. Sen A. Inequality Reexamined. Cambridge: Harvard University Press; 1992.

Wise Data References

1. Centers for Disease Control and Prevention. Infant mortality and low birth weight among black and white infants—United States, 1980-2000. *MMWR Morb Mortal Wkly Rep.* 2002;51(27):589-592. Available at: http://www.cdc.gov/mmwr/preview/mmwrhtml/mm5127a1.htm. Accessed May 21, 2004.

2. Guyer B, Johns Hopkins Bloomberg School of Public Health. Unpublished tabulations, 1900 to 1998 [Childhood mortality rates by age]. Washington, DC: National Center for Health Statistics; 2003.

3. Guyer B, Johns Hopkins Bloomberg School of Public Health. Published and Unpublished Calculations from National Vital Statistics Data, 1900 to 1998. Washington, DC: National Center for Health Statistics; 2003.

4. Murphy SL. *Vital Statistics of the United States.* Deaths: Final Data for 1998. Hyattsville, MD: National Center for Health Statistics; 2000:48(11).

5. Federal Interagency Forum on Child and Family Statistics. America's children: key national indicators of well-being, 2002. [Web site]. Available at: http://www.nichd.nih.gov/publications/pubs/childstats/report2002.pdf. Accessed May 13, 2004.

Chapter 45 McCabe & McCabe/Genetics

1. Cavalli-Sforza LL. *Genes, Peoples and Languages.* Berkeley: University of California Press; 2001.

2. Dipple KM, Phelan JK, McCabe ERB. Consequences of complexity within biological networks: robustness and health, or vulnerability and disease. *Mol Genetics Metab.* 2001;74:45-50.

3. Holve S, Hu D, McCandless SE. Metachromatic leukodystrophy in the Navajo: fallout of the American-Indian wars of the nineteenth century. *Am J Med Genetics.* 2003;101:203-208.

4. Khoury MJ, McCabe LL, McCabe ERB. Genomic medicine: population screening in the age of genomic medicine. *N Engl J Med.* 2003;348:50-58.

5. Leroy Hood. Quote at BIO (Biotechnology Industry Organization). 2003. Available at: www.futurepundit.com. Accessed May 13, 2004.

6. McCabe LL, McCabe ERB. Populations studies of allele frequencies in single gene disorders: methodologic and policy considerations. *Epidemiol Rev.* 1997;19:52-56.

7. Newborn Screening Task Force Report. Serving the family from birth to the medical home: a report from the Newborn Screening Task Force. *Pediatrics.* 2000;106S:383-427.

8. The National Human Genome Research Institute [Web site]. 2004. Available at: http://www.genome.gov. Accessed May 13, 2004.

9. Watson JD, Crick FHC. Molecular structure of nucleic acids: a structure for deoxyribose nucleic acid. *Nature.* 1953;171:737-738.

Chapter 46 Palfrey & Richmond/Health Services: Past, Present, and Future

1. Richmond JB. Child development: A basic science for pediatrics. *Pediatrics.* 1969;39:649-658.

2. US Bureau of the Census. *Historical Statistics of the United States. Colonial Times to 1970, Part 1.* Infant Mortality Rate for Massachusetts: 1851 to 1970. Washington DC; 1975. Series B 148.

3. Parmelee AH. Isaac Arthur Abt. In: Veeder BS, ed. *Pediatric Profiles.* St. Louis: C.V. Mosby Company; 1957:111.

4. Markel H. For the welfare of children. In: Stern AM, Markel H, eds. *Formative Years. Children's Health in the United States, 1880-2000*: University of Michigan Press; 2002:47-65.

5. Richmond JB. The Hull House Era. *Am J Orthopsychiatry*. 1995;65:10-20.

6. Follis RH. *The Pathology of Nutritional Disease*. Springfield, Illinois: Charles C. Thomas, Limited; 1948.

7. Fein R. *Medical Care, Medical Costs*. Cambridge, Massachusetts: Harvard University Press; 1986.

8. Hutchins VL, Hutchins JE. Public sector health services for children with special health care needs. In: Wallace HM, MacQueen JC, Biehl RF, Blackman JA, Saidoff DC, eds. *Mosby's Resource Guide to Children with Disabilities and Chronic Illness*: Mosby, Incorporated; 1996.

9. Taussig HB. *Congenital Malformations of the Heart*. New York: Commonwealth Fund; 1947.

10. American Board of Pediatrics.Certifying physicians for infants, children & adolescents. [Web site]. 2003. Available at: http://www.abp.org/abpfr.htm. Accessed January 15, 2004.

11. Baker JP. Technology in the nursery: incubators, ventilators and the rescue of premature infants. In: Stern AM, Markel H, eds. *Formative Years. Children's Health in the United States, 1880-2000*: University of Michigan Press; 2002:66-90.

12. Haggerty RJ, Roghmann KL, Pless IB, eds. *Child Health and the Community*. New York: John Wiley and Sons; 1975.

13. US Bureau of the Census. *Historical Statistics of the United States. Colonial Times to 1970, Part 1*. Birth rate total and for women 15-44 years old by race: 1800 to 1970. Washington DC: 1975. Series B 5-10.

14. US Bureau of the Census. *Statistical Abstracts of the United States: 2002*. Birth rates by live birth order and race: 1980 to 2000, Washington DC: US Bureau of the Census; 2001.73:62.

15. US Bureau of the Census. *Census 2000 Special Reports, Series CENSR-4. Demographic Trends in the 20th Century*. Washington, DC: US Bureau of the Census; 2000. Figure 2-3. 55.

16. Richmond JB, Stipek DJ, Zigler E. A decade of Head Start. In: Zigler E, Valentine J, ed. *Project Head Start: A Legacy of the War on Poverty*. New York: Free Press; 1979:35-152.

17. Office for Special Education and Rehabilitation Services. IDEA '97, the law [US Dept of Education Web site]. 1997. Available at: http://www.ed.gov/offices/OSERS/Policy/IDEA/the_law.html. Accessed January 24, 2004.

18. Smith PJ, Mathews KS, Hehir T, Palfrey JS. Educating children with disabilities: how pediatricians can help. *Contemp Pediatr*. 2000;9:102.

19. Zuckerman B, Frank DA, Hingson R, et al. Effects of maternal marijuana and cocaine use on fetal growth. *N Engl J Med*. 1989;320:762-758.

20. Prothrow-Stith D. *Deadly Consequences*. New York: Harper Collins; 1991.

21. Centers for Disease Control and Prevention. MMWR *Morb Mortal Wkly Rep*. [Centers for Disease Control and Prevention Web site] June 5, 1981. Available at http://www.cdc.gov/mmwr/preview/mmwrhtml/00043494.htm. Accessed May 14, 2004.

22. Robbins KE, Lemey P, Pybus OG, et al. US human immunodeficiency virus type 1 epidemic: date of origin, population history and characteristics of early strains. *J Virology*. 2003;77:6359-6366.

23. Kryder-Coe JH, Salamon LM, Molnar JM, eds. *Homeless Children and Youth: A New American Dilemma*. New Brunswick: Transaction Publishers; 1992.

24. Starfield B. Effects of poverty on health status. *Bull NY Acad Med*. 1992;68:17-24.

25. Palfrey JS, Walker D, Haynie M, et al. Technology's children: report of a statewide census of children dependent on medical supports. *Pediatrics*. 1991;87:611-618.

26. International Human Genome Consortium. Initial sequencing and analysis of the human genome. *Nature*. 2001;409:860-921.

27. Gortmaker SL, Must A, Sobol AM, Peterson K, Colditz GA, Dietz W. Television viewing as a cause of increasing obesity in the United States, 1986-1990. *Arch Pediatr Adolesc Med*. 1996;150:356-362.

28. Andrist LC. Media images, body dissatisfaction, and disordered eating in adolescent women. *Am J Mat Child Nurs*. 2003;28:119-123.

29. Fegusson D, Swain-Campbell N, Horwood J. Risky driving behavior: prevalence, personal characteristics and traffic accidents. *Aust N Z J Public Health*. 2003;27:337-342.

30. Hobbs F, Stoops, N. US Bureau of the Census. *Demographic Trends in the 20th Century*. Washington, DC: US Bureau of the Census; 2000. Census 2000 Special Reports, Series CENSR-4.Figure 5-17. 163.

31. Mrazek PJ, Haggerty RJ. *Reducing Risks for Mental Disorders, Report of the Committee on the Prevention of Mental Disorders of the Institute of Medicine*. Washington DC: National Academy Press; 1994.

32. US Bureau of the Census. *Statistical Abstracts of the United States 2002*. Immigration 1901 to 2000, Washington DC: US Bureau of the Census; 2001. No. 5:10.

33. Bass JL, Mehta KA, Eppes B. Parasitology screening of Latin American children in a primary care clinic. *Pediatrics*. 1992;89:279-283.

34. Enserink M. Breakthrough of the year. SARS: a pandemic prevented. *Science*. 2003;302:2045.

35. Fazel M, Stein A. The mental health of refugee children. *Arch Dis Child*. 2003;88:365-366.

36. Blaschke GS, Lynch J. Terrorism: its impact on pediatrics. *Pediatr Ann*. 2003;32(2,3,4).

37. Smedley BD, Stith AY, Nelson AR. *Unequal Treatment. Confronting Racial and Ethnic Disparities in Health Care*. Washington, DC: National Academies Press; 2003.

38. Centers for Disease Control and Prevention. *National Vital Statistics Report*. Deaths and death rates for the 10 leading causes of death in specified age groups: United States, preliminary 2000. Table 7. Washington, DC: Centers for Disease Control and Prevention. 2001;49(12):25.

39. March of Dimes. International comparisons of infant mortality rates, 1998 [March of Dimes Web site]. August 2002. Available at http://www.marchofdimes.com/files/international_rankings_1998.pdf. Accessed May 17, 2004.

40. National Center for Health Statistics. Infant deaths/mortality [Centers for Disease Control and Prevention Web site]. March 03, 2004. Available at: http://www.cdc.gov/nchs/fastats/infmort.htm. Accessed July 9, 2003.

41. Maternal and Child Health Bureau. *Child Health USA; 2002*. US Dept of Health and Human Services. [Health Resources and Services Administration Web site]. Available at http://www.ask.hrsa.gov/detail.cfm?id=MCH00066. Accessed May 14, 2004.

42. Centers for Disease Control and Prevention. Births: final data for 2000. *National Vital Statistics Reports* [Web site]. February 12, 2002. Available at: http://www.cdc.gov/nchs/data/nvsr/nvsr50/nvsr50_05.pdf. Accessed March 23, 2004.

43. American Academy of Pediatrics. Task force on infant sleep position and sudden infant death syndrome. Changing concepts of sudden infant death syndrome: implications for infant sleeping environment and sleep position [Web site]. March 2000. Available at: http://pediatrics.aappublications.org/cgi/content/full/105/3/650. Accessed March 23, 2004.

44. Office of Technology Assessment. Infant mortality [Woodrow Wilson School of Public and International Affairs Web site]. 1994. Available at: http://www.wws.princeton.edu/cgi-bin/byteserve.pr1/~ota/disk1/1994/9418/ (941806. PDF). Accessed February 1, 2004.

45. Deal LW, Gomby DS, Zippiroli L, Behrman RE. Unintentional injuries in childhood: analysis and recommendations. *Future of Child*. Spring/Summer 2000;10(1):4-22.

46. Connor EM, Sperling RS, Gelber R, et al. Reduction of maternal infant transmission of human immunodeficiency virus type 1 with zidovudine treatment. *N Engl J Med*. 1994;331:1173-1179.

47. Centers for Disease Control and Prevention. Profile of the nation's health. Major causes of mortality among 15-24 year olds. *CDC Fact Book 2000/2001*. Washington, DC: Dept of Health and Human Services; 2000:21.

48. Anne E. Casey Foundation. *KIDS COUNT*. Baltimore, MD: Annie E. Casey Foundation; 2003.

49. Centers for Disease Control and Prevention. Profile of the nation's health. Baseline 20th century annual morbidity and 1999 provisional morbidity from nine diseases with vaccines recommended before 1990 for universal use in children - United States. *CDC Fact Book 2000/2001*. Washington, DC: Dept of Health and Human Services; 2000:13.

50. Baskin MN, O'Rourke EJ, Fleisher GR. Outpatient treatment of febrile infants 28 to 89 days of age with intramuscularly administration of ceftriaxone. *Pediatrics.* 1992;121(5 Pt. 1):831-833.

51. Wise PH. Clinical innovation, social change and the dichotomization of pediatrics. Paper presented at: The Future of Education in Pediatrics Conference, the American Academy of Pediatrics and the Josiah Macy Foundation, June 2003; Half Moon Bay, Ca.

52. Whitney CG, Farley MM, Hadler J, et al. Increasing prevalence of multidrug-resistant streptococcus pneumoniae in the United States. *N Engl J Med.* 2000;343(26):1961-1963.

53. Auinger P, Lamphear BP, Kalkwarf HJ, Mansour ME. Trends in otitis media among children in the United States. *Pediatrics.* 2003;112(3 Pt 1):514-520.

54. Dowell SF, Marcy SM, Phillips WR, Gerber MA, Schwartz B. Principles of judicious use of microbial agents for pediatric upper respiratory tract infections. *Pediatrics.* 1998;101:163-165.

55. National Center for Health Statistics. National survey of children with special health care needs [Centers for Disease Control and Prevention Web site]. January 28, 2004. Available at: www.cdc.gov/nchs/about/major/slaits/cshcn.htm. Accessed February 1, 2004.

56. Blumberg SJ. Comparing states using survey data on health care services for children with special health care needs (CSHCN) [Centers for Disease Control and Prevention Web site]. December 12, 2003. Available at: http://www.cdc.gov/nchs/data/slaits/Comparing_States_CSHCNA.pdf. Accessed February 1, 2004.

57. National Center for Medical Home Initiatives for Children with Special Needs, American Academy of Pediatrics. National survey on children with special health care needs [American Academy of Pediatrics Web site]. February 6, 2004. Available at: http://www.medicalhomeinfo.org/about/cshcn.html. Accessed February 1, 2004.

58. McPherson M, Arango P, Fox H, et al. A new definition of children with special health care needs. *Pediatrics.* 1998;102(1 Pt 1):117-123.

59. Newacheck PW, Halfon N. Prevalence and impact of disabling chronic conditions in childhood. *Am J Public Health.* 1998;88(4):610-617.

60. Newacheck PW, Strickland B, Shonkoff JP, et al. An epidemiologic profile of children with special health care needs. *Pediatrics.* 1998;102(1 Pt 1):117-123.

61. Kuhlthau K, Perrin JM, Ettner SL, McLaughlin TJ, Gortmaker SL. High-expenditure children with supplemental security insurance income. *Pediatrics.* 1998;102(3 Pt 1):610-615.

62. Ireys HT, Henderson GF, Shaffer TJ, Neff TM. Expenditures for the care of children with chronic illnesses enrolled in the Washington State Medicaid program, fiscal year 1993. *Pediatrics.* 1997;100:197-204.

63. Liou TG, Adler FR, Fitzsimmons SC, Cahill BC, Hibbs JR, Marshall BC. Predictive 5-year survivorship model of cystic fibrosis. *Am J Epidemiol.* 2001;153(4):345-352.

64. Reisman J, Corey M, Canny G, Levison H. Diabetes mellitus in patients with cystic fibrosis: effect on survival. *Pediatrics.* 1990;86(3):374-377.

65. Englund M, Berg U, Tyden G. A longitudinal study of children who received renal transplants 10-20 years ago. *Transplantation.* 2003;76(2):311-318.

66. Smith M, McCaffrey R, Karl J. The secondary leukemias: challenges and research directions. *J Natl Cancer Inst.* 1996;88(7):407-418.

67. Ogden CL, Flegal KM, Carroll MD, Johnson CL. Prevalence and trends in overweight among US children and adolescents, 1999-2000. Table 4. Trends in Overweight for Children Birth Through 19 Years by Sex and Age Group (based on NHANES data). *JAMA.* 2002;288(14):1731.

68. Aye T, Levitsky LL. Type 2 diabetes: an epidemic disease in childhood. *Curr Opin Pediatr.* 2003;15:411-415.

69. Brown RT, Freeman WS, Perrin JM, et al. Prevalence and assessment of attention-deficit/hyperactivity disorder in primary care settings. *Pediatrics.* 2001;107(3):E43.

70. Ferris TG, Saglam D, Stafford R, et al. Changes in the daily practice of primary care for children. *Arch Pediatr Adolesc Med.* 1998;152::227-233.

71. Barbaresi WJ, Katusic SK, Colligan RC, et al. How common is attention-deficit/hyperactivity disorder? Incidence in a population-based birth cohort in Rochester, Minnesota. *Arch Pediatr Adolesc Med.* 2002;156:217-224.

72. Wolraich ML, Lindgren S, Stromquist A, Milich R, Davis C, Watson D. Stimulant medication use by primary care physicians in the treatment of attention deficit hyperactivity disorder. *Pediatrics.* 1990;86(1):95-101.

73. Robinson LM, Skaer TL, Sclar DA, Gallin RS. Is attention deficit hyperactivity disorder increasing among girls in the US? Trends in the diagnosis and the prescribing of stimulants. *CNS Drugs.* 2002;16(2):129-137.

74. Ris MD, Dietrich KN, Succop PA, Berger OG, Bornschein RL. Early exposure to lead and neuropsychological outcome in adolescence. *J Int Neuropsychol Soc.* 2004;10(2):261-270.

75. Stein J, Schettler T, Wallinga D, Valenti M. In harm's way: toxic threats to child development. *J Dev Behav Pediatr.* 2002;23(Suppl 1):S13-22.

76. Yeargin-Allsopp M, Rice C, Karapurkar T, Doernberg N, Boyle C, Murphy C. Prevalence of autism in a US metropolitan area. *JAMA.* 2003;289(1):49-55.

77. Bryson SE, Smith IM. Epidemiology of autism: prevalence, associated characteristics, and service delivery. *Ment Retard Dev Disabilities Res Rev.* 1998;4:97-103.

78. DeStefano F, Thompson WW. MMR vaccine and autism: an update on the scientific evidence. *Expert Rev Vaccines.* 2004;3(1):19-22.

79. Centers for Disease Control and Prevention. *National Vital Statistics Reports*; Infant mortality statistics from the 2000 period linked birth/infant death data set [Web site]. 2002. Available at http://www.cdc.gov/nchs/data/NVSR50/NVSR50_12.pdf. Accessed May 17, 2004.

80. Centers for Disease Control and Prevention. Division of HIV/AIDS Prevention. Young people at risk. HIV/AIDS among American youth [Web site]. March 11, 2002. Available at: http://www.cdc.gov/hiv/pubs/facts/youth.htm. Accessed February 1, 2004.

81. National Public Service Research Institute and National SAFE KIDS Campaign. Childhood injury: cost and prevention facts [Paraquad Web site]. 2003. Available at: http://www.paraquad.org/chldinj.htm. Accessed February 1, 2004.

82. National Public Service Research Institute and National SAFE KIDS Campaign. Estimated life expectancy of newborns by year of birth, race and gender. Selected years 1970-2001 [Child Trends Data Bank Web site]. 2002. Available at: http://www.childtrendsdatabank.org/figures/78-Figure-2.gif. Accessed February 1, 2004.

83. US Department of Health and Human Services. Healthy People 2010, Goals for the Nation [US Dept of Health and Human Services Web site]. 2000. Available at: http://www.healthypeople.gov/. Accessed March 6, 2004.

84. Olds DL, Eckenrode J, Henderson CR, et al. Long-term effects of home visitation on maternal life course and child abuse and neglect: fifteen-year follow-up of a randomized trial. *JAMA.* 1997;278(8):637-643.

85. Kitzman H, Olds DL, Henderson CR. Effect of prenatal and infancy home visitation by nurses on pregnancy outcomes, childhood injuries, and repeated childbearing: a randomized controlled trial. *JAMA.* 1997;278(8):644-652.

86. Karoly LA, Everingham SS, Hoube J, et al. *Benefits and Costs of Early Childhood Interventions: A Documented Briefing.* Santa Monica, CA: RAND; 1997.

87. Minkovitz CS, Hughart N, Strobino D, et al. A practice-based intervention to enhance quality of care in the first 3 years of life: the Healthy Steps for Young Children Program. *JAMA.* 2003;290(23):3081-3091.

88. Evans D, Mellins R, Lobach K, et al. Improving care for minority children with asthma: professional education in the public health clinic. *Pediatrics.* 1997;99(2):157-164.

89. Hymel MS, Greenberg BL. The Walden House young adult HIV project: meeting the needs of multidiagnosed youth. *J Adolesc Health.* 1998;23(Suppl 2):122-131.

90. Laraque D, Barlow B, Durkin M, Heagarty M. Injury prevention in an urban setting: challenges and successes. *Bull NY Acad Med.* 1995;72(1):16–30.

91. Yudkowsky B, Tang S. *Fact Sheet: Children's health insurance and Medicaid.* Division of Health Policy Research. American Academy of Pediatrics; 2003.

92. Elixhauser A, Machlin SR, Zodet MW, et al. Health care for children and youth in the United States: 2001 Annual Report on Access, Utilization, Quality, and Expenditures. *Ambulatory Pediatr*;2:419-437.

93. Green M, Palfrey JS, eds. *Bright Futures*. Washington DC: National Center for Education in Maternal and Child Health; 2000.

94. US Department of Health and Human Services, Health Resources and Services Administration, *All Aboard the 2010 Express: A 10-Year Action Plan to Achieve Community-Based Services Systems for Children and Youth with Special Health Care Needs and Their Families*. Washington, DC: Maternal and Child Health Bureau; 2001.

95. National Initiatives for Children's Healthcare Quality. Children deserve better care. NICHQ's goal is to make sure that they get it. [Web site]. 2003. Available at: www.nichq.org. Accessed March 6, 2004.

96. Palfrey JS, Sofis L, , Davidson E, Liu J, Freeman L, Ganz M. The pediatric alliance for coordinated care: evaluation of a medical home model. *Pediatrics*. 2004;113:1507-1516.

97. Satcher D. Closing the Gap [US Dept of Health and Human Services Web site]. September 16, 2003. Available at: www.healthgap.omhrc.gov. Accessed March 6, 2004.

98. Brunk D. Black-white gap in pneumococcal disease closing. *Pediatr News*. 2003;37:1,7.

Palfrey & Richmond Data References

1. Minino A, Smith B. *National Vital Statistics Report*. Deaths: Preliminary Data for 2000. Washington, DC: Centers for Disease Control and Prevention. 2001. Available at: http://www.cdc.gov/nchs/data/nvsr/nvsr49/nvsr49_12.pdf. Accessed on April 14, 2004.

Map Boundary File References

1. Environmental Systems Research Institute, Inc. (ESRI). U.S. States. Redlands, CA: ESRI; 2002.

2. Environmental Systems Research Institute, Inc. (ESRI). U.S. Counties. Redlands, CA: ESRI; 2002.

3. Environmental Systems Research Institute, Inc. (ESRI). U.S. States (Generalized). Redlands, CA: ESRI; 2002.

4. Environmental Systems Research Institute, Inc. (ESRI). U.S. Counties (Generalized). Redlands, CA: ESRI; 2002.

Photography Credits:

Internet Resources*

General Resources

1. Administration for Children & Families (ACF)
   www.acf.dhhs.gov
   An agency of the U.S. Department of Health & Human Services, the ACF funds programs such as family assistance, child support, child care, Head Start, and child welfare. Their Web site contains legislation, policy, publications, research, and statistics about the many topics the ACF encompasses. There are also answers to frequently asked questions and links to related agencies.

2. American Academy of Pediatrics (AAP)
   www.aap.org
   The AAP is the primary professional organization for pediatricians. Their Web site provides access to a wealth of information for professionals, parents, and anyone interested in the health of children. There are sections devoted to advocacy, research, family, professional education, and publications. There are also policy statements on many of the topics covered in this book located at http://aappolicy.aappublications.org.

3. American Public Health Association (APHA)
   www.apha.org
   The APHA is an organization of public health professionals. The APHA Web site has information about the association, recent news information, policy and advocacy information, and a listing of available books and journals.

4. Annie E. Casey Foundation (AECF)
   www.aecf.org
   The ACEF works to enhance the lives of disadvantaged children and their families by fostering public policies, human service reforms, and community supports. The foundation has programs, information, and resources on a wide array of topics including urban issues, education, mental health, and policy trends.

5. Child Trends DataBank
   www.childtrendsdatabank.org
   Child Trends is a nonprofit, nonpartisan children's research organization. Their databank provides access to research on key indicators of child and youth well-being. General areas in which research is available include health; social and emotional development; income, assets, and work; education and skills; demographics; and family and community.

6. Child Welfare League of America (CWLA)
   www.cwla.org
   CWLA is a membership-based organization dedicated to the well-being of children, youth, and their families. The Web site contains research, state and national facts, and information on topics including advocacy, child well-being, behavioral health, and juvenile justice.

7. Children's Defense Fund
   www.childrensdefense.org
   The Children's Defense Fund is a private, nonprofit organization devoted to children, with a particular interest in harm prevention and in poor, minority, or disabled children. Their Web site provides research reports and information on a host of children's issues including health, child care and Head Start, poverty, abuse, violence, and moral development.

8. The Commonwealth Fund
   www.cmwf.org
   The Commonwealth Fund is a private foundation that provides grants to improve health care practice and policy, and it supports independent research on health and social issues. Their Web site contains publications on a number of health and social issues including minority health, health insurance and the uninsured, child development and preventive care, Medicaid, and quality of care for underserved populations.

* Internet resources are provided to guide the reader pursuing further information about the topics covered in the *About Children*. This list is by no means exhaustive, and no criticism is implied of those not included. Inclusion on this list does not constitute an endorsement of these organizations or their programs by the Social Science Research Center at Mississippi State University, the Center for Child Health Research at the University of Rochester, the American Academy of Pediatrics, or any of the chapter authors, and none should be inferred. We do not take responsibility for the content of these Web sites.

9. Connect for Kids
www.connectforkids.org
Connect for Kids aims to provide meaningful information and solutions-oriented coverage of critical issues for children and families. The Web site has a weekly newsletter, an extensive information section arranged alphabetically, state information, and a searchable database of organizations working for children and families.

10. Federal Interagency Forum on Child and Family Statistics
www.childstats.gov
The Forum was set up by the Federal Office of Management and Budget and has both government and private members. Access to their annual report of the well-being of children and links to national and international data on children and families are available on the Web site.

11. Healthy People 2010
www.healthypeople.gov
Managed by the Office of Disease Prevention and Health Promotion of the U.S. Department of Health and Human Services, Healthy People 2010 identifies preventable threats to the health of Americans and sets national goals for reduction of those threats. The Web site provides access to Healthy People 2010 publications and data, information on how to make healthy choices, and a searchable database of health information.

12. KIDS COUNT
www.kidscount.org
KIDS COUNT is a project of the Annie E. Casey Foundation that tracks the status of U.S. children on the national as well as state level. Numerous publications are available, as is access to an interactive, online database.

13. The National Center for Health Statistics (NCHS)
www.cdc.gov/nchs
A division of the Centers for Disease Control and Prevention, the NCHS is the primary federal health statistics agency. Their Web site provides information about and access to numerous national surveys, including the National Health and Nutrition Examination Survey (NHANES). It also provides statistics and fact sheets on a range of health topics.

14. National Center for Youth Law
www.youthlaw.org
This private, nonprofit law office focuses on the legal needs of children and families. Extensive information, analyses, and links to state and federal governments, public policy organizations, and legislative resources can be found on this Web site.

15. U.S. Census Bureau
www.census.gov
The U.S. Census Bureau, a division of the U.S. Department of Commerce, is an excellent resource for census statistics. Maps and tables present information from Census 2000 as well as from numerous estimates and projections. Two helpful features include *American FactFinder* and *State & County QuickFacts*.

16. Zero to Three
www.zerotothree.org
Zero to Three is a research-based, nonpartisan, nonprofit national organization devoted to promoting healthy development for children in the first 3 years of life. Their Web site has sections for parents and professionals. There are parenting tips, fact sheets, policy initiatives, and partial access to a journal about early child development.

Part One: About Their Environments

Childhood "Affluenza"

1.1 Affluenza: PBS Program on the Epidemic of Overconsumption
www.pbs.org/kcts/affluenza
PBS Web site companion for the hour-long television special, *Affluenza*. This site has information about the show, an interactive quiz, a teacher's guide, a list of resources, and suggestions for simplifying your life.

1.2 Consumer Jungle
www.consumerjungle.org
Consumer Jungle, sponsored by the nonprofit organization Young Adult Consumer is a Web site targeting young adults with the goal of promoting consumer literacy. The Web site covers topics including appropriate credit card use, personal finance, and e-commerce fraud. There are a number of interactive activities as well as a large list of relevant resources.

1.3 PBS Kids: Don't Buy It, Get Media Smart
www.pbskids.org/dontbuyit
Funded by the Corporation for Public Broadcasting, this Web site on media awareness is geared toward children and adolescents. There are also sections for parents and teachers with information and suggestions for family activities and classroom lessons.

Advertising in Schools

2.1 Commercialism in Education Research Unit (CERU)
www.asu.edu/educ/epsl/ceru.htm
Located at the Education Policy Studies Laboratory of Arizona State University, CERU is a national academic research unit devoted to commercial activities in schools. The Web site provides information about CERU, publications by CERU staff and others, resources such as guidelines and legislation, and useful links.

2.2 Children Now: Children & the Media
www.childrennow.org/media/index.html
Children Now is an independent, nonpartisan research and action organization. The Children & the Media Program works to improve media for children and children's issues. It focuses largely on media images of race, class, and gender. The Web site provides articles, news briefs, a newsletter, and research reports.

2.3 Children Digital Media Center (CDMC)
www.digital-kids.net
As a consortium of universities founded by the National Science Foundation, the CDMC conducts research and disseminates information on the

impact of digital media on children. The Web site provides answers to frequently asked questions, publications, a media kit, and links to related Web sites. There are also links to the collaborating universities, whose Web sites contain further information including fact sheets, access to reports, and information about ongoing projects.

Interactive Media and Well-being

3.1 Children Digital Media Center
www.digital-kids.net   (See 2.3)

3.2 Children Go Online
www.children-go-online.net
Children Go Online is a project based in the Department of Media and Communications, London School of Economics and Political Science. They examine children's use of the Internet. The Web site provides information about the project, access to surveys used, and free reports.

3.3 Program for the Study of Entertainment Media and Health
www.kff.org/about/entmediastudies.cfm
As a program of the Henry J. Kaiser Family Foundation, the Program for the Study of Entertainment Media and Health conducts research, evaluations, and analyses on the effect of media on the public's health. The Web site has information on children and the media as well as access to relevant publications.

Children and Media

4.1 Children Now: Children & the Media
www.childrennow.org/media/index.html   (See 2.2)

4.2 Children Digital Media Center
www.digital-kids.net   (See 2.3)

4.3 Entertainment Industries Council, Inc. (EIC)
www.eiconline.org
The EIC is a nonprofit organization founded by entertainment industry leaders. Activities include work to promote accurate representations of social and health issues within entertainment. The Web site has sections devoted to media depiction of topics such as mental health and suicide; drugs, alcohol, and tobacco; HIV and AIDS; and conflict resolution.

4.4 Program for the Study of Entertainment Media and Health
www.kff.org/about/entmediastudies.cfm   (See 3.3)

4.5 Smoke Free Movies
www.smokefreemovies.ucsf.edu
Smoke Free Movies is a project of Stanton A. Glantz, PhD, professor of medicine at the University of California, San Francisco. The project's goal is to decrease the use of the U.S. film industry as a mechanism for tobacco marketing.

Violence in the Lives of Children

5.1 Harvard Youth Violence Center (HYVPC)
www.hsph.harvard.edu/hicrc/prevention.html
HYVPC is an interdisciplinary center located within the department of Health Policy and Management at the Harvard School of Public Health. HYVPC

partners with community-based organizations with the goal of advancing violence prevention science. The Center conducts research, training, and surveillance of youth violence and violence outcomes. The Web site provides publications, information about research, access to the National Violent Injury Statistics Program, and links to other Web-based resources.

5.2 National Institute of Mental Health (NIMH): Children and Violence
www.nimh.nih.gov/HealthInformation/violencemenu.cfm
The NIMH is a section of the National Institutes of Health, the Federal government's main biomedical and behavioral research agency. This section of the Web site provides booklets, fact sheets, and summaries on topics related to children and violence.

5.3 National Center for Children Exposed to Violence (NCCEV)
www.nccev.org
The U.S. Department of Justice, Office of Juvenile Justice and Delinquency Program established the NCCEV, located at the Yale Child Study Center. The Web site provides statistics on violence and children, signs and symptoms of violence exposure in children, publications, presentations, and an online library.

5.4 National Youth Violence Prevention Resource Center (NYVPRC)
www.safeyouth.org/scripts/index.asp
The NYVPRC, a partnership of the Centers for Disease Control and Prevention and ten other federal agencies, is a source for information on violence committed by and against youth. The Web site provides links to information developed by both federal agencies and private sector organizations for professionals, parents, and teens.

Children in a Post-9/11 World

6.1 Children, Terrorism, and Disasters, American Academy of Pediatrics (AAP)
www.aap.org/terrorism/index.html
This is a Web site created by the AAP's Task Force on Terrorism. This Web site covers a wide range of information, from biological and chemical agents to psychosocial aspects of terrorism and disasters. There is information for teachers, parents, and community planners, links to other helpful Web sites, and access to journal articles and reports.

6.2 Disaster Response, American Academy of Child and Adolescent Psychiatry (AACAP)
www.aacap.org/publications/DisasterResponse/index.htm
This Web site is from the AACAP, a professional organization for child and adolescent psychiatrists. The Web site has advice to parents from the AACAP president, facts for families, and additional resources including books and reports.

6.3 National Center for Children Exposed to Violence (NCCEV)
www.nccev.org/violence/children_terrorism.htm
(See 5.3)

6.4　National Center for Disaster Preparedness (NCDP)
www.ncdp.mailman.columbia.edu
Based at Columbia University's Mailman School of Public Health, the NCDP is a resource for national and international terrorism and disaster readiness. The Center's Web site contains publications, public and professional resources, news releases, and information about the Center's different programs, including the Program for Pediatric Preparedness.

Children of Incarcerated Parents

7.1　Bureau of Justice Statistics, U.S. Department of Justice
www.ojp.usdoj.gov/bjs/welcome.html
This Web site provides statistics on the justice system, which includes corrections, prosecution, and law enforcement.

7.2　The Center for Children of Incarcerated Parents (CCIP)
www.e-ccip.org
Fees earned for services, government contracts, research contracts, and grants support the CCIP. The Web site provides access to their journal, descriptions of their programs and training opportunities, and a catalog of publications.

7.3　Federal Resource Center for Children of Prisoners
www.cwla.org/programs/incarcerated/cop_03.htm
The Child Welfare League of America in collaboration with the National Institute of Corrections, the American Correctional Association, and the National Council on Crime and Delinquency runs the Resource Center for Children of Prisoners. The Web site has answers to frequently asked questions, information about current activities, program descriptions, and statistics.

Urban Housing

8.1　American Housing Survey (AHS)
www.census.gov/hhes/www/ahs.html
Conducted by the U.S. Census Bureau for the Department of Housing, the AHS is an excellent source of data on American housing, including homes and apartments, household characteristics, housing and neighborhood quality, housing costs, size of housing units, and recent movers. The Web site provides access to survey methodology as well as national data and data from 47 metropolitan areas.

8.2　U.S. Census Bureau, Housing Information
www.census.gov/hhes/www/housing.html
A part of the larger U.S. Census Bureau Web site, this section provides information about housing affordability, housing vacancy, homeownership, and many other topics. There are also links to related sites for housing data.

8.3　U.S. Department of Housing and Urban Development (HUD)
www.hud.gov
This is an extensive Web site with recent HUD news, information about applying for HUD programs, access to local information about homes and communities, and other information for citizens and the housing industry. There is a resource section with answers to common questions, an online library, and numerous handbooks and forms.

Homelessness and Its Consequences

9.1　National Alliance to End Homelessness
www.naeh.org
This nonprofit organization provides state and local plans to end homelessness along with resources, information, publications and statistics about homelessness. The section devoted to ending youth homelessness has an overview of the problem, research reports, best practices profiles, and federal policy updates.

9.2　National Center for Homeless Education at SERVE
www.serve.org/nche/index.php
The National Center for Homeless Education is a part of SERVE, an educational organization associated with the University of North Carolina at Greensboro's School of Education. The Web site has information about relevant legislation, state and local resources, publications and documents, and information about the homeless—organized by topic.

9.3　National Law Center on Homelessness & Poverty
www.nlchp.org
This Web site has general information about housing, income, education, and civil rights, with a focus on relevance to homelessness. There is an overview of homelessness, along with press releases, publications, and reports.

Tobacco and Health

10.1　American Lung Association, Tobacco Control
www.lungusa.org/tobacco
The Tobacco Control section of the American Lung Association's Web site contains information about smoking and tobacco, recent publications, suggestions for quitting smoking, and links to related sites.

10.2　Campaign for Tobacco-Free Kids[R], National Center for Tobacco-Free Kids
www.tobaccofreekids.org
This organization provides information on state, federal, and global tobacco initiatives as well as tobacco-related facts, special reports, recent tobacco publications, and research.

10.3　American Legacy Foundation
www.legacy.org
The American Legacy Foundation is a national, independent public health foundation working to eliminate disparities in access to tobacco prevention and cessation services and to impart to young people the knowledge and tools to reject tobacco. The Web site provides tobacco fact sheets, access to publications and tobacco industry documents, tobacco maps, and information about related surveys and studies.

10.4　National Latino Council on Alcohol and Tobacco Prevention (LCAT)
www.nlcatp.org/default.asp
Formed by Latino public health professionals and community advocates, LCAT is devoted to preventing or eliminating tobacco use and reducing alcohol abuse within the Latino community. The Web site has information about LCAT, access to their newsletter, an information clearinghouse, publications, answers to frequently asked

questions, and links to related Web sites.

10.5 Smoke Free Movies
www.smokefreemovies.ucsf.edu (See 4.5)

10.6 State Tobacco Activities Tracking & Evaluation System (STATE)
www2.cdc.gov/nccdphp/osh/state
Developed by the Centers for Disease Control and Prevention in the Office on Smoking and Health, National Center for Chronic Disease Prevention and Health Promotion, STATE has data on state-level tobacco prevention and control. Topics covered include behaviors, demographics, health consequences and costs, economics, legislation, and funding.

10.7 Tobacco Information and Prevention Source (TIPS)
www.cdc.gov/tobacco/index.htm
TIPS is a division of the National Center for Chronic Disease Prevention and Health Promotion, Centers for Disease Control and Prevention. This Web site is geared toward a variety of audiences from children to professionals and contains Surgeon General's reports, tobacco control program guidelines and data, research data and reports, youth tips, and tobacco industry documents.

Substance Abuse

11.1 Center for Substance Abuse Research (CESAR), University of Maryland
www.cesar.umd.edu
CESAR focuses on the problems substance abuse creates for individuals, families, and communities. The Web site has drug profiles, statistics, and information on topics including criminal justice, policy, prevention, education, and treatment.

11.2 The National Center on Addiction and Substance Abuse at Columbia University (CASA)
www.casacolumbia.org
This Web site provides CASA publications, a newsroom with editorials and news releases, information about ongoing research and programs, and an extensive list of resources and links. There is a section on family and youth information.

11.3 National Institute on Drug Abuse (NIDA)
www.nida.nih.gov
NIDA is a part of the National Institutes of Health, U.S. Department of Health and Human Services. There is information including statistics, research reports, newsletters, and fact sheets geared toward researchers, health care professionals, parents, and teachers. The Web site provides a link to the newly created NIDA site for teenagers and other Web sites focused on substance abuse.

11.4 Substance Abuse & Mental Health Services Administration
www.samhsa.gov
This is an agency of the U.S. Department of Health and Human Services. The Web site contains access to publications, news releases, and addiction treatment and prevention information. There is information about funding as well as a section containing statistics and data and links to numerous information clearinghouses.

Part Two: About Their Family Life and Well-being

Turbulence: The Effects of Change

12.1 Child Trends DataBank
www.childtrendsdatabank.org (See 5)

12.2 Federal Interagency Forum on Child and Family Statistics
www.childstats.gov (See 10)

12.3 KIDS COUNT
www.kidscount.org (See 12)

Children of the Fortress: America's Most Invisible Culture

13.1 Military Children and Youth
www.mfrc-dodqol.org/MCY
Developed by the Department of Defense's Military Family Resource Center, this Web site has information on issues, programs, and initiatives for military children. There is a searchable documents database with information on the following topics: military child care, youth, and parenting programs; legislation and policies within and outside of the military; and a number of child topics.

13.2 Military Family Resource Center
www.mfrc-dodqol.org/index.htm
Sponsored by the Department of Defense, the Resource Center provides statistics on military families, surveys, a document database, and military quality of life programs and policy information. There is a section on family resources with answers to frequently asked questions.

The Consequences of Divorce

14.1 National Center for Health Statistics (NCHS), Divorce Fast Stats
www.cdc.gov/nchs/fastats/divorce.htm
The NCHS is a part of the Centers for Disease Control and Prevention. This Web site has annual divorce statistics, comprehensive data, and links to other relevant Web sites.

14.2 U.S. Census Bureau
www.census.gov (See 15)

Grandparents Raising Grandchildren

15.1 AARP: Grandparenting
www.aarp.org/life/grandparents
The AARP is a membership organization for persons ages 50 years or older. This section of their Web site contains information about and for grandparents. There are statistics from Census 2000, access to a newsletter for grandparents raising children, and information about finding health insurance for grandchildren and finding help to raise grandchildren.

15.2 Administration on Aging (AoA): Grandparents Raising Grandchildren
www.aoa.gov/prof/notes/notes_grandparents.asp
The AoA is a part of the federal Department of Health and Human Services. This section of the Web site provides both general and specific

information about grandparents raising grandchildren and subsequent legal issues, policy and research articles, state programs and reports, governmental and foundations programs, and informational Web sites.

15.3   Generations United (GU)
www.gu.org
GU is a national organization that promotes intergenerational policies, programs, and strategies. The GU Web site contains resources for policymakers and the public on intergenerational cooperation, including legislation and kinship care information and multiple GU publications.

15.4   U.S. Census Bureau
www.census.gov   (See 15)

Foster Care

16.1   Adoption & Foster Care Analysis & Reporting System (AFCARS)
www.acf.dhhs.gov/programs/cb/dis/afcars
As a part of the Children's Bureau of the U.S. Department of Health and Human Services' Administration for Children and Families, AFCARS collects case-level information on children in foster care and on foster and adoptive parents. Relevant information including state-by-state statistics is available at the Web site.

16.2   Casey Family Programs
www.casey.org/Home
Casey Family Programs is a national foundation dedicated to providing, improving, and preventing the need for foster care. The Web site has information for the media, foster families, communities, and professionals working with children in foster care.

16.3   National Foster Parent Association (NFPA)
www.nfpainc.org
NFPA is a national organization that supports foster parents and advocates for children. Information available on the Web site covers foster parenting, legislation, advocacy, and training.

16.4   National Resource Center for Foster Care and Permanency Planning (NRCFCPP)
www.hunter.cuny.edu/socwork/nrcfcpp
Located at the Hunter College School of Social Work, NRCFCPP provides training, technical assistance, and information services to child welfare agencies that make permanent child placements. The Web site has information about NRCFCPP and its programs, links to statistics, access to their newsletter, as well as fast facts about foster parenting, kinship care, special needs adoption, and youth in transition.

16.5   North American Council on Adoptable Children (NACAC)
www.nacac.org
Founded by adoptive parents, NACAC strives to assist the needs of children waiting for adoption and the families who adopt them. This Web site includes information about children in foster care, public policies surrounding adoption, adoption issues, and recruitment of foster and adoptive families.

Children of Immigrants

17.1   Center for Immigration Studies (CIS)
www.cis.org
CIS is an independent, nonpartisan, nonprofit research organization that focuses on U.S. immigration research and policy analysis. The Web site provides reports, papers, background information, news articles, answers to common questions, and transcripts of testimony about immigration.

17.2   U.S. Census Bureau
www.census.gov   (See 15)

17.3   U.S. Citizenship and Immigration Services (USCIS)
www.uscis.gov/graphics/index.htm
The USCIS is a bureau of the U.S. Department of Homeland Security. The Web site provides information on immigration procedures, full-text reports and studies, and sections on history, genealogy, and education.

Experiences in the After-school Hours

18.1   Afterschool.gov
www.afterschool.gov
Afterschool.gov is a federal program housed and supported by the General Services Administration and the Interagency Federal Child Care Council. The Web site provides links to government programs supporting after-school programs and includes news and research studies about after-school programs.

18.2   Afterschool Alliance
www.afterschoolalliance.org
The Afterschool Alliance is a nonprofit organization that champions after-school programs and advocates for quality, affordable programs for all children. The Web site provides issue briefs, polling data, publications, and links to research.

18.3   Child Care Bureau (CCB)
www.acf.hhs.gov/programs/ccb
A part of the U.S. Department of Health and Human Services, the CCB administers federal funds to assist low-income families in accessing quality child care. This Web site is geared primarily toward administrators who manage funded programs, but it also has general information, including data and policy documents appropriate for parents, care providers, and researchers.

18.4   National Association of Child Care Resource and Referral Agencies (NACCRRA)
www.naccrra.org
NACCRRA supports community child care resources and referrals and promotes national policies and partnerships devoted to the development and learning of all children. Information about their programs, public policy updates, access to an online resource list, and access to a national dataset are available on the Web site.

18.5   National Network for Child Care (NNCC)
www.nncc.org/homepage.html
Supported by the the Cooperative State Research, Education and Extension Service, U.S. Department of Agriculture, and the Cooperative Extension

System's Children, Youth, and Family Network, NNCC provides more than 1,000 research publications and resources at this Web site.

Challenges of Child Care

19.1   Child Care Aware
www.childcareaware.org
This is a nonprofit program of the National Association of Child Care Resources and Referral Agencies funded through the Child Care Bureau of the U.S. Department of Health and Human Services. The Web site is geared primarily toward parents looking for child care and child care resources and provides a series of publications, a child care newsletter, and information on parenting and finding quality child care.

19.2   Child Care Bureau (CCB)
www.acf.hhs.gov/programs/ccb   (See 18.3)

19.3   Child Care and Early Education Research Connections (CCEERC)
www.childcareresearch.org/discover/index.jsp
The CCEERC is a partnership among the National Center for Children in Poverty at the Mailman School of Public Health, Columbia University; the Inter-university Consortium for Political and Social Research at the Institute for Social Research, the University of Michigan; and the Child Care Bureau, Administration for Children and Families of the U.S. Department of Health and Human Services. The Web site is designed for researchers and policymakers and includes data sets for secondary analysis, a searchable research collection, a state policy data tool, and specially designed syntheses.

19.4   National Association of Child Care Resource and Referral Agencies (NACCRRA)
www.naccrra.org   (See 18.4)

19.5   National Association for the Education of Young Children (NAEYC)
www.naeyc.org
The NAEYC is an organization of early childhood educators and others dedicated to improving programs for children from birth through grade 3 and is the only accrediting body for child care centers. A search for accredited child care centers can be performed at the Web site.

19.6   National Child Care Information Center (NCCIC)
www.nccic.org
As a project of the Child Care Bureau of the Department of Health and Human Services, NCCIC links people and information. The Web site has information about NCCIC, publications and resources, a searchable database, and state profiles.

19.7   National Head Start Association (NHSA)
www.nhsa.org
NHSA is a nonprofit organization dedicated to meeting the needs of Head Start children and their families. The Web site provides substantial information about Head Start, advocacy services, and child care research as well as links to relevant resources.

19.8   National Network for Child Care
www.nncc.org/homepage.html   (See 18.5)

Gender Roles

20.1   Families and Work Institute (FWI)
www.familiesandwork.org/index.html
FWI is a nonprofit research center that focuses on the changing workforce, the changing family, and the changing community. Among their research projects are the *Ask the Children*[R] *Series*, studies looking at child and youth views of issues such as violence, employment, and learning. The Web site includes publications and answers to frequently asked questions.

Poverty

21.1   Children's Defense Fund
www.childrensdefense.org   (See 7)

21.2   Institute for Research on Poverty (IRP)
www.ssc.wisc.edu/irp
IRP is a nonprofit, nonpartisan institute based at the University of Wisconsin, Madison. The Web site has information about IRP, IRP publications, answers to frequently asked questions about poverty, and links to poverty-related Web sites.

21.3   National Center for Children in Poverty (NCCP)
www.nccp.org
A part of Columbia University's Mailman School of Public Health, the NCCP has a searchable Web site containing recent news releases, fact sheets summarizing poverty topics, and a newsletter. There is an archive of publications organized by publication title and by publication date as well as specific sections devoted to demographics, economic security, early care and learning, and family stability.

21.4   National Poverty Center
www.npc.umich.edu
This nonpartisan research center is based at the University of Michigan, Ann Arbor's Gerald R. Ford School of Public Policy with major funding through the Assistant Secretary for Planning and Evaluation, U.S. Department of Health and Human Services. The Web site contains publications, recent news and events, poverty facts, and links to related Web sites.

Food Insecurity

22.1   Center on Hunger and Poverty
www.centeronhunger.org
The Center is located at the Heller School of Public Policy of Brandeis University, with its programs carried out by the Asset Development Institute and the Food Security Institute; both can be accessed from this Web site. Web site resources include publications, state- and national-level data, and links to related organizations.

22.3   Food and Nutrition Service (FNS)
www.fns.usda.gov/fns
The FNS administers the nutrition assistance programs of the U.S. Department of Agriculture. The Web site has information about FNS programs including School Meals, the Food Stamp Program, the Child and Adult Care Food Program, and Women, Infants and Children Program. There is also access to research and publications, many of which focus on children.

22.4 Food Research and Action Center (FRAC)
www.frac.org/html/all_about_frac/about_index.html
FRAC is a nonprofit, nonpartisan research and public policy center improving public policies to eradicate hunger and under-nutrition. The Web site provides an overview of hunger in the United States, information about federal food programs, current news and analyses, and publications.

22.5 Food Security in the United States, Economic Research Service (ERS)
www.ers.usda.gov/briefing/FoodSecurity
ERS is a part of the U.S. Department of Agriculture. This Web site provides an overview of food security in the United States, data products including a Food Stamp Map Machine, and links to reports and resources on related topics.

Part Three: About Their Health

Child Health: An Evaluation of the Last Century

23.1 American Academy of Pediatrics (AAP)
www.aap.org   (See 2)

23.2 Bright Futures
www.brightfutures.aap.org
The Maternal and Child Health Bureau of the U.S. Department of Health and Human Services began Bright Futures, and the American Academy of Pediatrics is currently updating the Bright Futures health supervision guidelines for children and youth. The Web site provides relevant literature and access to related newsletters as well as sections for health care professionals, public health professionals, families, and communities.

23.3 Centers for Disease Control and Prevention: Infants and Children
www.cdc.gov/health/nfantsmenu.htm
The Centers for Disease Control and Prevention has information and resources regarding infant and child health listed alphabetically by topic.

23.4 Healthy People 2010
www.healthypeople.gov   (See 11)

23.5 KidsHealth
www.kidshealth.org
Run by the Nemours Foundation's Center for Children's Health Media, KidsHealth has health information about children and youths of all ages and has separate sections for parents, teens, and children. The Web site hosts thousands of articles, resources, games, and animations.

23.6 Maternal and Child Health Bureau
www.mchb.hrsa.gov
The Maternal and Child Health Bureau is part of the Health Resources and Services Administration, U.S. Department of Health and Human Services. The Web site has recent news and publications, information on health topics arranged alphabetically, and information about funding opportunities.

23.7 National Institute of Child Health & Human Development
www.nichd.nih.gov
The National Institute of Child Health and Human Development is a part of the National Institutes of Health. The Web site has health information, news and events, publications, and links to research resources.

23.8 National Center for Health Statistics (NCHS)
www.cdc.gov/nchs   (See 13)

Tooth Decay: The Best of Times, the Worst of Times

24.1 American Academy of Pediatric Dentistry (AAPD)
www.aapd.org
The AAPD is a membership organization for pediatric dentists. The Web site has resources for professionals as well as laypersons, care policies and guidelines, recent news, dental health resources, and access to articles and publications.

24.2 American Association of Public Health Dentistry (AAPHD)
www.aaphd.org
AAPHD is a membership organization for individuals concerned about the oral health of the public. The AAPHD newsletter and an extensive list of links to relevant documents, dental organizations, education programs, oral health data, and medical information are available on the Web site.

24.3 American Dental Association
www.ada.org
The American Dental Association is a professional association of dentists. The Web site has information geared toward dentists and non-dentists alike. There is an information section on oral health arranged alphabetically as well as recent news releases.

24.4 Association of State & Territorial Dental Directors (ASTDD)
www.astdd.org
The ASTDD is a national nonprofit organization for directors and staff of state public health agency programs for oral health. The Web site includes best practices for public health dentistry, publications, and links to Web-based resources.

24.5 Children's Dental Health Project (CDHP)
www.cdhp.org
The CDHP is a nonprofit organization that assists policymakers, health care professionals, advocates, and parents to improve children's oral health. The Web site contains media information, Congressional resources, publications, and other resources, including the Surgeon General's National Call to Action to Promote Oral Health.

24.6 CDC Oral Health Resources: Children's Oral Health
www.cdc.gov/OralHealth/topics/child.htm
A section of the Center for Disease Control and Prevention's Web site on Oral Health Resources, this site provides a summary of children's oral health, fact sheets, answers to frequently asked questions, and links to relevant publications. General oral health resources include state-by-state reports, guidelines, and a resource library.

24.7 Dental, Oral, and Craniofacial Data Resource Center (DRC)
drc.nidcr.nih.gov/default.htm
Cosponsored by the National Institute of Dental and Craniofacial Research and the Division of Oral Health, Centers for Disease Control and Prevention, the DRC provides dental, oral, and craniofacial data to researchers, practitioners, policymakers, and the general public.

24.8 National Maternal and Child Oral Health Resource Center
www.mchoralhealth.org
The Resource Center is based at Georgetown University and receives funding from the Maternal and Child Health Bureau, U.S. Department of Health and Human Services. The Web site provides fact sheets on oral health, links to relevant resources, and information about how oral health pertains to Head Start.

Overweight: An Epidemic

25.1 Knowledge Path: Obesity in Children and Adolescents
www.mchlibrary.info/KnowledgePaths/ kp_obesity.html
This Web site is from the Maternal and Child Health Library, a part of the National Center for Education in Maternal and Child Health at Georgetown University. It provides a summary of the topic along with links to Web sites and electronic publications, journal articles and other publications, databases, discussion groups, and electronic newsletters. The site has links to "Knowledge Paths" about physical activity and nutrition in children and adolescents.

25.2 The National Center for Health Statistics (NCHS)
www.cdc.gov/nchs   (See 13)

25.3 Nutrition and Physical Activity, National Center for Chronic Disease Prevention and Health Promotion, Centers for Disease Control and Prevention
www.cdc.gov/nccdphp/dnpa/index.htm
This Web site contains information and publications about child and adult overweight, nutrition, and physical activity. There are public health programs, recommendations from governmental agencies, data and statistics, training and software tools, and links to related Web sites.

25.4 Overweight and Obesity, The Office of the Surgeon General
www.surgeongeneral.gov/topics/obesity
The Web site of the Office of the Surgeon General contains access to full-length reports of the Surgeon General, along with resources for overweight education, nutrition, and activity.

Asthma

26.1 American Academy of Allergy, Asthma, and Immunology (AAAAI)
www.aaaai.org
The AAAAI is an organization of medical professionals focused on asthma. There is a section for patients and consumers with information on allergic conditions including pediatric asthma, a section geared towards children, access to Asthma Magazine as well as a medication guide. The section for professionals is extensive, and statistics and recent new releases are included.

26.2 American Lung Association, Asthma
www.lungusa.org/asthma
This Web site has sections on general asthma information, asthma in adults, asthma in children, and recommended readings.

26.3 Asthma and Allergy Foundation of America[R]
www.aafa.org
This patient advocacy organization provides asthma and allergy information, including general information, facts and figures, answers to frequently asked questions, and a multimedia asthma library. Information about chapters, support groups, and available grants are also provided.

26.4 SLAITS National Asthma Survey
www.cdc.gov/nchs/about/major/slaits/nsa.htm
This is the section of the National Center for Health Statistics Web site for the national asthma survey. The survey is available for viewing at this time, and the survey data will be available in late 2004.

Special Health Care Needs

27.1 The Center for Children with Special Needs
www.cshcn.org
The Center is a program of Children's Hospital and Regional Medical Center in Seattle, Washington. The Web site is geared towards parents and professionals involved with children with special health care needs and contains relevant presentations, articles, a newsletter, and resources.

27.2 Family Village
www.familyvillage.wisc.edu
Based at the University of Wisconsin, Madison, Family Village provides local, state, and international resources, information, and communication opportunities for people with disabilities, their families, and their supporters. Information on specific diagnoses, health issues, disability-related literature, adaptive technology, recreational activities, education, and worship are among the resources at this Web site.

27.3 National Center of Medical Home Initiatives for Children with Special Health Care Needs
www.medicalhomeinfo.org
The National Center, a project of the AAP, works with federal agencies to ensure that children with special needs have access to a medical home. The National Center provides access to educational, resource, and advocacy materials, guidelines for care, evaluation tools, and technical assistance to parents, physicians, and other health care professionals.

27.4 The National Policy Center for Children with Special Health Care Needs
www.jhsph.edu/Centers/cshcn
The Center is a collaboration between The Johns Hopkins School of Hygiene and Public Health, Health Systems Research, and Family Voices. The Web site provides online publications and links to relevant organizations.

27.5 SLAITS National Survey of Children with Special Health Care Needs
www.cdc.gov/nchs/about/major/slaits/cshcn.htm
This section of the National Center for Health Statistics Web site is devoted to the national survey on the special health care needs of children. The availability of the dataset enables original analyses to be performed. In addition, fact sheets, publications, and presentations using the data are available.

27.6 Family Voices
www.familyvoices.org
Family Voices serves as a clearinghouse for information about the health care of children with special health care needs. The Web site provides information and publications relevant to children with special health care needs, information about national and local Family Voices projects, and links to other resources. One of the site's most important assets is its list of state contacts for information and resources for children and youth with special health care needs.

Impact of Injuries

28.1 Center for Injury Prevention Policy and Practice (CIPPP)
www.cippp.org/index.htm
CIPPP is a part of San Diego State University Graduate School of Public Health. The Web site contains CIPPP publications and access to SafetyLit.org, a weekly updated source of injury literature, and SafetyPolicy.org, with policy recommendations and Healthy People 2010 objectives. There is a section with injury prevention books and links.

28.2 National Center for Injury Prevention and Control (NCIPC)
www.cdc.gov/ncipc/ncipchm.htm
A part of the Centers for Disease Control and Prevention, the NCIPC is the primary federal agency for injury prevention. The Web site has injury fact sheets and information on unintentional injury, violence, and injury care. There are also links to Web sites containing publications, funding opportunities, mass trauma information, and injury maps.

Maltreatment

29.1 National Clearinghouse on Child Abuse and Neglect Information
nccanch.acf.hhs.gov
Established by the Administration for Children & Families, U.S. Department of Health and Human Services, this is the ultimate resource for finding information about child abuse and neglect. There is information about issues associated with child abuse and neglect, resources for professionals, and links to agencies and clearinghouses with information on child abuse.

29.2 National Data Archive on Child Abuse and Neglect (NDACAN)
www.ndacan.cornell.edu/index.html#top
A project of the Family Life Development Center of the College of Human Ecology at Cornell University, NDACAN facilitates secondary analysis of research data relating to child abuse and neglect. The Web

site provides a list of available datasets, publications, a list serve, information on relevant workshops, and links to other resources.

Immunization Delivery

30.1 American Academy of Pediatrics: Immunization Initiatives
www.cispimmunize.org
The AAP is the primary professional organization for pediatricians. This Web site contains extensive information about immunizations, including immunization initiatives, questions and answers for families, information and support for clinicians, and resource links.

30.2 Immunization Action Coalition (IAC)
www.immunize.org
The IAC organization strives to decrease disease and increase vaccination rates through the creation and distribution of educational materials. The Web site contains many practical tools for the office and for parents, including vaccine information statements in multiple languages, vaccine administration records, patient screening tools, and an immunization techniques video.

30.3 National Immunization Program (NIP)
www.cdc.gov/nip
A part of the Centers for Disease Control and Prevention, the NIP is involved in the planning, coordination, and conduction of immunization activities nationwide. The Web site provides links to related organizations and information for the public, the media, and professionals.

30.4 National Immunization Survey
www.cdc.gov/nis
This survey is sponsored by the National Immunization Program and conducted by the National Center for Health Statistics. The Web site provides official estimates of vaccination coverage rates, reports, publications, and public-use data files.

30.5 Teaching Immunization Delivery and Evaluation (TIDE)
www.musc.edu/tide
Funded by the Centers for Disease Control and Prevention's National Immunization Program and the Medical University of South Carolina, TIDE is a Web-based interactive educational program for providers and educators. The Web site contains educational modules for immunization delivery and evaluation.

Health Insurance

31.1 Centers for Medicare and Medicaid Services (CMS)
www.cms.hhs.gov
A federal agency within the U.S. Department of Health and Human Services, CMS oversees Medicaid and SCHIP, along with numerous other programs. The Web site has Medicaid consumer information providing general information about Medicaid and specific information categorized by state. The Web site also provides significant information about SCHIP, including legislative information and access to current CMS publications.

31.2 Health Insurance Coverage, National Center for Health Statistics
www.cdc.gov/nchs/fastats/hinsure.htm
The National Center for Health Statistics is a part of the Centers for Disease Control and Prevention. This section of the Web site has insurance coverage facts and access to publications, reports, and primary data from multiple surveys.

31.3 The Kaiser Commission on Medicaid and the Uninsured
www.kff.org/medicaid/index.cfm
This commission is a health care access and coverage research and policy institute and is the largest operating program of the Henry J. Kaiser Family Foundation. The Web site contains an archive of publications; recent news about Medicaid, SCHIP, and the uninsured; Medicaid data organized by state; fact sheets; and sections devoted to topics including managed care, children, and the uninsured.

31.4 U.S. Census Bureau
www.census.gov   (See 15)

Mental Health

32.1 AboutOurKids.org
www.aboutourkids.org
AboutOurKids is a product of the Child Study Center of New York University's School of Medicine. The Web site has information on a range of topics including parenting and child mental health, access to a newsletter, information about ongoing research, and a list of suggested books.

32.2 American Academy of Child and Adolescent Psychiatry (AACAP)
www.aacap.org
The AACAP is a professional organization for Child and Adolescent Psychiatrists. This Web site has information for practitioners and laypersons alike, including articles on recent topics in psychiatry, press releases, a section devoted to advocacy, and facts and resources for families.

32.3 The Federation of Families for Children's Mental Health
www.ffcmh.org
Funded by the federal government as well as non-governmental organizations, this federation helps children with behavioral and mental health needs and their families through policy, technical assistance, and training. The Web site includes issue briefs, newsletters, presentations, and resources suitable for a variety of audiences.

32.4 National Institute of Mental Health (NIMH)
www.nimh.nih.gov
The NIMH is a section of the National Institutes of Health (NIH), the federal government's main biomedical and behavioral research agency. The Web site has extensive information for researchers, practitioners, and the general public. Fact sheets, research reports, statistics, and news releases are included.

32.5 SAMHSA'S National Mental Health Information Center
www.mentalhealth.org
The National Mental Health Information Center is a

service of the Center for Mental Health Services, U.S. Department of Health and Human Services. The Web site has news releases, current reports, and a listing of mental health services, resources, and statistics searchable by state.

Maternal Depression

33.1 American Psychiatric Association
www.psych.org
The APA is an internationally recognized medical society. This Web site offers information about depression and other illnesses, psychiatric medications, mental health coverage, ethics, and research for physicians and the public. There is access to the APA library and contact information for mental health resources.

33.2 National Institute of Mental Health (NIMH)
www.nimh.nih.gov   (See 32.4)

33.3 SAMHSA'S National Mental Health Information Center
www.mentalhealth.org   (See 32.5)

Youth Suicide

34.1 American Academy of Child and Adolescent Psychiatry (AACAP)
www.aacap.org   (See 32.2)

34.2 American Association of Suicidology (AAS)
www.suicidology.org/index.cfm
The AAS is a not-for-profit organization working to understand and prevent suicide. The Web site provides information about suicide, including information specific to youth and suicide. There are publications, a recommended book list, prevention resources, and information about research.

34.3 The Federation of Families for Children's Mental Health
www.ffcmh.org   (See 32.3)

34.4 National Institute of Mental Health (NIMH)
www.nimh.nih.gov   (See 32.4)

34.5 SAMHSA'S National Mental Health Information Center
www.mentalheallth.org   (See 32.5)

34.6 Youth Risk Behavior Surveillance System (YRBSS)
www.cdc.gov/nccdphp/dash/yrbs
The YRBSS is a study funded by the Centers for Disease Control and Prevention. This Web site has information about the study, fact sheets generated from the study, study publications, and access to questionnaires and data.

Attention Deficit Hyperactivity Disorder

35.1 AboutOurKids.org
www.aboutourkids.org   (See 32.1)

35.2 American Academy of Child and Adolescent Psychiatry (AACAP)
www.aacap.org   (See 32.2)

35.3 Children and Adults with Attention Deficit/Hyperactivity Disorder (CHADD)
www.chadd.org

CHADD is a nonprofit organization for children and adults with ADHD and their families. This site contains a national ADHD resource center funded by the Centers for Disease Control and Prevention, fact sheets, information about ongoing research projects, policy information, and information about local chapters.

35.4   National Institute of Mental Health (NIMH)
www.nimh.nih.gov   (See 32.4)

Part Four: About Their Roles, Hopes, and Rights

Religion Among American Teens: Contours and Consequences

36.1   American Academy of Religion (AAR)
www.aarweb.org
The AAR is an association for researchers and teachers of religion that neither endorses nor rejects any particular religious beliefs or practices. Their Web site provides online access to the *Journal of the American Academy of Religion*, limited access to newsletters, a searchable database, and links to related Web sites.

36.2   National Study of Youth and Religion
www.youthandreligion.org
The National Study of Youth and Religion is a research project being conducted at the University of North Carolina, Chapel Hill. The Web site provides information about the study, news releases, access to articles and publications, and an extensive list of links to relevant Web sites.

Adolescent Sexuality: Beyond the Numbers

37.1   Adolescent & School Health: Sexual Behaviors
www.cdc.gov/nccdphp/dash/sexualbehaviors/
_index.htm
This section of the Centers for Disease Control and Prevention, National Center for Chronic Disease Prevention and Health Promotion's Web site contains information about adolescent sexual behavior. It contains data and statistics, information about national and state programs, and links to related Web sites.

37.2   Reproductive Health Information Source: Unintended Pregnancy
www.cdc.gov/reproductivehealth/up_adolpreg.htm
This section of the Centers for Disease Control and Prevention, National Center for Chronic Disease Prevention and Health Promotion's Web site is devoted to unintended pregnancy as it pertains to adolescent pregnancy and births. The site contains reports and statistics on adolescent pregnancy, along with links to other reproductive health sites.

37.3   Health Care Information Resources: Adolescent Sexuality Links
www-hsl.mcmaster.ca/tomflem/teensex.html
This Web site was developed by the McMaster University Health Sciences Library in Canada. It consists of Web site links about adolescent sexuality and also provides access to links about adolescent pregnancy, contraception, sexual health, sexually transmitted disease, and gay, lesbian, and bisexual health.

37.4   National Longitudinal Study of Adolescent Health
www.cpc.unc.edu/addhealth
The National Longitudinal Study of Adolescent Health is a study of the health and behavior of students in grades 7 to 12, funded by the National Institute of Child Health and Human Development (NICHD) and 17 other federal agencies. The Web site gives background about the study and explains how to obtain codebooks and data.

37.5   Resources for Adolescent Providers (RAP)
www.arhp.org/rap
RAP, formerly the National Adolescent Reproductive Health Partnership, is an outgrowth of a project coordinated by the Association of Reproductive Health Professionals, a nonprofit membership association for professionals working in the field of reproductive health. Their Web site contains a database of related resources, a bookstore, and health assessment tools for clinicians.

Adolescence: Youth as a Resource

38.1   Family and Youth Services Bureau (FYSB)
www.acf.hhs.gov/programs/fysb/index.html
The FYSB, a part of the U.S. Department of Health & Human Services, awards funding to help communities provide opportunities to youths and their families. The Web site contains a section on positive youth development.

38.2   National Adolescent Health Information Center
www.youth.ucsf.edu/nahic
Based at the University of California, San Francisco, the Center strives to be a national resource for adolescent health information and research and provides online access to a number of their publications.

38.3   National Education Longitudinal Survey of 1988
www.nces.ed.gov/surveys/nels88
Implemented by the National Center for Education Statistics, this longitudinal survey of students focuses on academic topics but also contains information about work, educational, and occupational aspirations and extracurricular activities. Publications based on this data are available, as is information regarding accessing the data directly.

38.4   The National Longitudinal Study of Adolescent Health
www.cpc.unc.edu/projects/addhealth   (See 37.4)

38.5   Youth Info
www.acf.hhs.gov/programs/fysb/youthinfo/index.htm
Maintained by the Family and Youth Services Bureau, U.S. Department of Health & Human Services, this Web site contains much information regarding the development of U.S. youth. The site has youth data and information on the positive youth development approach to supporting and partnering with young people. There are resources geared toward youth, parents, professionals, and policymakers.

38.6   The William T. Grant Foundation
www.wtgrantfoundation.org
This foundation is a longstanding nonprofit
charitable organization that currently focuses on the
positive aspects of youth. Foundation publications
on relevant topics are available.

Access to Postsecondary Education

39.1   Educational Resources Information Center (ERIC)
www.eric.ed.gov
ERIC, an education literature and resources
information system, is funded by the U.S.
Department of Education. There is a searchable
database of journal articles, research reports,
books, and other education resources. There are
also 16 subject-specific clearinghouses, including
the ERIC Clearinghouse on Higher Education, and
access to more over 2,400 ERIC digests.

39.2   National Center for Education Statistics (NCES)
www.nces.ed.gov
This federal center collects and analyzes
educational data in the United States and abroad.
The Web site provides general education statistics,
tables and figures, fast facts, and direct links to
numerous educational databases. For many of
these databases, access to the original data is
available.

39.3   The National Center for Public Policy and Higher
Education
www.highereducation.org
The National Center for Public Policy and Higher
Education is an independent, nonprofit, nonpartisan
organization that promotes public policies to
promote education and training beyond high school.
This Web site provides news reports, publications,
and links to higher education and policy Web sites.

39.4   U.S. Department of Education
www.ed.gov/index.jhtml
This Web site contains information for students,
parents, teachers, and administrators. There are
links to news articles and a section on research and
statistics.

Children and the Law

40.1   Justice Research and Statistics Association (JRSA)
www.jrsa.org
JRSA is a nonprofit organization of state statistical
analysis center directors, researchers, and
practitioners. The Web site provides a
clearinghouse of publications and research, access
to reports, a newsletter, and a journal, along with
notices about grant opportunities. The Web site
also provides links to JRSA's many projects,
including the Juvenile Justice Evaluation Center
Online.

40.2   National Center for Juvenile Justice
www.ncjj.servehttp.com/NCJJWeb site/index.html
The National Center for Juvenile Justice is a
private, nonprofit organization striving for justice for
children and families through research and
technical assistance. The Web site provides
access to publications and answers to frequently
asked questions concerning juvenile justice in the
United States.

40.3   National Center for Youth Law
www.youthlaw.org
This private, nonprofit law office focuses on the
legal needs of children and families. Extensive
information, analyses, and links to public policy,
legislative, and state and federal governments can
be found on this Web site.

40.4   Office of Juvenile Justice and Delinquency
Prevention (OJJDP)
www.ojjdp.ncjrs.org
The OJJDP is an agency of the U.S. Department of
Justice. The Web site provides statistics and
information about topics that include juvenile
justice, delinquency prevention, violence, and
victimization. There is access to publications and
an OJJDP journal as well as links to other justice
organizations.

Part Five: About Their Demography and Diversity

Families: Diversity and Change

41.1   Federal Interagency Forum on Child and Family
Statistics
www.childstats.gov   (See 10)

41.2   National Bureau of Economic Research
www.nber.org
The National Bureau of Economic Research is a
private, nonprofit, nonpartisan research
organization. The Web site provides information on
and links to a host of economic topics.

41.3   National Indian Child Welfare Association (NICWA)
www.nicwa.org
NICWA is a private, nonprofit membership
organization whose members include tribes, private
organizations, and individuals concerned about
Indian children and families. Information about the
Indian Child Welfare Act and a catalog of
publications are included on the Web site.

41.4   Population Reference Bureau (PRB)
www.prb.org
This organization provides information on U.S. and
international population trends and their
implications. Statistics and PRB reports on a wide
range of national and international population topics
are accessible from the Web site.

41.5   Office of the Assistant Secretary for Planning and
Evaluation, U.S. Department of Health and
Human Services
www.aspe.hhs.gov
This Web site has information on human services
policy issues, including income and poverty, welfare
and work, family formation, special populations, and
indicators and databases.

Minority Child Population Growth

42.1   Center for Family and Demographic Research
www.bgsu.edu/organizations/cfdr/main.html
Located at Bowling Green State University, the
Center conducts demography research about the
health and development of children, adolescents,
and families. The Web site has a section on
statistical data and coding and access to a data
archive.

42.2 Center for International Earth Science Information Network's (CIESIN) U.S. Demography Home Page
www.ciesin.org/datasets/us-demog/us-demog-home.html
This Web site is from the CIESIN at Columbia University. The Web site consists of links to national data resources, online supporting documentation such as codebooks, and options for obtaining data.

42.3 National Indian Child Welfare Association (NICWA)
www.nicwa.org   (See 41.3)

42.4 Population Reference Bureau
www.prb.org   (See 41.4)

42.5 U.S. Census Bureau
www.census.gov   (See 15)

Changes in the Well-being of Children

43.1 Child Trends Databank
www.childtrendsdatabank.org   (See 5)

43.2 Federal Interagency Forum on Child and Family Statistics
www.childstats.gov   (See 10)

43.3 KIDS COUNT
www.kidscount.org   (See 12)

43.4 U.S. Census Bureau
www.census.gov   (See 15)

43.5 Office of the Assistant Secretary for Planning and Evaluation, U.S. Department of Health and Human Services
www.aspe.hhs.gov (See 41.5)

Part Six: Looking Toward Their Future

Medical Progress and Inequalities in Child Health

44.1 Agency for Healthcare Research and Quality (AHRQ): Healthcare Informatics
www.ahcpr.gov/data/infoix.htm
The AHRQ is a part of the U.S. Department of Health and Human Services. This section of their Web site provides information about and data sources for topics within health care informatics.

44.2 International Network of Agencies for Health Technology Assessment
www.inahta.org
These networks are comprised of nonprofit organizations that assess technology in health care and are related to regional or national government and receive at least half of their funding from public sources. The Web site provides access to relevant publications, newsletters, reports, a database, and links to information sources.

44.3 The National Center for Health Statistics (NCHS)
www.cdc.gov/nchs   (See 13)

44.4 National Information Center on Health Services Research and Health Care Technology (NICHSR)
www.nlm.nih.gov/nichsr/nichsr.html
The NICHSR at the National Library of Medicine is a part of the National Institutes of Health. The NICHSR is involved with the distribution of health services research, including health care technology assessments. The Web site provides large amounts of information and access to databases, publications, and Web sites.

Genetics

45.1 National Human Genome Research Institute (NHGRI)
www.genome.gov
The NHGRI is a research institute of the National Institutes of Health. The Web site contains significant amounts of information about genetics organized into three broad sections: research, health, and policy and ethics.

45.2 Center for Society, the Individual and Genetics
www.arc2.ucla.edu/csig
The Center is located at the University of California, Los Angeles. The Web site provides information on the field of genetics and its impact on society, including articles, news updates, presentations, and links to other genetics Web sites.

45.3 American College of Medical Genetics (ACMG)
www.acmg.net
The ACMC is a professional organization for geneticists, genetic counselors, and other health care professionals involved with medical genetics. The Web site provides articles and updates about medical genetics as well as ACMG policy statements.

45.4 National Center for Biotechnology Information: Online Mendelian Inheritance in Man (OMIM™)
www.ncbi.nlm.nih.gov/entrez/query.fcgi?db=OMIM
OMIM™ is a database of human genes and genetic disorders containing information, pictures, and references. The Web site also provides links to OMIM™-allied resources.

Health Services: Past, Present, and Future

46.1 American Academy of Pediatrics (AAP)
www.aap.org   (See 2)

46.2 Center for Disease Control and Prevention: Infants and Children
www.cdc.gov/health/nfantsmenu.htm   (See 23.3)

46.3 Healthy People 2010
www.healthypeople.gov   (See 11)

46.4 The National Center for Health Statistics (NCHS)
www.cdc.gov/nchs   (See 13)

46.5 National Library of Medicine (NLM), History of Medicine
www.nlm.nih.gov/hmd
Located at the National Institutes of Health, the NLM is the world's largest medical library. The History of Medicine Division contains resources for historical scholarship in medicine.

46.6 U.S. Census Bureau
www.census.gov   (See 15)

Index

G